Presidents Under the Knife

Presidents Under the Knife

Surgical Successes, Failures and Deceptions

Per-Olof Hasselgren

McFarland & Company, Inc., Publishers
Jefferson, North Carolina

Library of Congress Cataloging-in-Publication Data

Names: Hasselgren, Per-Olof author
Title: Presidents under the knife : surgical successes, failures and deceptions / Per-Olof Hasselgren.
Description: Jefferson, North Carolina : McFarland & Company, Inc., Publishers, 2025. | Includes bibliographical references and index.
Identifiers: LCCN 2025013431 | ISBN 9781476692876 paperback ♾
ISBN 9781476654201 ebook
Subjects: LCSH: Presidents—United States—Surgery—History | Presidents—United States—Health—History | BISAC: HISTORY / United States / General | MEDICAL / Surgery / General
Classification: LCC E176.1 .H36 2025 | DDC 973.09/9—dc23/eng/20250327
LC record available at https://lccn.loc.gov/2025013431

ISBN (print) 978-1-4766-9287-6
ISBN (ebook) 978-1-4766-5420-1

Front cover images: Ronald Reagan, 1981 (National Archives); portrait of Andrew Jackson, 1856 (Library of Congress); George Washington, painting by Gilbert Stuart, oil on canvas, 1821 (Library of Congress); Franklin D. Roosevelt (collection-FDR Photos; Franklin D. Roosevelt Library Photographs); Lyndon B. Johnson (Lyndon B. Johnson Presidential Library and Museum); surgical team © Gorodenkoff/Shutterstock.

Printed in the United States of America

McFarland & Company, Inc., Publishers
Box 611, Jefferson, North Carolina 28640
www.mcfarlandpub.com

Table of Contents

Acknowledgments

Many people gave me help and support when writing this book. Grace Freedson, my literary agent for the last several years, provided enthusiastic encouragement and wise advice throughout the project. Robert Skole (deceased) and Monika Skole, both with impressive careers as journalists and authors, provided numerous comments with regard to style, English grammar, and factual errors in my early drafts.

Dr. Harry S. Goldsmith, an academic surgeon and one of the world's most prominent experts on President Franklin D. Roosevelt's medical history, in particular when it comes to Roosevelt's suspected malignant melanoma, shared his knowledge and passion for the subject in multiple long telephone conversations.

Several of my colleagues in the Department of Surgery at the Beth Israel Deaconess Medical Center in Boston kindly reviewed parts of my manuscript and provided generous factual checks in the areas of their expertise: Dr. James Naples in the Department of Otolaryngology, Head and Neck Surgery gave me valuable comments regarding the chapters on George Washington (and the alleged epiglottitis that killed him partly because he was denied a tracheotomy) and the daring surgery of Grover Cleveland (removal of a major part of the left upper jaw) performed under less than optimal conditions; Dr. Richard Whyte, chief of thoracic surgery, provided insightful comments about President Ronald Reagan's emergency thoracotomy after the attempted assassination in 1981; and Dr. Thomas Cataldo, a busy colorectal surgeon with a leadership role in the training of future colorectal surgeons, gave me thoughtful comments regarding two of the presidents who had intestinal surgery, Dwight D. Eisenhower and Ronald Reagan.

Arlene Shaner, historical collections librarian at the New York Academy of Medicine, not only helped me in getting permission to reproduce some of the images of artifacts from Grover Cleveland's surgery held by the New York Academy of Medicine but also generously shared her time and knowledge (and enthusiasm) about President Grover Cleveland and his New York connections when it comes to his surgery regarding the tumor of his mouth. Timothy Horning at the Archives of the University of Pennsylvania, Logan Daly at the *Journal of the American College of Surgeons*, Tony Dudek at the Tribune Content Agency Network, Annissa Zak at the *Journal of the American Medical Association Network*, and Matthew Lutts at Associated Press Images supported me in obtaining permissions to reprint images from their institutions and journals. Matthew Levine was particularly accommodating when arranging for permission to use the cartoon created by his late father, David

Levine, showing Lyndon Johnson exposing his scar after the removal of his gallbladder. David Leopold, archivist at the David Levine Archives, gave additional support.

Last but not least, I am grateful to my wife for putting up with me during yet another book project, taking time away from our time together and our walks around Boston. She (almost) never complained, even when I left her alone for many hours.

Introduction

Background

Even the country's first president had surgery. In June 1789 only a couple of months into his presidency, George Washington had surgery for a "tumor" on his left leg. It turned out to be a large abscess giving rise to immense pain and "threatening" fevers. The cutting open of the abscess and drainage of its content may have saved the president from dying of sepsis.

Washington was less fortunate a decade later when he developed what many recent medical historians believe was epiglottitis. The swelling in his throat choked the ex-president to death. His life might have been saved by a tracheotomy (the opening of the windpipe with a knife), as was proposed by one of the physicians attending Washington's sickbed. However, instead of lifesaving surgery, the president was subjected to those days' standard treatments of inflammation: bleeding and purging. Washington was bled repeatedly, which, if anything, hastened his demise. To make things worse, he also received drugs that caused diarrhea and vomiting, purging that most likely also contributed to his death less than forty-eight hours after getting sick.

Several presidents have had surgery at some point during their lifetime. In this book, we will focus on nine presidents who had surgeries while in office. For those presidents, operations performed before or after their terms are also described. In contrast, presidents who have had surgeries exclusively outside their occupancy of the White House are not in the book. Examples of such presidents include Joe Biden, who had surgery before he was elected president, and Jimmy Carter, Bill Clinton, and George W. Bush, who underwent surgeries after leaving office.

The decision not to include presidents on whom surgeries were performed exclusively before or after their terms was based on several considerations. First, even if those operations generated public interest, they had no political and economic ramifications as surgeries on presidents in office have had. Second, the argument that information about a president's health should be made public is not valid if the president had surgeries only as a private citizen. Third, much less information is (rightfully) available regarding presidents whose surgeries took place exclusively when they were private citizens.

With regard to criteria used to decide whether or not to include a president in the book, President John F. Kennedy warrants a special mention. Despite the fact that a tracheotomy was performed in the emergency room at the Parkland Memorial Hospital in Dallas on November 22, 1963, that procedure is not included here because it was performed on a president who had already expired. In addition, Kennedy's nonsurvivable head injury, his condition when arriving at the hospital and the frantic efforts by surgeons and other physicians to resuscitate the president have been described in numerous books and articles and continue to be the subject of writers today.

As implied in the subtitle of the book, we will find successes, failures, and deceptions when learning about the surgeries on American presidents. One of the greatest successes from a surgical standpoint was the saving of President Ronald Reagan's life following his shooting on March 30, 1981. After he was rushed to the George Washington University Hospital, it became obvious that the president was actively bleeding in his chest and that his life was threatened. He was swiftly taken to the operating room, where the surgeons opened his chest and stopped the bleeding. Reagan returned to the White House twelve days after the attempted assassination.

In light of the success in saving Reagan's life, the failures surrounding the surgeries of two other presidents who were shot stand out as tragic failures. James Garfield was shot by a deranged political opponent in 1881. Although the injuries caused by the bullet were not life-threatening, Garfield died seventy-nine painful days later by widespread infections caused by the surgeons' dirty fingers. At the trial the president's assassin claimed, "Yes, I shot the president, but his physicians killed him."

It would be only twenty years before another U.S. president was assassinated. In September 1901, William McKinley was shot while visiting the Pan-American Exposition in Buffalo. The killer, an anarchist, shot the president in the abdomen. Despite an operation attended by several renowned surgeons, McKinley died from a nonfatal injury a week later. The failure of the surgeons has been claimed to be the reason the president died; it has been said that McKinley "got the wrong operation by the wrong surgeon."

Deception is not uncommon in politics and has also been employed in the reporting of presidents' health. A prime example is the circumstances surrounding the surgery on Grover Cleveland. Shortly after President Cleveland was inaugurated for his second term, he felt a rough spot on the roof of his mouth. His doctors discovered a tumor, and fearing it was cancer, they recommended surgery. Cleveland reluctantly agreed but only if the operation could be done in secrecy. His voice needed to be unchanged (he was getting ready for an important message to Congress), and no visible scars would be tolerated. And the mustache needed to stay!

In July 1893, Cleveland underwent a daring operation by a team of surgeons sworn to secrecy. The procedure was done aboard a private yacht sailing along the coast of Long Island. Cleveland was a morbidly obese, high-risk patient who loved his cigars, lager beer, and whiskey. When the yacht and the recovering president were delayed arriving at Cleveland's summerhouse at Buzzards Bay in Massachusetts, the press was lied to and informed that the delay was caused by good fishing areas found by the president and his company. Although the deception initially worked, it would be less than a week before there was a leak and newspapers all over the country reported that the president had undergone secret surgery for cancer.

Why Was This Book Written?

People have always been interested in U.S. presidents' health. In an article published in the *Washington Post* in 2016, the writers commented that "the history of the presidency includes a running thread of illness and incapacity, much of it hidden from the public out of political calculation."[1] The well-being of the country's leader is important for political stability. A president's illness can have economic consequences and can certainly influence the financial markets. "When the president sneezes, the country catches a cold." The press has often spent large amounts of energy and ink on presidents' medical and surgical care.

Although a plethora of books and articles have dealt with the health of American presidents, with some of them describing presidents' surgical procedures, there is a lack of comprehensive work describing details of the surgeries and how presidents' operations may have influenced the political and economic landscape of the country. Most biographies of U.S. presidents have been authored by historians, with relatively little attention being paid to the details of presidents' medical and surgical care.

In this book, a more extensive description of surgeries performed on American presidents is provided. For that purpose, I have reviewed numerous original articles published in medical and surgical journals, often authored by surgeons involved in the procedures, to make it possible to give a more detailed description of the operations from a surgeon's perspective. In addition, I have attempted to paint the political and economic background influencing the decision-making surrounding the surgeries.

Does the President Have the Right to Keep Information About His Health Private?

It is a given that the doctor-patient relationship should be confidential and that physicians should not disclose private medical information without the patient's permission. Breaking this rule is viewed as not only unethical but may also be unlawful and result in lawsuits.

When it comes to the president of the United States, the rules appear to be different.[2] The media have a seemingly unstoppable appetite for information about the president's medical condition, and any affliction of the country's leader quickly generates screaming headlines and brisk sales of newspapers and clicks on the internet. News spreads rapidly and easily goes viral on social media.

It may be argued that people have a right to be informed about changes in the president's health, since presidential illnesses may have significant national as well as international implications from a political, economic, and even military standpoint.

Modern presidents seem to have accepted the fact that there are no limits to public curiosity, people's right to know, and the media's intrusive coverage of health issues. This was not always the case. The history of U.S. presidents is replete with examples of illnesses concealed to the public and surgeries carried out in secrecy, as we will see in this book.

Not only is it now accepted that the president's health is everyone's business, but the same argument has been extended to cover presidential candidates during election campaigns. It is often insisted that voters have a right to know if they are electing someone healthy enough to do this demanding job.

Closely related to the issues discussed here are the regulations of the Health Insurance Portability and Accountability Act of 1996 (HIPAA). The law includes rules regarding privacy protection designed to shield personal health information from disclosure without a patient's consent. Although there are instances when the act does not prevent disclosure, in general the law is clear and includes the president as well. The HIPAA regulations, of course, do not prevent the president from authorizing the disclosure of publicly relevant information, and U.S. presidents can either inform the public themselves or can tell their doctors to share the information.

Who Takes Over When the President Is Killed, Dies from Illness, or Is Otherwise Incapacitated?

Closely related to the details of presidential surgeries is the question of what happens if the commander in chief dies (from illness, during surgery, or by the hands of an assassin), is incapacitated from illness, or is "put under" during a surgical procedure.[3]

Before the 25th Amendment was added to the U.S. Constitution in 1967, the Presidential Succession Act regulated what would happen if the president was killed, died from illness, or became incapacitated for any other reason. Naturally, the first person in line to assume the responsibilities of the presidency is the vice president. An important question is what happens if both the president and vice president died (on September 11, 2001, there was real concern that both the president and vice president might be killed).

The founding fathers realized that the transfer of power from a president who can no longer fulfill his or her obligations was a question that needed to be regulated. The first Presidential Succession Act was passed in 1792. It stipulated that after the vice president, the president pro tempore (elected by the Senate and commonly, but not always, the most senior senator in the majority party) was next in line, followed by the Speaker of the House of Representatives.

A new Presidential Succession Act was passed in 1886. There were concerns about having politicians in Congress in line for the presidency despite their lack of executive experience. In the new Presidential Succession Act, the congressional officers were substituted by the president's cabinet members by rank. The rank order reflected the time since the department was created. Given that the State

Department is the oldest department, the secretary of state had (and still has) the highest rank followed by the secretary of the treasury, with the rank order going further down the list if needed.

In July 1947, President Harry S. Truman signed a new revised Presidential Succession Act. With the revised act, the Speaker of the House and the president pro tempore of the Senate, in that order, were inserted between the vice president and cabinet members.

When President Kennedy was assassinated in November 1963 and Vice President Lyndon Johnson was sworn in as president, the need for a more solidified protocol for presidential succession became clear. This resulted in the 25th Amendment, signed into law by President Johnson in February 1967. The amendment confirmed the obvious rule that if the president is removed from office, dies, or resigns, the vice president becomes president. This and other rules of the 25th Amendment are spelled out in four sections.[4]

Section 1: If the President Is Removed, Dies, or Resigns, the Vice President Becomes President

"In case of the removal of the President from office or of his death or resignation, the Vice President shall become President."

Section 2: The President Can Nominate a New Vice President

"Whenever there is a vacancy in the office of the Vice President, the President shall nominate a Vice President who shall take office upon confirmation by a majority vote of both Houses of Congress."

Section 3: If the President Is Ill, the Vice President Becomes Acting President

"Whenever the President transmits to the President Pro Tempore of the Senate and the Speaker of the House of Representatives his written declaration that he is unable to discharge the powers and duties of his office, and until he transmits to them a written declaration to the contrary, such powers and duties shall be discharged by the Vice President as Acting President."

In 1988, a special commission was formed to address the question of how to proceed when anesthesia is administered to the president. The commission advised that any U.S. president scheduled to receive general anesthesia should use Section 3 of the 25th Amendment and that "this mechanism should be made part of a routine course of action so that its invocation carries no implications of instability or crisis."

Section 4: If the President Is Declared Unfit to Serve, the Vice President Will Become Acting President

"Whenever the Vice President and a majority of either the principal officers of the executive departments or of such other body as Congress may by law provide, transmit to the President Pro Tempore of the Senate and the Speaker of the House of Representatives their written declaration that the President is unable to discharge the powers and duties of his office, the Vice President shall immediately assume the powers and duties of the office as Acting President."

The third section of the 25th Amendment has been invoked four times: during President Reagan's surgery for colon cancer in 1985, when President George W. Bush underwent colonoscopies with sedation in 2002 and 2007, and, more recently, when President Biden underwent a colonoscopy with sedation. In 1985, Vice President George H.W. Bush became the first acting president in U.S. history (on July 13 between 11:28 a.m. and 7:29 p.m.). In 2002 and 2007, Vice President Dick Chaney was acting president during the President George W. Bush's colonoscopies. During President Biden's colonoscopy in November 2021, Vice President Kamala Harris became the first female acting president.

Although Reagan's staff allegedly considered invoking Section 4 of the 25th Amendment when the president's mental health was questioned during the Iran-Contra scandal, the section was never invoked. Demands that Section 4 should be invoked after January 6, 2021, were raised, mainly by Democrats, but that did not happen.

Why Do Presidential Surgeries Fascinate?

Presidents' health in general, and surgeries in particular, have always intrigued the public, and there are several reasons for that fascination. Surgery on the country's leader can have multiple both political and economic consequences. Stories told in this book illustrate both these aspects of presidential surgeries. In addition, we will review aspects of surgical procedures that have previously been described only in articles published in surgical and medical journals and will be made more accessible here to a broader audience.

The repercussions of surgery on a president will depend on the reason for the surgery, the magnitude of the operation, and whether or not the president bounces back after the procedure without complications. Surgery performed because of injuries caused by an assassination attempt naturally will create the largest headlines. Unfortunately, our country has more than once had to live through the anxiety of having a president under the knife after being shot. As we will find, the outcome of such procedures can be extremely gratifying but may also be disastrous because of incompetent surgeries.

It is well established that surgery on a president can cause ripple effects on the stock market and result in financial turmoil. The surgery may also have other associations with the economy. For example, the timing of President Cleveland's surgery for his oral cancer was heavily influenced by the economic conditions in the country at the time and his upcoming message to Congress in which he would defend his position as a conservative "sound money man."[5]

When a president needs surgery for a condition that any regular citizen can be afflicted with, such as gallstones necessitating the removal of the gallbladder, this may also be interesting and even reassuring because it proves the obvious: that the president, even though being the most powerful person in the world, is human and just like us.

Details about surgical procedures on presidents may be particularly interesting for surgeons. It is fortunate that presidential surgeries have been described in many professional articles, making it possible for colleagues to analyze details of the operations. Reports written by surgeons present in the operating room are especially valuable—and educational—and make us understand that the outcome may not always be favorable even when expert surgeons are involved. Surgery performed on a high-profile person such as the president of the United States, with the whole world watching, may certainly be very stressful. The fear of being criticized publicly for surgical decisions and performance, especially if complications occur, must weigh heavily on the surgeon's shoulders.

It is the purpose of the present book to highlight these and other aspects of presidents' surgeries. Hopefully, the stories told will be captivating to surgeons as well as nonmedical readers interested in the history of our country.

Chapter One

George Washington

"Cut away—deeper, deeper still"

The First President

April 30, 1789–March 4, 1797

The year was 1789. Less than two months after the country's first presidential inauguration, the commander in chief couldn't take it any longer. He had developed a large abscess ("the size of two fists") on his left thigh and was having "threatening" fevers and severe pain.[1] He called for a surgeon to get some relief. The doctor arrived together with his father, also a surgeon, and sharpened his knife and cut open the carbuncle.

Diseases and Caring for the Sick and Injured in America at the Time of Washington

George Washington was no stranger to disease. He had seen plenty of illness and suffering among his fellow Americans. During his time as leader of the Continental Army, he had been challenged by epidemics as well as war injuries among his soldiers.

When Washington arrived at Cambridge, Massachusetts, in early July 1775 to take command of the Continental Army, he realized that he had a big problem at hand. How were sick and injured soldiers to be taken care of?

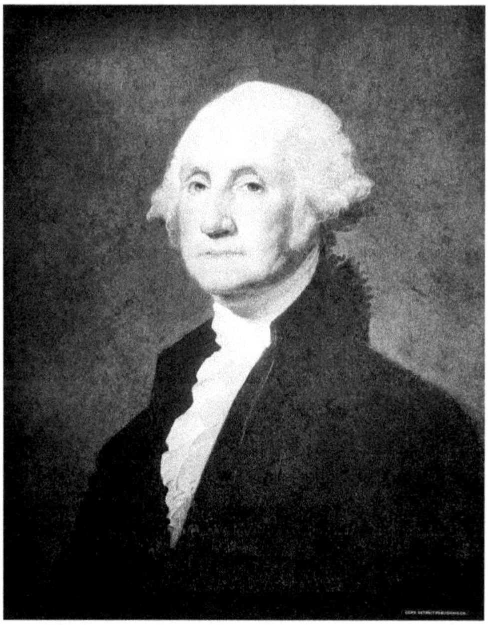

George Washington. Painting by Gilbert Stuart, oil on canvas, 1821. Library of Congress, Prints and Photographs Division, Washington, D.C.

With the Continental Congress in Philadelphia planning for an army of 20,000 or more, Washington was frustrated by the slow progress in organizing a hospital and medical system that would be able to care for the warriors. In his desperation he fired off an angry letter to the Congress on July 20, 1775, requesting an immediate creation of a "Hospital" (here meaning a hospital system rather than a building designed to admit and treat patients). He wrote, "I have made inquiry with respect to the Establishment of the Hospital, and find it a very unsettled Condition. There is no Principal Director, nor any Subordination among the Surgeons; of consequence Disputes and Contentions have arisen and must continue until it is reduced to some System." He then went on to emphasize why this was an extremely important issue. The warriors' survival was at stake: "I could wish it was immediately taken into consideration as the Lives and Health of both Officers and Soldiers so much depend upon a due regulation of this Department."[2]

Washington's understanding of the need for a medical system and his involvement in the medical affairs resulted in the decision by the Continental Congress on July 27, 1775, to create "a hospital for an army consisting of 20,000 men" and how this "Hospital Department" (later to be called the "Medical Department") should be structured with regard to its surgeons, their duties and their pay scale.[3] Military hospitals during the American Revolutionary War, at least initially, were almost always constructions not erected for sick and injured soldiers but rather to serve as meetinghouses, living quarters, churches, barns, and other building that could be retrofitted to put up soldiers as need arose.[4]

Although Washington for obvious reasons was mainly engaged in the affairs of military hospitals, civilians also needed health care in America during the 1700s. The Pennsylvania Hospital in Philadelphia was the first hospital built on the continent. It was founded in 1751 by Dr. Thomas Bond and Benjamin Franklin "to care for the sick—poor, and insane who were walking the streets of Philadelphia."[5] The second hospital erected in the colonies was the New York Hospital, the construction of which began in 1773. Because a fire destroyed the initial building just before its completion, the hospital in New York could not be fully opened until 1791. The Massachusetts General Hospital was erected in Boston almost seventy years after the Pennsylvania Hospital and saw its first patient admitted in 1821.

The conditions in the hospitals, both military and civilian, were miserable. They were unsanitary, crowded, and dangerous (with many dying from infections acquired in the hospitals or following surgeries). The role of bacteria and the need for sterility were still at least a century in the future. Even the common sense to clean and wash one's hands before operating on patients was often disregarded. A lack of hospitals and hospital beds was an additional strain on any attempt to provide healing. There was a lack of food and equipment, including medicine and surgical instruments. Importantly, especially in times of war, there was a lack of competent surgeons.

The lack of surgical instruments during the American Revolution was frustrating. At one point when the field surgeons ran out of scalpels, Dr. John Warren lost his patience. John Warren was the younger brother of Joseph Warren, the hero Patriot and surgeon who had died too young at the Battle of Bunker Hill in June

1775. During the spring of 1776 John Warren, awaiting a British onslaught on New York, was in charge of the General Hospital at Long Island. He could no longer keep quiet about the situation and complained in a letter to the general director of the Medical Department, John Morgan, about the fact that the surgeons could not perform their tasks because they had no scalpels available. Morgan responded in a letter to Warren penned in May 1776, just a couple of months before the disastrous Battle of Long Island in which Washington saw nearly two thousand of his soldiers being killed, injured, or taken prisoner. In the letter, which has gone down in history as the "Razor Letter," Morgan explained that he understood that surgeons often had "no scalpels, as whatever I have committed to the hospitals has always been lost. I send you two, in which case, if you want more, use a razor for an incision knife."[6]

It was not only the hospital conditions that were miserable; the patients themselves were also in a deplorable state. The soldiers lacked warm and clean clothing. They frequently were even without shoes and stockings and had to march barefoot. It was not uncommon that the march of men over ice and frozen snow could be tracked from blood left by their naked and lacerated feet. Tragically, amputations of feet for frostbite were not rare, in particular during the first winters of the American Revolutionary War.

Washington's experience with the poor conditions of his soldiers and their health care was at its worst during the winter camp of 1777–1778 at Valley Forge. The warriors marching toward the camp looked like "an army of skeletons … naked, starved, sick and discouraged."[7] When arriving at the camp, the soldiers were quartered in tents and hastily constructed huts. They had to sleep on straw spread out on cold and damp dirt floors. The lodgings had no toilets, and when nature called, the men had to run out and relieve themselves and run back in as fast as they could to escape the cold. If the weather was too ugly, it was easier to take care of their nature calls inside the tents or huts than to go outside. The stench from human waste, aggravated by the smell from rotting carcasses of dead horses (about fifteen hundred horses died from starvation at Valley Forge) and other refuse, spread all over the encampment and became unbearable. No wonder Washington was disgusted and angry about the unsanitary conditions.

Soldiers who were not already sick when entering Valley Forge ran a high risk of becoming afflicted by illness. Contagious diseases were rampant, in particular influenza, typhus, typhoid, and dysentery. Venereal diseases, spread by prostitutes who followed the army during its many campaigns, were common. The constantly feared enemy, smallpox, continued to be a threat. Many of the surgeons at Valley Forge were busy inoculating between three thousand and four thousand of the more than twelve thousand soldiers against the dreaded disease.

Washington's Own Illnesses

In addition to seeing war injuries and diseases among his soldiers and health struggles among civilians, Washington had his own health challenges throughout his life. Some of Washington's early maladies were severe and even life-threatening, but somehow he beat them all until, when at the age of sixty-seven, he succumbed to a condition that would choke him to death.

Tuberculosis and smallpox were two of the most feared threats to life in the colonies during the 1700s. Washington had been afflicted in early life by both. In addition, at the age of seventeen, he had contracted malaria. The humid climate and marshes of Virginia created large mosquito populations, and malaria was common. As is typical for the disease, Washington would suffer intermittent bouts of fever during the rest of his life. Bark from the cinchona tree containing quinine became one of Washington's favorite medicines to help him fight the recurrent fevers.

In 1751, Washington accompanied his thirty-three-year-old half brother Lawrence on a voyage to Barbados.[8] The purpose of sailing to Barbados was to give Lawrence a chance to improve from his tuberculosis in the mild Caribbean climate. Because Lawrence's wife had recently delivered a baby, George, nineteen years old at the time, was sent along as a companion. Not only was the visit to Barbados a failure when it came to healing Lawrence (he died from consumption only a couple of months after returning to Virginia in July 1752), but it also resulted in George getting infected with the feared disease. When he returned to Mount Vernon, he had to fight symptoms of pulmonary tuberculosis. It would take him several years to fully recover.

When Lawrence and George arrived in Barbados, they were invited to dinners at the home of Gedney Clarke, a wealthy merchant on the island and a relative of Lawrence's wife. Historians have speculated that Mrs. Clarke at the time had smallpox (she was "much indisposed"), and since George was "strongly attacked with the small Pox" a couple of weeks into his stay at Barbados,[9] it is possible that he was infected at Clarke's home. Regardless of the source, the "speckled monster" had George bedridden for three weeks before he could return to Virginia. He left Barbados a marked man: the pockmarks on his face would stay with him for the rest of his life. More importantly and on the upside, Washington's encounter with the dreaded disease made him immune against smallpox, something that would become important two and a half decades later when, as the newly appointed commander of the army, he had to face outbreaks of smallpox threatening the Continental Army.

In 1755, Washington joined the British general Edward Braddock in the French and Indian War. During the campaign, in which Braddock was killed, Washington contracted dysentery. He experienced violent diarrheas and rectal pain. He needed a pillow to be able to sit on his horse. The combination of the war and the disease took its toll. On the way back home, an exhausted Washington had to recuperate at Fort Cumberland in Maryland. In a letter to his mother on July 18, 1755, Washington wrote, "I was not half recovered from a violent illness that had confined me to my bed and a wagon for above ten days. I am still in a weak and feeble condition, which induces me to halt here two or three days in the hope of recovering a little strength, to enable me to proceed homewards."[10]

Add to these ailments bad teeth and bouts of influenza and pneumonia, and it is easy to understand that Washington had experienced many challenges to his health before 1789.

Washington and the Smallpox Epidemics

Smallpox was the disease that had the greatest impact on Washington's political and military career, in particular during his time as commander of the Continental Army. Smallpox may have put an end to the revolution had Washington not taken decisive actions.

Recurring smallpox epidemics were common in America during the 1700s. Repeated outbreaks in Boston in 1721, 1752, 1764, and 1775 were severe and accompanied by extremely high death rates. In the epidemic that hit Boston in 1721, nearly 15 percent of those who contracted the malady died.

It was an ancient observation that people who survived an attack of the scourge seldom got the disease again. This had led to the centuries-old practice of inoculation in places such as Greece, Armenia, and northern Africa. The inoculations were performed by introducing matter from ripe pustules of patients into superficial skin incisions on individuals to be inoculated, resulting in "mild" controlled cases of smallpox and, importantly, lifelong immunity against the disease.

The method arrived in England in the early 1700s and was introduced in the colonies shortly thereafter. During the 1721 epidemic, Dr. Zabdiel Boylston, the first American-born surgeon on the continent, started inoculations in Boston on the suggestion of the Reverend Cotton Mather.[11] Initially, the procedure provoked anger and outrage among Bostonians mainly because it was considered dangerous, occasionally even killing the inoculated subject. In addition, Puritan opponents, including members of the clergy, felt that it was wrong to interfere with a disease they thought was God's punishment for sinful living. Soon, the anger between people on the different sides of the issue spilled over to the press and even resulted in violence. The vitriol frequently focused on Mather and Boylston, who were harassed in newspaper and pamphlet headlines that would make even today's banners look timid. On one occasion Mather's home was firebombed, with a message attached to the missile: "Cotton Mather, You Dog, Dam you. I'll inoculate you with this, with a Pox to you."[12]

Despite overwhelming evidence of the effectiveness of the inoculations, the procedure remained controversial for decades even among physicians. In 1776, the Continental Congress issued a proclamation that prohibited inoculation in the military. Washington was well aware of the threat of smallpox to his troops and realized that an outbreak among his soldiers would probably mean the end of the revolution. Initially and with the Congress's ban on inoculations, Washington had to rely on isolation and quarantines to prevent spread of the disease. He also relied on the protection from the disease among individuals who had contracted smallpox infection earlier in life.

When Washington took command of the Continental Army, Boston was suffering a new outbreak of the scourge. The city, occupied by the British at the time, was soon under siege by Washington's army. There were rumors that the occupying power was smuggling infected Bostonians out from the town to spread the malady among the rebel soldiers, using what today would be called biological warfare. When the British finally evacuated Boston, Washington only allowed soldiers who had previously had the disease to enter the city; soldiers with facial pockmarks qualified as protected.

Boston was not the only place where smallpox would play a role during Washington's first year as commander of the rebellious warriors. A historian described how the infection "seemed to be everywhere" and listed several examples: "In Massachusetts during the siege of Boston, in Virginia during the mobilization of Lord Dunmore's Ethiopian Regiment, and in Canada during the siege of Quebec" where, as the author pointed out, "smallpox wreaked havoc as people and microbes came together in explosive combinations."[13]

Although Washington initially was skeptical about inoculations and prevented by the politicians to use it, it would not take long until he realized that he would have to resort to the method to protect his army. Early in 1777, Washington ordered the surgeon general of the Continental Army to inoculate all soldiers coming through Philadelphia. Later during the winter camp at Valley Forge, Washington ordered all unprotected soldiers to undergo the procedure. In mid–March 1778, "the commander in chief's mood was … lifted by the news that every [unprotected] man in camp had been inoculated against smallpox."[14] Historians have argued that Washington's decision to mandate the mass inoculation at Valley Forge may have saved the Continental Army and ultimately the revolution.

Even if most soldiers had now been inoculated or had contracted and recovered from the infection, the worry that the disease would resurface remained on Washington's mind throughout the Revolutionary War. The fear that the enemy would use infected individuals, even slaves, to spread the disease remained of great concern. During the final major battle of the war in 1781, a military surgeon reported that "the British have sent from Yorktown a large number of negroes sick with the smallpox, probably for the purpose of communicating the infection to our army."[15]

It is obvious that Washington had to fight not only the British but smallpox as well from the beginning to the end of the Revolutionary War and in addition had to face the scourge among civilians.

Washington's "Malignant Carbuncle" in 1789

When George Washington was sworn in as the first president of the United States, New York City was the capital. The new president was inaugurated on the balcony of Federal Hall on April 30, 1789. Less than two months later, Washington was ill with a condition that could have killed him. He had developed a tender and extremely painful swelling on his left thigh accompanied by chills and high fever. Although most historical accounts indicate that the president's ailment was a huge abscess on his left thigh, the exact nature and even its location have remained somewhat of a controversy among biographers. Some have called it "a large and painful tumor on his left thigh,"[16] while others have called it "a fast-growing tumor,"[17] a "carbuncle," or a "malignant carbuncle."[18] In a book published about seventy years after the event, the lesion was described as a "painful tumor … upon his thigh," and a reason was proposed as to why the illness had developed, explaining that "it was brought on by the excitements and labors which he had undergone since his inauguration."[19]

Although the various ways to describe Washington's lesion (abscess, carbuncle, tumor) may seem contradictory, that may not need to be the case. A large abscess is often described as a carbuncle. The term "tumor" doesn't always imply a malignant tumor but may also be caused by a nonmalignant swelling, such as an abscess.

Whereas most writings suggest that the abscess was on Washington's left thigh,[20] recently some historians have suggested that it was "an irritation on his left buttock that began as a minor saddle-sore (Washington was an avid horseback rider) and became a painful infected boil," which ultimately developed into a "very large tumor."[21] The same authors suggested that most previous accounts, placing the abscess on the president's leg rather than on the buttock, did so to spare Washington from the embarrassment of being reported to have a medical problem close to his private parts.

Regardless of the exact location and cause of the malady, taken together, most previous accounts seem to support the notion that the newly inaugurated president suffered from immense pain and "threatening" fever from a large abscess on his left thigh.

When the citizens of New York realized that their president (and hero) was ill, they worried. Their concern increased when they found the street in front of Washington's residency blocked off with a "chain ... stretched across the street" and the sidewalk being "laid with straw" to give Washington as much quiet as possible and improve his recuperation.[22] The people felt increasingly convinced that "the President's case was ... extremely dangerous."[23] Washington was also concerned and understood that he might die from the condition. On one occasion he asked his doctor about "the probable termination of his disease" and instructed him, "Do not flatter me with vain hopes; I am not afraid to die and therefore can bear the worst." Stoically, he added, "Whether to-night or twenty years hence, makes no difference; I know that I am in the hands of a good Providence."[24]

The pain and fevers grew worse, and finally not even the stoic Washington could stand it any longer. He requested that a surgeon be called in. When asked whether his old friend and long-standing personal physician, Dr. James Craik, should be sent for, the president, realizing that Craik was too far away from New York to make it to his bedside in a short time, answered that he would have been gratified to have his old friend with him, but in lieu of that, Washington felt fortunate to be in such good hands as Dr. Bard's.

Drs. John and Samuel Bard

Dr. John Bard and his son Dr. Samuel Bard were surgeons, well known and busy physicians in New York during the mid–1700s. John Bard had moved to New York from Philadelphia in 1746 after being advised by his friend Benjamin Franklin to leave his practice in the City of Brotherly Love for better opportunities in New York City. Bard was missed in his old hometown, where he was known as "a man who will not be quickly forgotten where he was once known."[25] His skills as a surgeon and his reputation as a good and honorable individual served him well in his new hometown.

John Bard gained international fame for performing one of the first laparotomies on the American continent in 1759. The patient was "Mrs. Stagg, the wife of a mason, about 28 years of age," who was suffering from a tumor in her lower abdomen. When she had her belly cut open by Bard (without anesthesia, of course), the surgeon found a dead fetus, the result of an ectopic pregnancy. He described his findings in a letter dated December 25, 1759, to the famous London physician John Fothergill, who reported the case to the Society of Physicians of London on March 4, 1760. Fothergill later published Bard's letter in its entirety in 1762 in *Medical Observations and Inquiries of the Society of Physicians in London.*[26] In his letter, Bard described in detail what he discovered during the laparotomy, including "a vast quantity of extremely fetid matter, together with the third phalanx of a finger of a child." In addition, he found "the child's elbow" and the remainder of "a foetus of the common size, at the ordinary time of delivery."[27]

John's son, Samuel, was fortunate to have generous parents. They paid for an expensive five-year medical and surgical training in England and Scotland that ultimately resulted in an MD degree from the University of Edinburgh. His degree was well earned. Not only had he been studying hard under the tutelage of some of the world's most famous surgeons and anatomists, such as John and William Hunter, William Cullen, and Alexander Monro, but he had also had to fight homesickness and the feeling of being among unfriendly and hostile people. Although Samuel had been warned before his voyage to Europe that "you are going to a part of the world where you will be surrounded with allurement,"[28] he was overwhelmed by unfriendliness when he arrived at the English capital and reported back to his father that "I never found one so unsocial [place] as London. Nothing is minded here but businesses; every one you meet is in a hurry, and if you do not work with circumspection, you run the risk of being shoved into the gutter. I assure you I am most heartily tired of it."[29]

When Samuel returned from Europe in 1766 he joined his father, and together they built a busy and successful medical practice. In addition to following in his father's footsteps as a skillful surgeon, Samuel also became involved in the founding of the second medical school in America in 1767 (the Medical Department of King's College in New York, preceded only by the medical school at Philadelphia) and the building of New York Hospital. So, it was indeed an accomplished pair of surgeons who were called to Washington's bedside in the summer of 1789.

The Surgeons Coming to the Rescue

When Washington's condition came to a head, Samuel Bard was already aware of the president's situation. Samuel had attended the patient "night and day" for several days.[30] When he was called upon on June 17, he understood that more drastic measures would be needed. He brought his knife for the handiwork and his father (who had retired more than ten years earlier) for moral support. Both surgeons understood that it was important to open and drain the abscess to ease Washington's suffering but were also anxious when facing the need to cut into the flesh of the newly inaugurated president. Just imagining the terrible pain they were about to inflict on the patient made them very uncomfortable, but they felt that they had no choice.

Bard senior was probably the most nervous of the two surgeons. "The elder being somewhat doubtful of his nerves, gave the knife to his son, bidding him to 'cut away—deeper, deeper still; don't be afraid; you see how well he bears it.'"[31] Opening the abscess and draining it of the pus was probably what saved the president's life. Luckily enough, the operation proved successful, and the patient's recovery removed "all cause of alarm." It would be a while, however, before Washington was back to normal. For a couple of weeks after the surgery, he could not lie on his left side. To calm the New Yorkers, the president was driven around in a wagon lying on his right side on a mattress and was able to wave to the cheering crowds. Soon he was able to take up plans for more extensive travel and set out for a tour through New England. The nation could take a deep breath, being relieved from the fear of losing their first president already a couple of months into his term.

Although the surgery had been successful, it would only take two years before Washington had a relapse, as described by Thomas Jefferson in a letter to James Madison. "The President is indisposed with the same blind tumour, & in the same place which he had the year before last in New York."[32] Most likely, however, surgery did not have to be employed this time because, as Jefferson explained, although the president "has at times a little fever," the carbuncle "does not promise to suppurate."[33]

It would be almost a decade before Washington would need another operation. This time, however, he was less lucky and did not get the necessary surgery. Before describing that event and to put things in perspective, it may be worthwhile to reflect upon the state of surgery at the time of Washington.

Surgeries in America During the 1700s

Surgeons in the eighteenth century were rapidly and aggressively expanding the boundaries of their profession. This happened despite the absence of anesthesia and despite the dangers involved. Surgeries at this time were brutal, fast, dirty, and all too commonly deadly. Operations were performed for injuries, either civilian caused by accidents or war-related incurred on the battlefields. Among civilians, there were many opportunities to get injured: people fell off horses and carriages and fractured legs and skulls, and they sustained injuries when working on farms and ships and in the harbors. Several conditions unrelated to trauma were also managed by surgeons. Those conditions included bladder stones, hernias, breast tumors, and tumors of the abdomen.

On the battlefields, surgeons saw gruesome injuries caused by swords, bayonets, guns, and canons, and the eighteenth century had its share of wars. Multiple conflicts on the European continent resulted in bloody battles with ghastly injuries that required the involvement of knifemen. The American Revolutionary War added to the need for physicians on the American continent, with surgeons participating on both sides of the conflict. Surgeries performed for injuries suffered on the battlefields, such as amputations, disarticulations, and treatment of fractures and wounds, were great in number.

Many circumstances related to surgeries during the 1700s are remarkable. Surgeries were performed without anesthesia (the first operation under general anesthesia in America would not take place until in the 1840s), and although large quantities of wine and laudanum (opium dissolved in alcohol) reduced pain and suffering somewhat, it is almost impossible to comprehend how people would agree to have major surgery while being awake and experiencing indescribable horror. The pain and risks were staggering, and many people chose to continue to suffer from their conditions and ultimately die rather than submit themselves to the terrifying pain inflicted by being cut upon.

Complications after surgical procedures were common. Bleeding occurred frequently, and the ways to stop bleedings were primitive and cruel. Infectious complications were plentiful if not the rule. Formation of pus in the wound was considered laudable and a sign of proper healing. In other less happy situations, the infections became overwhelming and caused the death of patients who had survived the surgery itself.

Even if Washington's surgery performed by Samuel Bard must have been utterly painful, more extensive surgeries giving rise to even greater agony took place in America during the 1700s. Amputations were some of the most horrific procedures. Not only were the patients awake, realizing that an arm or a leg was being cut off, but feeling the horrendous pain must have been an indescribable experience. Speed was of essence to shorten the suffering; surgeons were known to clock the time needed for an amputation and bragged about being able to cut a leg off in a few minutes. Sometimes accuracy took a backseat to speed; there were stories about not only a leg being amputated but also fingers of assistants holding down the patient's leg being sacrificed as well. Dr. John Jones, the "Father of American Surgery," warned against amputations that were too rushed. "Never affect great expedition, by which very capital and even fatal errors have been committed."[34] Interestingly, the same Dr. Jones participated in the care of Washington in 1790 when he was critically ill from a condition of an "inflammatory nature,"[35] most likely pneumonia following a bout of influenza.[36] Although Thomas Jefferson at the time was concerned that "we have been very near losing the President," Washington survived. In his gratitude to Jones for saving his life, the president appointed Jones his family physician.

Washington's Final Disease

The morning of December 12, 1799, was cold and windy and offered rain and snow showers around Mount Vernon. Washington described the conditions in the following way: "Morning snowing, about 3 inches deep, wind at N.E. and mercury at 30.0. Continuing snowing til 10 o'clock and at about 4 P.M. it became perfectly clear.

Wind in the same place, but not hard."[37] Despite the miserable weather, Washington, true to his habits, got on his horse and rode out to inspect his property. When the ex-president returned for dinner, he was cold and freezing and sat down for the meal without taking the time to change into warm and dry clothes.

The following morning, Washington woke up with a cold and a sore throat. Despite not feeling well, he went out in the afternoon to mark some trees that needed to be cut down. In the evening, his symptoms worsened. His longtime friend and secretary, Tobias Lear, encouraged Washington to take something for his cold. Washington refused, reminding Lear, "You know I never take anything for a cold; let it go as it came."[38] Between two and three o'clock the next morning, Saturday, December 14, Washington awoke his wife and told her that he was "very unwell, and had an ague."[39] Alarmed, Martha found her husband scarcely being able to speak and breathing with great difficulty. Lear was called to Washington's chamber and tried to help him by providing a "mixture of molasses, vinegar, and butter, to try its effects in the throat; but he could not swallow a drop."

Martha and Lear were growing increasingly anxious and sent for Albin Rawlins, one of the overseers of the estate and Washington's accountant and secretary, and Dr. Craik. Washington requested that Rawlins bleed him before Craik arrived. Rawlins had learned the technique of bloodletting on animals at the farm but was understandably nervous attempting it on his boss, the famous ex-president and commander in chief. When Washington noticed that Rawlins "appeared to be agitated," he comforted him. "Don't be afraid," Washington said.[40] As Martha saw the blood flowing freely out of her husband's arm, she started to have second thoughts and requested that the bloodletting be stopped. Washington, however, was a strong believer in the procedure and raised his hand to prevent the bleeding from being interrupted and instead said, "More, more."[41] All in all, Washington would lose eighty ounces (almost 2.4 liters) of blood on his deathbed.

Dr. Craik arrived around nine o'clock. Meanwhile, Mrs. Washington had sent for an additional physician, Dr. Gustavus Richard Brown of Port Tobacco, to be available "if any case should ever occur that was seriously alarming." Brown was another lifelong friend of Washington and had participated in the founding of the Medical (Hospital) Department of the Continental Army during the Revolutionary War. When Craik arrived, he put a blister of cantharides (Spanish fly) on Washington's neck and "took some more blood from him." He also prepared a mixture of vinegar and hot water and instructed Washington to inhale the steam from the decoction.

Dr. Brown had not yet made it to Washington's sickbed, so Craik sent for yet another colleague, Dr. Elisha Cullen Dick, "as he feared Dr. Brown would not come in time." About this time, "the General was bled again." Nothing seemed to help, and panic started to develop. Finally, around four o'clock in the afternoon the whole team of doctors was assembled: Drs. Craik, Dick, and Brown. Add to the picture Martha, Lear, Rawlins, and slaves and servants running back and forth and in the center of it all the patient gasping for air and having terrible pain when trying to swallow, and it is easy to imagine the scene of threatening disaster. Supplementing the repeated bleedings with calomel to induce diarrhea and antimony tartrate to provoke vomiting clearly did not help.

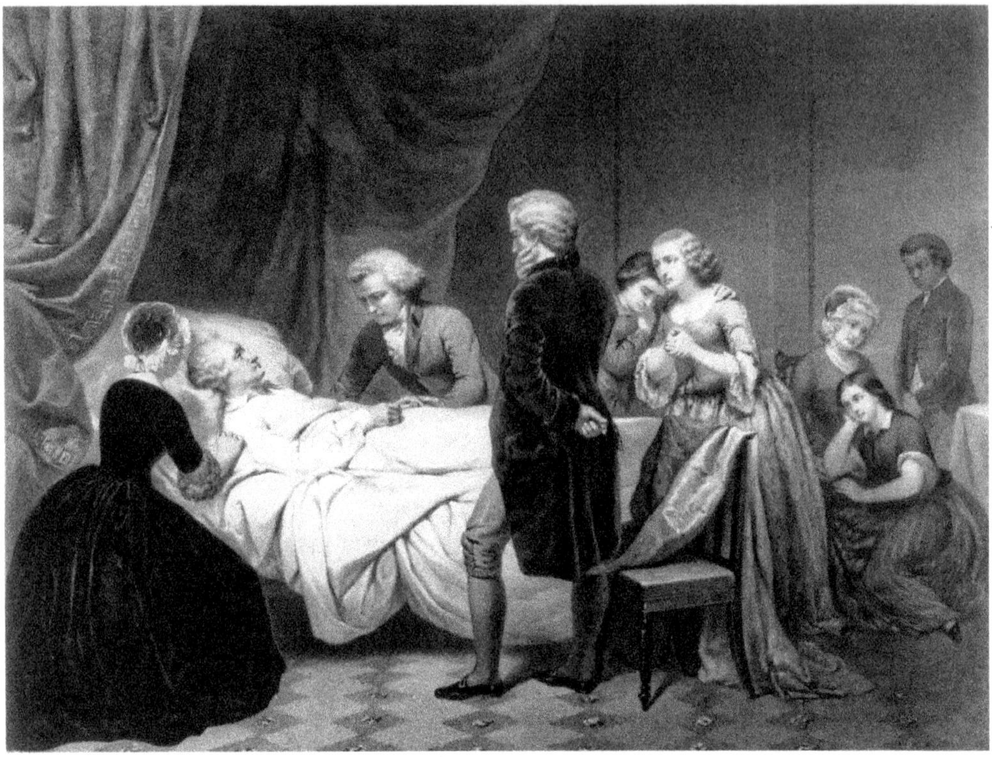

Washington's deathbed. Lithograph by Claude Regnier, after Junius Brutus Stearns, 1853. Library of Congress, Prints and Photographs Division, Washington, D.C.

Later in the afternoon, Washington started to fear that he may not survive. Not being able to breathe was horrifying, and understanding that the doctors were unable to help him was alarming. At around five o'clock, Washington sent for Martha to review his will. He said to Lear, "I find I am going. My breath cannot last long."[42] He instructed Lear to "arrange my accounts and settle my books." To Craik, the dying ex-president said, "Doctor, I die hard, but I am not afraid to go." Between five and six o'clock Washington bid farewell to Drs. Brown and Dick. "I feel myself going; I thank you for your attentions; but I pray you to take no more trouble about me. Let me go off quietly. I cannot last long."[43]

Washington lasted until between ten and eleven o'clock in the evening. His final words were "Tis well."[44]

The Physicians at Washington's Deathbed

The team of doctors attending Washington during his last struggle were all well-educated and accomplished physicians and longtime friends of the ex-president and his family.

Dr. Craik was the first physician to arrive at Mount Vernon on December 14, 1799. At the age of sixty-nine, he was the oldest of the colleagues who would ultimately surround the dying Washington. Craik was born in Scotland in 1730. His medical training was at Edinburgh where the premier academic medical school of the time was located. Craik started his career as a surgeon in the British Army, moved to the colonies in the early 1750s, and settled in Norfolk, Virginia.

As we have seen, Craik was the surgeon Washington initially would have preferred when he needed the abscess on his left thigh cut open in 1789. Craik's and Washington's friendship was deep and had lasted for decades. They had fought together in the French and Indian War and later in the American Revolutionary War and had remained close personal friends ever since. Craik was a frequent guest at the president's Mount Vernon estate and also served as Washington's personal physician. As proof of his admiration of Washington, Craik had named one of his sons George Washington. Craik attended Martha Washington at her demise two years after her husband passed away.[45]

Elisha Cullen Dick was the youngest among the physicians attending Washington. He was thirty-seven years old and, like Craik, had gone through a solid medical education and had graduated from the University of Pennsylvania School of Medicine in 1782. Dick had studied under Benjamin Rush and William Shippen, Jr., both prominent physicians and surgeons during the American Revolution with close ties to Washington. In addition to being an eminent surgeon, Dick was also involved in politics and had served as a member of the Virginia House of Delegates in the mid–1790s.

When Dick arrived at Mount Vernon on December 14, he was not only the youngest among his colleagues but was also probably more up-to-date with treatment options and recent literature than the other doctors. He certainly seemed to be the most daring of the surgeons. He proposed a tracheotomy to be performed, but his fellow physicians objected to that idea and overruled him. In particular, Craik was vehemently opposed to the idea and vetoed Dick's suggestion. Craik did not want to perform a risky procedure that was still extremely rare and unknown to many surgeons at the time despite being known since "long before the dawn of modern scientific medicine."[46] Tracheotomy was accepted in Europe since the early 1700s in the treatment of acute upper airway obstruction caused by foreign body ingestion, aspiration, and inflammation, but at the time of Washington's death it had not yet been performed in America.[47] As one historian explained, "Undoubtedly, the specter of failure with a grisly, painful (in the absence of anesthesia) and untried surgical experiment on the former president weighed heavily in Craik's decision to veto this radical suggestion."[48]

When reflecting on the events surrounding Washington's death, Dick stated that "I shall never cease to regret that the operation was not performed."[49] Later when Dick criticized his colleagues for preventing him from performing the tracheotomy, he sarcastically wrote that they had fallen victims to "age-related caution."[50]

The last physician who joined the doctors trying to save Washington was Gustavus Richard Brown, "a wealthy, 52-year-old physician from Port Tobacco, Maryland."[51] He arrived at around four o'clock in the afternoon, one hour after Dick had reached Mount Vernon. Brown, like Craik, had studied medicine at Edinburgh, where he graduated in 1768.

Akin to his colleagues, Brown was also a longtime close friend of Washington.

They had worked closely together during the American Revolution. Brown's skills as a physician were well known and respected among his peers. It was on Craik's suggestion that Brown was summoned by Martha to Washington's sickbed.

Having the three physicians work together in the care of the critically ill Washington must have been reassuring. The colleagues could share the responsibility and find support in each other's assessment of the patient's condition. They seemed to be in agreement of Washington's diagnosis, *cynanche trachealis,* now most commonly referring to as childhood croup. At the time of Washington, however, *cynanche trachealis* referred to nonspecific inflammation and swelling of the throat, causing pain on swallowing and difficulties in breathing. Different disorders can result in these symptoms, including epiglottitis (inflammation of the epiglottis).

In contrast to the agreement on Washington's diagnosis, the doctors were not in agreement regarding treatment. In particular, Dr. Dick was an outlier. Not only did he propose a tracheotomy to help Washington's breathing, but he also felt that the bloodlettings favored by his colleagues were too aggressive.

When Washington died, his doctors understood that they would be at risk of being criticized for the care of their patient. To preempt the criticism, Craik and Dick published an account of the circumstances around Washington's illness and demise in the *Alexandria Times* five days after Washington's passing.[52] Despite their efforts, Washington's physicians were not able to divert criticism. "Furious attacks were directed against them, and they came from physicians as well as laymen."[53] A century later, one biographer used harsh words when criticizing Washington's doctors: "there can scarcely be a doubt that the treatment of his last illness by the doctors was little short of murder."[54]

Could Washington's Life Have Been Saved by a Tracheotomy?

Biographers have debated both the disease that killed Washington and the care he received. Importantly, it has been speculated whether a tracheotomy, the surgical opening of the windpipe below the swelling that prevented the breathing, could have saved Washington's life.

The list of ailments that have been suspected to have caused Washington's death is long and include diphtheria, *cynanche trachealis*, quincy (peritonsillar abscess), and streptococcal laryngitis. More recent medical historians seem to favor the diagnosis of epiglottitis as explaining the patient's symptoms and the ultimate outcome.[55] When a specialist in otolaryngology (ear, nose, and throat surgery) carefully reviewed signs and symptoms experienced by Washington, he concluded that "all this can mean only one thing—acute epiglottitis."[56]

Historians have also speculated about how much the treatments, in particular the bloodletting and purging, may have contributed to Washington's death. Even if the remedies that his doctors used did not help the condition but may actually have hastened the patient's demise, the treatments were not forced upon Washington; he even asked for "more, more" when he was bled. Bleedings and purging, of course, were part of the standard treatment for anything that was ascribed to "inflammation" at the time.

If indeed Washington died from epiglottitis, the blockage that prevented him from breathing could probably have been bypassed by performing a tracheotomy. Dick, the youngest among Washington's doctors, was eager to remind people in later statements that he had recommended a tracheotomy on that fateful evening of December 14, 1799: "I proposed to perforate the trachea as [a] means to prolonging life and affording time for the removal of the obstruction to respiration in the larynx."[57] Although it may be easy in hindsight to be critical of Dick's colleagues for preventing him from performing a tracheotomy, it is important to remember that they were under immense pressure and were horrified that something might go wrong. Dr. Craik proclaimed that the procedure was "a grisly, painful, and untried surgical experiment."[58]

Although it will never be known what might have happened if Washington had had a tracheotomy, it may be speculated that in contrast to what happened a decade prior when the president's life was saved by a surgical procedure, he now died because he was denied a potentially lifesaving intervention.

Chapter Two

Andrew Jackson

Red-Haired Hothead

The Seventh President

March 4, 1829–March 4, 1837

Born in the Waxhaw District of South Carolina in 1767 to a Scotch-Irish family, Andrew Jackson grew up "a tall, lean, remarkably agile, freckle-faced boy with bright blue eyes, a shock of tousled hair that was almost red and a temper in keeping."[1] He was described as having "a habit of 'slobbering' which he was unable to control until almost grown."[2] Important for his future health, already as a young boy he was known to have a character that "spelled combat, whatever the odds."[3]

Jackson was merely an eight-year-old boy when the American Revolutionary War erupted. Five years into the war, Jackson and one of his elder brothers, Robert, joined a local militia to serve as couriers. Their eldest brother, Hugh, had joined the fight for freedom a year prior and had died after an engagement in June 1779. Andrew and Robert were captured by the British in April 1781 while breakfasting at the home of their cousin Lieutenant Thomas Crawford. Redcoats stormed the house, wrecked some of the furniture, disrupted the morning meal, and took the brothers prisoners. To show his power and superiority, a British officer ordered Andrew to polish his boots. True to

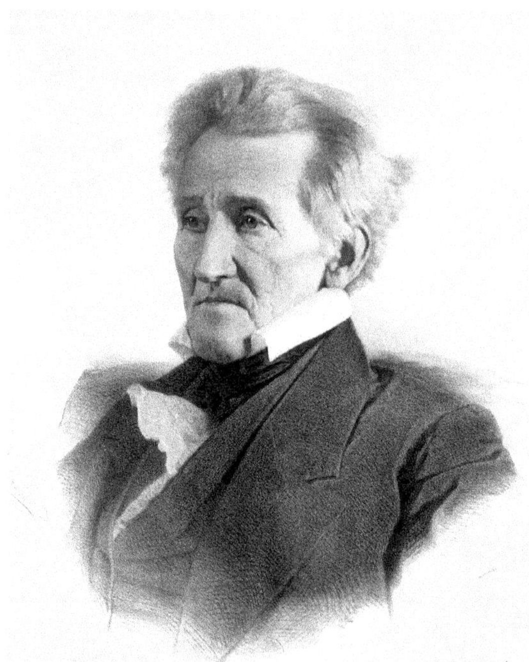

Portrait of Andrew Jackson, 1856. Library of Congress, Prints and Photographs Division, Washington, D.C.

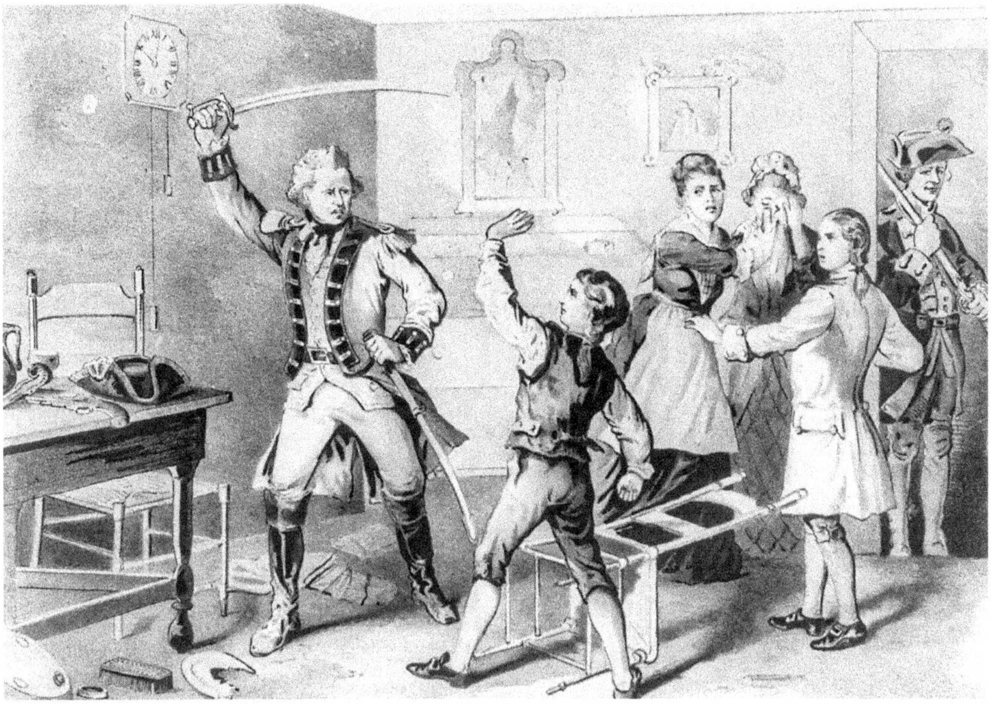

"The Brave Boy of the Waxhaws." A print by Nathaniel Currier (1813–1888) and James Ives (1824–1895) appearing in 1876 and depicting the young Andrew Jackson defying a British officer and sustaining a saber wound on his left wrist and the left side of his head. Library of Congress, Prints and Photographs Division, Washington, D.C.

his character, Andrew refused and obstinately informed the officer that as prisoners of war, he and his brother had certain rights. This, not surprisingly, did not sit well with the officer, who angrily drew his sword, aiming at Andrew's head. Andrew used his left arm as protection, resulting in a deep cut of his wrist extending down to the bone. Robert, who also refused to obey the officer, was subjected to a similar abuse as his younger brother. Together with twenty other captured colonial soldiers, the brothers were marched off to the military prison at Camden, some forty miles away.

The brothers were in for a rough time at the prison camp. They were crammed together with more than two hundred other Patriots. The conditions were horrific: no beds, no medicine, no dressings for the wounds, and not enough food. The prisoners were nearly starved to death. Smallpox was ravaging the jail, and the brothers contracted the scourge. After several months of deplorable conditions, the boys' widowed mother, Elizabeth, managed to secure the release of her sons with the help of an American militia captain through a prisoners' exchange. When heading home to the Waxhaw area, both Andrew and Robert were severely ill. Andrew, drenched with heavy rain, had to walk "barefooted, bareheaded, and without a coat."[4] Robert was close to dying when leaving the prison camp, and despite being allowed to ride on the only available horse, he survived for only two days after arriving home. Elizabeth kept nurturing Andrew and was able to save his life.

After seeing the terrible conditions in the British prison at Camden and experiencing her sons' suffering and, in addition, realizing that her sister's son was a prisoner on one of two ships kept by the British in the harbor of Charleston, Elizabeth volunteered to help American prisoners on the British ships. Sadly, she contracted "ship fever" (typhus) and "after a short illness, died."[5] Andrew, whose father had died in a logging accident three weeks before his son was born, was now a fourteen-year-old orphan, bitterly blaming the British for the loss of his brothers and mother. He never learned where his mother had been buried, adding to his agony.

The Dickinson Duel in 1806

During the early 1800s disputes were sometimes resolved by duels, even though they were illegal in some states. The nation had seen Alexander Hamilton killed in a duel with Aaron Burr in 1804. That same year Jackson, then a justice on the bench of the Tennessee Supreme Court, had challenged the governor of the same state, John Sevier, to a duel, a craziness that "could only happen in the west."[6] The practice, which had been condemned by George Washington and Benjamin Franklin, would continue for many more years. Being a hotspur, it is not surprising that Jackson ended up challenging or being challenged by enemies on several occasions. One reason for many of Jackson's heated arguments and pistol duels was his efforts to protect the honor of his wife, Rachel.

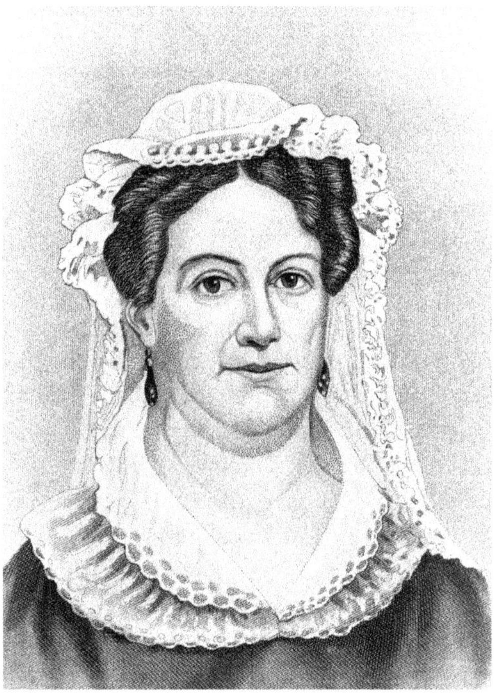

A miniature portrait of Rachel Jackson engraved by John Chester Buttre, ca. 1883, from oil painting on ivory by Louisa Catherine Strobel (according to Robert Remini on page inserted after p. 238) or by Anna C. Peale in Washington, December 1815 (according to Marquis James on page inserted after p. 88). The original miniature portrait was worn by Jackson over his heart after Rachel's death in 1828. Library of Congress, Prints and Photographs Division, Washington, D.C.

When Andrew and Rachel tied the knot the first time in 1791, they assumed that Rachel was legally divorced from her previous husband, Lewis Robards of Kentucky. That turned out not to be correct, and the marriage technically was bigamous; Andrew and Rachel remarried in 1794 after Rachel's legal status had been resolved. The fact that Rachel may still have been married to another man when she initially married Andrew generated many gleeful comments from enemies. Jackson was understandably upset by the gossip spread by his foes and ended up challenging many of them to duels. Reportedly, Jackson fought about one hundred duels to defend Rachel's honor.

In the spring of 1806, it happened again; Jackson challenged Charles Dickinson. Dickinson was a young lawyer in Nashville, "a man of fashion and success,"[7] but also a well-off horse breeder and plantation owner. In addition, Dickinson was a famous duelist and superb marksman; his reputation alleged that "he could put four balls in a mark twenty-four feet away, each ball touching each another."[8] When Jackson heard that Dickinson had made "an allusion to Rachel Donelson's matrimonial history,"[9] he was outraged. Although Dickinson apologized and was forgiven by Jackson, the bad blood between them persisted. Jackson could not forget that Dickinson had taken "the sacred name" of Rachel Jackson into his "polluted mouth."[10] It therefore did not take much to reignite the fight, and after a dispute related to a horse race, Jackson challenged, and Dickinson accepted. During the days leading up to the duel, the opponents kept hurling insults at each other. Jackson called his enemy a "cowardly talebearer."[11] Dickinson responded by publishing his assessment of Jackson in the *Nashville Impartial Review and Cumberland Repository,* Nashville's only newspaper, on May 24, 1806, and called him "a worthless scoundrel, ... a poltroon and a coward."[12]

The duel took place on May 30, 1806. Because dueling was illegal in Tennessee at the time, the combatants were to meet at Red River in Kentucky, just across the border with Tennessee. The day before the fight, Jackson "rose at five o'clock and after breakfast told Rachel that he would be gone for a couple of days and meanwhile he might have some trouble with Mr. Dickinson."[13] Jackson and his entourage, including his second, General Thomas Overton, arrived at a tavern on the banks of the Red River and checked in for an overnight stay. Even if Jackson was nervous about next morning's duel, he did not let it show; he "ate heartily at supper that night, conversing in a lively, pleasant manner, and smoked his evening pipe as usual."[14]

The thin and lanky Jackson came to the fight dressed in an oversized dark blue frock, referred to by one historian as "an enormous black overcoat, which he did not remove."[15] When Jackson arrived at the appointed place someone asked him, "How do you feel about it now, General?" A confident Jackson replied, "Oh, all right, I shall wing him, never fear."[16]

Jackson had decided "not to compete with Dickson for the first fire" and let his opponent have the opening shot.[17] Although being a feared duelist, Dickinson missed his target. It is possible that Jackson's large overcoat confused Dickinson, explaining why "the bullet went wide of the mark" and missed the heart. It still caused significant damage and "tore the chest muscles, broke a rib or two and settled in the chest cavity, where it remained the rest of Jackson's life."[18] The large overcoat may have saved Jackson's life.

Bleeding and in pain from a fresh wound, Jackson managed to raise his pistol and fire, hitting Dickinson below the ribs and causing "a furrow through his bowels."[19] Dickinson's assistants "stripped off his clothes" and noticed that the blood "was gushing from his side in a torrent."[20] Later that evening, "poor Dickinson bled to death."[21] After the shooting, Jackson wanted to downplay his own injury. When he left the area together with a group of supporters, someone noted that Jackson's left boot was filling up with blood. When Jackson was alerted to the bleeding, he replied, "Oh, I believe that he has pinked me a little!"[22]

The slug left behind in Jackson's chest would haunt him the rest of his life. Medical historians have suggested that Jackson's recurring episodes of bloody coughs and need for periods of bed rest may have been caused by a chronic lung abscess related to the Dickinson duel in 1806. A more immediate consequence of Dickinson's death was an outrage among the citizens of Nashville, increasing the number of Jackson's enemies in the city.

The Barroom Brawl in Downtown Nashville, September 1813

The circumstances ultimately resulting in the barroom brawl in downtown Nashville on September 4, 1813, are "a bit cloudy."[23] What is known about the events has been told by several Jackson biographers. Parts of the narratives read like scripts for a Wild West movie.

Pertinent for the background was the U.S. declaration of war on Britain on June 18, 1812, signaling the beginning of the War of 1812. To Jackson's great disappointment, it would take half a year until he was called upon to throw himself into the conflict and secure a commission to bring his Tennessee volunteers to New Orleans. They left Nashville on January 7, 1813, after a "particularly brutal winter." Among the troops, Jackson had appointed two individuals who would become part of the story behind the barroom brawl. William Carroll, "a bright and energetic young man,"[24] was appointed brigade inspector, and Thomas Hart Benton, a "clever young lawyer" whom Jackson had met previously during deliberations in the Tennessee Supreme Court,[25] was appointed aide-de-camp.

After thirty-nine freezing days, the troops arrived at Natchez on the east bank of the Mississippi River, north of New Orleans, and awaited further orders as to how and when to march south to New Orleans. No instructions came; instead, after waiting for several weeks, Jackson was ordered by Secretary of War John Armstrong to dismiss the troops and return home. Jackson refused to abandon his soldiers and declared that because the troops had "followed me to the field; I shall carefully march them back to their homes."[26] The difficult footslog back from Natchez to Nashville in the spring of 1813 was full of agony. It was during this march that Jackson's soldiers realized that the he was "tougher than most anything imaginable. Tough as hickory,"[27] and this is how he earned his nickname "Old Hickory."

The origin of the barroom debacle has been traced back to Jackson's march homeward from Natchez. During the march, a dispute had erupted between Carroll and a "wild young fellow of the anti–Carroll faction" named Littleton Johnston.[28] The disagreement between the two men resulted in Johnston challenging Carroll to a duel. Carroll felt that Johnston was below his definition of "gentleman" and did not accept the challenge. Johnston engaged Jesse Benton to deliver a new challenge, hoping that Jesse's social status, brother of General Jackson's aide-de-camp, would make it difficult for Carroll to refuse the challenge. Again, however, Carroll declined. Not until Jesse had offered himself to substitute for Johnston did Carroll feel that the challenge was worthy acceptance.

Carroll, now in the need of a second, rode out to Jackson's home, the Hermitage, and asked for help. General Jackson, however, initially turned down the request, commenting that "I am too old. The time has been when I should have gone out with pleasure; but, at my time of life, it would be extremely injudicious."[29] Carroll kept pleading his case and explained to Jackson that he was afraid there was a conspiracy "among certain young men to run him out of the country." This turned out to be pushing the right button, because when Jackson heard Carroll's concern of being run "out of the country," Old Hickory got mad and said, "Well, Carroll, you may make your mind easy on *one* point: they sha'n't run you out of the country as long as Andrew Jackson lives in it."[30]

The duel between Carroll and Jesse Benton was scheduled for June 14, 1813, at six o'clock in the morning.

Jesse Benton was a better marksman than Carroll and a more feared duelist. Negotiating the rules for the duel, Carroll managed to reach an agreement to have the firing distance between the opponents reduced to ten feet (rather than thirty) to "equalize" their skills.[31] In addition, they agreed that the duel would start with a back-to-back position. Understanding that Carroll may be nervous about meeting a superior duelist, Jackson tried to reassure him: "You needn't fear him, Carroll; he'd never hit you, if you were as broad as a barn-door."[32] When "Fire!" was called, the combatants quickly wheeled around and unloaded their pistols. Jesse hit Carroll in the thumb, whereas Carroll managed to hit Jesse "in the ... part of his person ... covered by the seat of his trousers,"[33] inflicting "a long, raking wound across both cheeks of his buttocks."[34] The wound was painful and embarrassing; "it did far more injury to the spirit than the flesh,"[35] and "poor Jesse became the object of much laughter in Nashville."[36]

The humiliation of Jesse outraged his brother. Thomas, who up until recently had been a close friend of Jackson, told anybody in Tennessee who wanted to listen how much he now despised Jackson for being "a party of his brother's humiliation" and accused Jackson of showing "very poor business in a man of your age and standing to be conducting a duel about nothing between young men who had no harm against each."[37] Being bad-mouthed by Thomas Benton in this way outraged Old Hickory, who commented, "The trouble with Benton ... [is] ... his inability to keep his mouth shut," and Jackson promised that "he would horsewhip Tom Benton the first time he saw him."[38] The excitement started to build. Everyone in Nashville, including the Benton brothers, soon knew that Jackson had promised to whip Thomas Benton "on sight."

The time for horsewhipping came in early September. Jackson, together with his friend the militia general John Coffee, rode into Nashville to pick up the mail and spend a night in town. They checked in at the Old Nashville Inn. The following morning, they went to the post office to pick up their letters. On the way, they spotted Thomas Benton in the doorway to the nearby City Hotel.[39] When seeing Jackson's enemy, Coffee whispered, "Do you see that fellow?" Without turning his head, Jackson replied, "Oh, yes. I have my eye on him."[40]

When Jackson and Coffee walked back from the post office, the Benton brothers were waiting at the City Hotel with loaded pistols. Closing in on Thomas, Jackson suddenly turned around, wielded his horsewhip and a short sword, and shouted, "Now, you d-d rascal, I am going to punish you. Defend yourself."[41] Jackson, threatening with his pistol, forced Thomas to retreat into the hotel. Jesse rushed through the barroom into a hallway leading onto a rear porch from where he unloaded his pistol at Jackson, who was hit in his left upper arm by two bullets. One of the slugs shattered his shoulder, and the other "buried itself near the bone,"[42] where it would remain for almost two decades. Old Hickory had been severely injured. "The shock of the wounds was such, that Jackson fell across the entry, and remained prostrate, bleeding profusely."[43]

Stockley Hays, Jackson's nephew who was also in Jackson's party and was "a man of a giant's size, and a giant's strength," rushed into the hotel, wrestled Jesse to the floor, and stabbed him repeatedly with a dagger. Coffee joined the tumult, firing his pistol at Thomas (but missing) and throwing Thomas down the stairs on the back side of the hotel. "And with that, the gunfight ended."[44]

The Aftermath of the Barroom Brawl

Still hemorrhaging heavily, Jackson was carried across the square to the Old Nashville Inn. Meanwhile, the Benton brothers paraded in front of the people gathered at the square outside the City Hotel and loudly denounced Jackson as an assassin. Triumphantly, they broke the sword that Jackson had dropped during the debacle and expressed their disdain of him in a "thundering voice."[45] The triumph, however, would not be long-lasting. The Nashville people did not appreciate seeing Jackson—who after his courageous march of his soldiers back from Natchez and was now a celebrated hero—wounded and humiliated, and the Benton brothers started to feel the wrath from the citizens. Thomas Benton wrote, "I am literally in hell here; the meanest wretches under heaven to contend with—liars, affidavit-makers, and shameless cowards."[46] He continued, "All the puppies of Jackson are at work on me." The Benton brothers did not feel safe in Nashville any longer, and Thomas complained, "My life is in danger."[47]

To escape Jackson's "puppies," the brothers left town. Thomas moved back to his home in Franklin, Tennessee. It would be ten years before Thomas Benton and Jackson met again to make friends as U.S. senators. Jesse, in contrast, remained bitter the rest of his life and could never forgive Jackson (or his brother for calling a truce with Jackson).

Over at the Nashville Inn, Jackson continued to bleed from his fresh wounds. Before the hemorrhage could be stopped, two mattresses had been soaked through. The injured general attracted the attention of the entire Nashville medical community. "All the doctors in Nashville were seen in attendance,"[48] and all except one recommended amputation of the arm. Jackson overheard the physicians' discussions, and before he lost consciousness, he declared, "I'll keep my arm."[49] When he woke up, he still had his arm. The doctors had not dared to contradict him.

Jackson was weakened by the blood loss and remained bedridden for three weeks. The wounds were dressed with "poultices of slippery elm, and other products of the woods," following "the simple manner of the Indians and pioneers."[50] The time of recuperation would not last much longer. Already a month after the events at the City Hotel in Nashville, General Jackson was called into action.

The Creek War

On August 30, 1813, Creek Indians who were fighting other Indian tribes, hated whites in general, and had taken the side of the British in the War of 1812, massacred hundreds of settlers at Fort Mims in Mississippi Territory (now Alabama). The attack was led by William Weatherford, also known as Chief Red Eagle, and was utterly brutal. The onslaught resulted in the deaths of 250 settlers, who were "butchered in the quickest manner."[51] The Creeks' rage did not spare children or women. "The children were seized by the legs, and killed by batting their heads." The women were scalped, and "those who were pregnant were opened, while they were alive, and the embryo infants were let out of the womb."[52] The violence was so repulsive that even their commander tried to stop the savagery, but when Red Eagle tried to interfere, "many clubs were raised over his head and he was forced to withdraw to save his own life."[53]

The news of the massacre "burst like a thunderclap over Tennessee."[54] The governor mobilized five thousand volunteers for a three-month tour of duty. In Nashville, a committee on public safety was formed and rushed to the Hermitage, pleading with Jackson to help save them. Although still bedridden, Old Hickory promised to come to their rescue. "By the eternal, these people must be saved."[55] Jackson reassured the anxious citizens of Tennessee that "the health of your general is restored" and promised that he would "command in person."[56] A biographer commented that "Jackson was too weak to leave his bed but was strong enough to make war."[57]

Jackson now had a chance to live up to his epithet, Old Hickory. On October 7, with his left arm still in a sling, he led his troops on a thirty-two-mile, nine-hour-long march to join Coffee and his cavalry. On the morning of November 3, 1813, the village of Tallushatchee, deep in the eastern part of the Mississippi Territory, was encircled by a thousand cavalry and mounted riflemen who massacred most of the Indian warriors. Davy Crocket, the famous frontiersman, reported that "we shot them like dogs."[58] Jackson triumphantly said, "We have retaliated for Fort Mims."[59]

Even being a tough and merciless general, Jackson also had a soft side. During the campaign at Tallushatchee, a slain Indian mother was found on the battlefield, still embracing her living infant son. When the child was brought to Jackson together with other captives, Jackson asked some of the Creek women to take care of the boy. They refused and stated that "all his relations are dead, kill him too."[60] The statement made Jackson remember his own childhood when he had lost his family. He sent the women away and ordered that the child be taken to his tent, where he "dissolved a little brown sugar and coaxed the boy to drink."[61]

Jackson, at his own expense, arranged for the boy to be taken to a nearby town to be nursed, clothed, and housed. When the military campaign was finished, he sent the boy to the Hermitage, where he ordered his wife to treat the child "not like a servant nor an orphan."[62] He continued by telling Rachel that "I therefore want him well taken care of; he may have been given to me for some valuable purpose—in fact when I reflect that he as to his relations is so much like myself I feel an unusual sympathy for him."[63]

The boy was given the name Lincoyer and was brought up at the Hermitage as a son of the family. "He grew to be a finely formed and robust youth, and received the education usually given to the planters' sons in the neighborhood."[64] Sadly, Lincoyer contracted consumption to which he succumbed, not yet having turned seventeen years old. Jackson sincerely mourned his loss and often spoke of the boy "as a parent speaks of a lost child."[65]

The killing of Native Americans did not end with Tallushatchee. On March 27 the following year, Jackson encircled eight hundred Creek warriors with his field army of two thousand men at the Horseshoe Bend of the Tallapoosa River. Even if Jackson allowed women and children to be carried across the river for safety before he ordered the final assault on the Creeks, the battle turned into yet another brutal tragedy. In a letter to Rachel, Jackson wrote that "the carnage was dreadful."[66] At the end of the day, the battleground was covered with 557 dead Indian warriors, and "the river held two hundred more."[67] Chief Red Eagle surrendered three weeks later, and the Creek War was over. But the War of 1812 was not.

The War of 1812, the Battle of New Orleans, and Jackson's Health

After the end of the Creek campaign, Jackson had the defeated enemy pay a high price. As part of the Treaty of Fort Jackson, the Creeks were forced to surrender more than twenty million acres of their land to the United States. Jackson showed no mercy for the Indians; his treatment of them was characterized by "retaliation and vengeance."[68]

Jackson, who had risen in the ranks to major general in the U.S. Army, could now turn his attention toward the British and the Spanish. He accused Spain of arming Native Americans against the United States and breaking the agreement of neutrality by allowing the British forces into the Floridas. At the Battle of Pensacola on November 7, Jackson defeated both adversaries. The Spanish surrendered, and the British, together with hundreds of their Indian allies, fled to their ships and sailed away into the Gulf of Mexico. Jackson was pleased "to see the whole British force leave the port and their friends to our Mercy."[69]

Jackson soon became aware of the British plan to capture New Orleans, which, located at the outlet of Mississippi River, had extraordinary strategic and commercial importance. It was not difficult for the general to make the decision to rush his forces to defend the city.

Jackson arrived with his army at New Orleans on December 1, 1814. The British arrived three weeks later. By then, Jackson had enforced the defenses of the city with multiple effective fortifications. The decisive battle took place on January 8, 1815. The day ended in disaster for the British; they saw 291 of their soldiers killed, as opposed to 13 among Jackson's army. The British had to withdraw in defeat. Unbeknownst to the warring parties on the day of the battle, the War of 1812 had already ended by the signing of the Treaty of Ghent on Christmas Eve 1814. Had they known, lives could have been saved.

The victorious defense of New Orleans would help make Jackson not only the "Hero of New Orleans" but also a national hero, factors that would help him when he ultimately decided to seek the presidency. This, however, was still almost fifteen years in the future.

Historians agree that "Jackson's reputation as general, as westerner, as frontiersman, as symbol, was made by the Creek War."[70] Additional campaigns during the War of 1812 certainly contributed to putting Jackson's name on the map. As one of his biographers pointed out, Old Hickory "mirrored in splendid excess the westerners' yearning for heroics, drama, storm."[71] The military achievements, however, had their price; they would ruin Jackson's health.

Of course, mounting his horse in early October 1813 and taking command of an army with an injury to his left arm and shoulder not yet healed, with the arm still in a sling, was a challenge. He understood that Rachel, left behind at the Hermitage, was worried about him, and in an effort to calm her fears, he downplayed his sufferings. In a letter written about a week after starting the march to the south, he wrote to his wife, "My health is good and my arm mending fast. The little place on my shoulder gives me more pain than my arm. Both, I hope, will soon be well."[72] His hope, however, would not be fulfilled. Jackson would continue to have problems with his left arm for almost two decades. During that time, he would continue to have pain and see the scar open up and drain pus and bone fragments on several occasions. Not until Jackson had been under the knife to have the bullet removed did his wound heal and his agony resolve.

Although Jackson had experienced occasional stomach pains for many years, they grew worse during the military campaigns of 1813–1815. Sometimes they were so severe that they forced him to sit on a chair "with his chest against the back of it and his arm dangling forward."[73] He could be seen in that position for hours before he got relief from the pain. The abdominal agony was often accompanied by diarrhea and likely, Jackson was suffering from dysentery.

As if the torments from his arm and belly were not enough, Jackson also had severe pulmonary symptoms. Ever since the Dickinson duel in 1806, Jackson had experienced suffocating coughing spells, often combined with hemorrhages and production of "great quantities of flime."[74] The coughing attacks were frequently preceded by chills and fevers, so Jackson knew when he was in for another episode of terrible chest symptoms. Some historians have interpreted Jackson's symptoms (fevers, coughing, and hemoptysis) as evidence that Jackson suffered from pulmonary tuberculosis. Others have questioned that assumption and ascribed the symptoms to a chronic abscess resulting from the bullet retained in Jackson's chest since Dickinson put it there at the duel. Because the slug was buried deep in the chest, no attempts had been made to remove it. Occasional attempts to perform surgery of the chest had been made earlier, but thoracotomies would not be more commonly performed until the late 1800s and early 1900s. William Conrad Roentgen's discovery of X-rays was also almost a century in the future.

Regardless of the cause of Jackson's pulmonary symptoms, they would stay with him for the rest of his life and get worse as time went by.

Similar to earlier centuries, bloodletting remained a remedy used frequently well into the 1800s. Jackson was a true believer of bleeding as a cure for almost anything, even to the point of bleeding himself. When he had nobody else around and felt a fever coming on, he would bare his arm, take out his penknife, and "call his servant to hold the bowl, and bleed himself freely."[75] He was known to continue the self-bleedings even into his presidency. During his military campaigns, Jackson was bled on several occasions.

Jackson's continuous suffering from various ailments kept getting worse during the War of 1812. He pleaded with Rachel to come and join him at New Orleans; "he needed her desperately because he was close to total physical collapse."[76] A couple of weeks before reaching New Orleans, Jackson wrote in a letter to his wife, "I was taken very ill ... and there was Eight days on the march that I never broke bread."[77]

When reaching New Orleans, Jackson looked haggard, thin, and exhausted. Dr. Frederick May, who was with Jackson during the Creek War and at New Orleans, described the general in the following way: "The rigors of border warfare had left him a perpetual indigestion which was starving him into a shadow, a case of diarrhea that all but disemboweled him, ... and ... tuberculosis ... finding its way into his lungs."[78] Despite being an "emaciated shell," Jackson carried himself with pride and determination. His manner "radiated confidence, stern decision, and enormous energy,"[79] features that impressed people around him, not least the women in town. Newly arrived, Jackson was invited to dinner at the mayor's house, where "the ladies were astonished at his poise and gratified by his grand manner." When Jackson left the dinner party, the female guests flocked around the lady of the house and commented, "Is *this* your back woods-man? Why, madam, he is a prince."[80] Of course, it helped that Jackson, under the threat of a British attack, assured the ladies that "he would save the city, ... urging them not to trouble themselves about the matter."

And save the city Jackson did. The victory signaled the end of what some have called the "Second American Revolution" and "decisively changed the course of American history."[81]

Jackson and Slavery

Even having a soft side and being able to be compassionate from time to time, the complexity of Jackson's character, and indeed the character of the nation at the time, was shown by the treatment of slaves. During several decades, Jackson kept increasing the number of slaves he owned. Beginning in 1794, he was reported to own 10 slaves. By the time he became president there were 95 slaves at the Hermitage, a number that had grown to 150 a couple of years later. At the Hermitage, the slaves were essential for the farming of cotton, corn, and wheat. When Jackson was away, Rachel stepped in to supervise the work of the slaves.

Although Jackson "for the most part ... treated his slaves decently and tried to make certain they were not abused by overseers,"[82] he would deliver severe punishments, including whipping and shackling slaves, when he felt that such treatment was merited. A biographer commented that Jackson's "behavior on occasion can only be described as barbaric" and exemplified that statement with an advertisement placed by Jackson in the *Nashville Tennessee Gazette* on September 26, 1804, when one of his slaves had run away; Jackson promised "ten dollars extra, for every hundred lashes any person will give him, to the amount of three hundred."[83]

Having large numbers of Black slaves in the country not surprisingly created tensions and a constant fear among whites about what would happen if the slaves were to revolt. This fear also extended to freed slaves. When Jackson supported the engagement of free Blacks in the defense of New Orleans, he was criticized by many Louisianans who feared uprising if weapons were placed in the hands of colored men. Jackson, who understood that any help would be important in the defense of the country, did not take the critique against his hiring of Blacks lightly. When one official questioned Jackson's right to enlist Blacks, the general basically asked him to shut up: "Be pleased to keep to yourself your opinions upon the policy ... without inquiring whether the troops are white, black, or tea."[84]

Had Jackson lived today, his ownership and sometimes cruel treatment of Black slaves are things he would probably not be proud of. Likewise, his view of Native Americans, culminating in the Indian Removal Act of 1830, is something he would not want to repeat.

Winning the White House but Losing Rachel

Jackson had started to show political ambitions already before the War of 1812, but historians agree that his involvement in the Creek War and, in particular, his victory in the Battle of New Orleans were main factors in the advancement of his political career. Jackson was elected to the U.S. Congress and served both in the House of Representatives and the Senate for short periods in the 1790s. He had been admitted to the North Carolina Bar in 1787 and practiced law in the part of North Carolina that would later become Tennessee. After six years as a justice on the Tennessee Supreme Court and a shorter period as the military commissioner of Florida, he returned to the U.S. Senate for a two-year period starting in 1823.

In 1824, Jackson was running for president for the first time. His opponent was John Quincy Adams, who despite losing the electoral vote (but winning the popular vote) was elected president. Four years later in a rematch between the two opponents, Jackson won both the electoral vote and the popular vote and was sworn in as the country's seventh president in 1829. Adams would never get over his loss to Jackson and kept holding a grudge toward his political enemy. When Jackson was visiting Boston in 1833, he was awarded an honorary degree at Harvard. One of the university's most famous alumni, John Quincy Adams, did not like the honor bestowed on Jackson but made the belittling comment that "Jackson could hardly write his own name."[85]

Jackson's win of the presidential race in 1828 was bittersweet. During the election campaign, Rachel was subjected to vicious attacks by the supporters of her husband's opponent. In a newspaper a writer asked, "Ought a convicted adulteress and her paramour husband to be placed in the highest offices of this free and Christian land?"[86] When Rachel realized "the full range of the slander leveled against her, … the language, the implications, the outright accusation of adultery and bigamy," she broke down and "wept hysterically."[87] No wonder Rachel was depressed and hated the idea of moving to the capital. She lamented, "I would rather be a doorkeeper in the house of God than live in that palace in Washington."

On December 17, 1828, doctors were hastily summoned to the Hermitage to find Rachel's face "contorted with pain" and with "spasmodic affection of the muscles of the chest and left shoulder, attended with an irregular action of the heart."[88] Despite repeated bleedings, Rachel's condition deteriorated quickly, and after five days' struggle, "Rachel Jackson's long flight from fame was over."[89] Most medical historians believe that Rachel died from a massive heart attack.

Jackson was devastated by the loss. He blamed his political enemies for the death of Rachel and at her funeral he said, "May God Almighty forgive her murderers. I never can."[90] Jackson arrived in Washington for his first inauguration a broken man without a first lady. He never remarried. Rachel's niece, Emily Donelson, served as President Jackson's private secretary in the White House but also functioned as a substitute first lady. After a falling-out between Jackson and Emily, she left the White House in 1834. She was replaced by Sarah Yorke Jackson, who was married to Jackson's adopted son and served as first lady through the remainder of Jackson's presidency. When Jackson retired in 1837, Sarah and her husband moved with the president to the Hermitage.

Jackson's "Operations" for Hydrocele, 1831 and 1833

A hydrocele is caused by the accumulation of water-like fluid around the testicle, typically resulting in swelling of the scrotum. It usually does not give rise to pain or other symptoms but may become bothersome if the swelling grows big. Hydrocele is not uncommon in newborn boys and disappears without any treatment within a year in most cases. It may also develop in adult men, commonly as a result of trauma or inflammation.

Jackson underwent an "operation" for hydrocele by Dr. James Crowdhill Hall of Washington, D.C., in 1831 and needed a second procedure by the same surgeon two years later.[91] The modern surgical treatment (if needed) for a hydrocele is removal of the fluid-filled sac surrounding the testicle, a "hydrocelectomy," but that is not what Jackson got; hydrocelectomy did not become a standard procedure until the end of the nineteenth century.[92] During the days of Jackson, the physicians just drained the fluids by either opening the sac with a small trocar or making a small incision with a scalpel. The famous eighteenth-century London surgeon/anatomist John Hunter, in one of his surgical lectures, called this the "temporary cure" or "palliative" operation for hydrocele.[93] The risk for recurrence of the hydrocele after this type of procedure was high. The fact that Jackson needed a second operation after two years indicates that his initial procedure in 1831 was a "temporary cure."

In his lecture on hydrocele, Hunter discussed other operations used to achieve "radical cure," such as inducing inflammation or scarification of the sac after removal of the fluid. This resulted in obliteration of the sac and prevented reaccumulation of fluid. Different agents were used for that purpose, including a zinc solution or a mixture of "equal parts of port wine and water."[94] For the surgeons' billing purposes, the different procedures were classified as "operations" for hydrocele. Interestingly, the Library of Congress has preserved Dr. Hall's surgical bills sent to Jackson for the procedures performed in 1831 and 1833 and for follow-up consultations in 1834–1836.[95] A review of similar bills sent to other less famous patients led to the conclusion that "Dr. James Hall ... appropriately billed the 7th President for what would be now described as a hydrocele drainage and scarification."[96] Apparently Jackson's second operation was successful, since there are no historic records of additional procedures for hydrocele in Jackson.

Cutting Out the Bullet in Jackson's Left Arm

If Jackson thought he could forget about the bullet remaining in his left arm after that fateful day at the City Hotel in Nashville in 1813, he was wrong. The wound became infected, and, worse, the nearby bone also became infected. Bone infection (osteomyelitis) is a serious condition causing fevers, pain, and disability. Even with today's antibiotics, the condition can be difficult to treat, and not infrequently it turns into a chronic problem. It is caused by bacteria (the role of bacteria was not understood in Jackson's days) commonly brought close to (or into) the bone by a dirty object. The bullet hitting Jackson's left upper arm was of course not sterile, and when left behind close to the humerus (the bone of the upper arm), it caused an infection of the bone.

One common feature of osteomyelitis, in addition to its chronicity, is the recurrent episodes of drainage of pus from the infected bone. Sometimes a necrotic fragment of the bone can break away and migrate to the surface of the skin. In such cases, a piece of bone may be felt under the skin or can even penetrate through the skin and be expulsed. This is what happened to Jackson about a year after the barroom brawl. In the fall of 1814, a sequestrum (bone fragment) worked its way from the infected bone and sloughed through the skin.[97] Jackson sent the piece of bone to Rachel "as a souvenir" (a somewhat macabre gift), adding,[98] "I hope all the loose pieces of bone is out, and I will no longer be pained with it."[99] Unfortunately, the bullet was not expulsed at the same time; it would remain in Jackson's arm and continue to cause problems for another eighteen years.

During all those years, Jackson continued to have pain and discomfort in his arm, at times making "the arm almost useless."[100] The problems would culminate in 1831, two years after Jackson assumed the presidency of the United States for his first term. The bullet fired by Jesse Benton had started to migrate and could now be felt under the skin close to the wound in the left upper arm. In April 1831, with the pain intensifying, Jackson considered traveling to Philadelphia to see a surgeon but canceled the trip when he realized the political ramifications caused by seeing the president needing surgery. Instead, he tried to cope with it.

When the pain ultimately became unbearable, he decided to have the bullet removed. This time the surgeon, Thomas Harris of Philadelphia, was summoned to Washington for the operation.[101] The procedure took place on January 12, 1832.[102] Of course, anesthesia was not available, so Old Hickory "simply bared his arm, gritted his jaws, grasped his walking stick," and told his surgeon to "go ahead."[103] Dr. Harris made an incision, squeezed the arm, and "out popped a 'half ball' of the ordinary pistol size."[104] After the wound had been dressed, the President "went right back to work,"[105] and he was able to attend "a small dinner party that evening."[106]

Both the bullet in Jackson's arm and the ball in the chest (stuck there since the Dickinson duel in 1806) contained lead, and historians have speculated that some of the many medical problems Jackson developed over the years (such as excessive salivation, rapid loss of teeth, abdominal colic, diarrhea, pallor, hand tremor, irritability, paranoia, mood swings, and probable renal failure) may have been caused by lead poisoning. The fact that some of Jackson's symptoms improved after the surgeon had cut out the bullet in the arm has supported such speculations.

Further support for the theory that Jackson suffered from plumbism was reported following forensic investigations in which lead concentrations in hair samples from Jackson dating back to 1815 and 1839 were determined.[107] Sophisticated measurements revealed significantly elevated concentrations of lead in the hair collected from Jackson in 1815. The levels were lower in 1839 (possibly reflecting the removal of the bullet in the arm in 1832) but still above normal, perhaps because the bullet in Jackson's chest was still there. The authors of the report concluded that the bullets embedded in Jackson's lung and left arm for many years were "likely candidates as the source of plumbism."[108] Jackson's elevated lead levels were also not helped by his habit of using sugar of lead (lead acetate) on a frequent basis for various symptoms. He used it freely both internally and externally. He drank it for intestinal cramps, poured it onto his wounds, and bathed his eyes with the solution when his vision started to deteriorate. He even took total body baths in sugar of lead when recommended to do so by his doctors.

Ironically, some of the symptoms for which Jackson ingested lead may actually have been worsened by the presumed remedy. For example, lead poisoning may result in abdominal pain and changes in bowel habits.[109]

Another heavy metal that has been suspected as a cause of Jackson's medical problems is mercury. Mercury-containing calomel was used for centuries as a treatment for a variety of maladies, in particular diarrhea. Jackson used it frequently, but even if elevated mercury levels were discovered in a hair sample from him, the levels were not high enough to explain the more severe health problems he experienced.[110] The decay of his teeth, ultimately resulting in extraction of all his teeth in 1828, however, may have been caused or at least worsened by the calomel.

After removal of the bullet in the left arm, Jackson would serve as president for another five years. He lived for eight years after his two terms in the White House. Some medical historians suspect that Jackson died of chronic renal failure,[111] although other causes of his death have also been suggested, including heart failure. Both of these conditions may explain why Jackson developed pronounced dropsy (edema) toward the end of his life. In a letter written to President James Polk in April 1845, Jackson expressed his frustration with the swelling of his body: "My disease has assumed an alarming type of dropsy, how soon this with my other combined afflictions may take me off, that all-wise god ... only knows."[112] In May, Jackson wrote to his foster son that "I am swollen from my toes to the crown of my head and in bandages to my hips."[113]

One of Jackson's biographers felt convinced that the bullet retained in Old Hickory's chest after the duel in 1806 was a major contributor to his demise and stated that "it was Dickinson's bullet that killed Andrew Jackson at last."[114] Others have provided multiple arguments that tuberculosis may have been an important factor in Jackson's demise.[115] The possibility that Jackson had developed amyloidosis, an unusual disease associated with prolonged and chronic infections and by the infiltration of several organs, including the heart and kidneys, by an abnormal protein has been proposed by some medical historians.[116]

Regardless of the cause of death, Jackson was a sick man for several years prior to his passing. When Old Hickory ended his "grisly last years," his "beautiful mind rested in a body which was nothing more than a decaying mass."[117] On his deathbed, Jackson was surrounded by family and slave servants. When they realized that he was slipping away from them, they sobbed and cried. Old Hickory exclaimed, "What is the matter with my Dear Children, have I alarmed you?"[118] He then added, as if to atone for the harsh treatment of his slaves, "I want to meet you all in heaven, both white & black."[119]

The end came on June 8, 1845. One of Jackson's doctors lamented, "Thus died the greatest and best man of the age, or, perhaps of any age."[120] Jackson was laid to rest at the Hermitage beside his beloved Rachel.

Chapter Three

James A. Garfield

"Yes, I shot the president, but his physicians killed him"

The Twentieth President

March 4, 1881–September 19, 1881

James Abram Garfield was certainly not born silver spoon in hand. He entered this world in a log cabin in Orange Township in northern Ohio on November 19, 1831, and grew up a poor farmer boy. Later in life, Garfield would comment, "I lament that I was born to poverty."[1] That he ended up as president of the United States attests to the American Dream that anything is possible if you work for it hard enough. One of Garfield's biographers highlighted this remarkable life journey by titling his work *From Canal Boy to President.*[2]

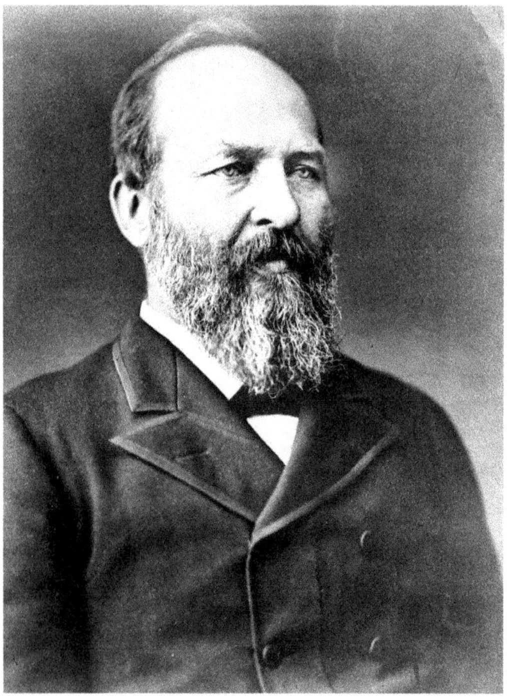

Portrait of James Garfield. Library of Congress, Prints and Photographs Division, Washington, D.C.

Early Life

The financial struggle of the family did not improve when James's father, Abram, died from pneumonia, leaving his two-year-old son fatherless and his widowed wife in charge of the farm and the upbringing of the children. The mother had strict rules and would not allow anything "that approached impurity of life and speech, in any degree," and enforced her rules with "a sort of flaming sword swinging constantly against all forms of indecency and immorality."[3]

James Garfield was a robust boy already from the outset. When remembering the birth of her son, James's mother, Eliza, commented that "James A. was the largest Babe I ever had, he looked like a red Irishman."[4] Garfield retained his sturdy appearance when growing up. A friend recalled that his "first impression of him as a young man" was that he was "about six feet in height, powerfully built, with a head of bushy hair, and weighing about 185 pounds."[5] There is no doubt that Garfield had to pay his dues, helping his mother around the farm, so when he told her he wanted to leave home and look for work outside the farm, she was "aghast and bitterly opposed to her son's leaving."[6]

As a teenager Garfield dreamt about becoming a sailor, but when he left home at age sixteen, the closest he came to a sailing career was the edge of Lake Eire. He remained close to water, however, and found employment as a canal boy, towing barges along the Ohio Canal. He had good use of his strong muscles, driving horses and mules to pull the flatboats along the canal. However, he could not swim, and when he fell into the muddy, mosquito-infested water (which he did on multiple occasions), he was near drowning several times. When he later in life recalled his experience, he mentioned that he "had fourteen almost miraculous escapes from drowning."[7] Because of his bad experience along the Ohio Canal, made even worse by contracting malaria, he called it quits already after six weeks and went back home in the fall of 1847.

Education

It was now time to think about learning. Garfield's mother sent him off to the nearby Geauga Seminary to study religion, grammar, mathematics, and philosophy. Perhaps as an indication of his future career, Garfield joined the debate club, and he loved it! He commented that "it creates some excitement," and he then explained, "I love agitation and investigation and glory in defending unpopular truth against popular error."[8]

In the autumn of 1851, Garfield enrolled at the Western Reserve Eclectic Institute at Hiram. At the time, the institute was not accredited as a college (it would be another four years before it became Hiram College), but the years at Hiram prepared Garfield for continued education at a licensed college. Hiram became like a second home for Garfield, and he poured everything into his time there. He proved that he was able to work extremely hard to achieve his goals; one of his biographers described how "Garfield rose at four of five in the morning, attended classes for ten hours a day … mastered Greek and Latin, managed to learn geometry on his own."[9] Notwithstanding the early mornings, Garfield "often stayed up until midnight, ensuring that his carrel's candle was the last to be extinguished."[10]

Despite his love for debates and addressing an audience from a lectern, Garfield had not yet embraced the idea of going into politics. In fact, what he saw of politicians during the presidential campaigns of 1852 made him repulse the political process. In his diary he wrote, "I am exceedingly disgusted with the wire pulling of politicians and the total disregard for truth in all their operations."[11]

After three years at Hiram, Garfield turned his eyes eastward. In September 1854, he matriculated at Williams College in Williamstown, Massachusetts. The leader of Williams College, Mark Hopkins, "a compelling and energetic educator,"[12] was one of the most respected college presidents in the country. The college was famous for its libraries, containing 25,000 volumes, and for its faculty, providing in-depth and demanding experiences for its students.

It did not take long for Garfield to become one of Hopkins's favorite students not only as an outstanding debater but also for academic achievements. When Hopkins recalled Garfield's time at Williams, he wrote that "there was a large general capacity applicable to any subject" and added that "there was no pretense of genius, or alternation of spasmodic effort, but a satisfactory accomplishment in all directions."[13] The admiration was mutual; Garfield commented on Hopkins in his diary that "I think he is a great man."[14]

During his time at Williams College, Garfield not only acquired academic knowledge but also matured as a person and started to form opinions about societal and political movements. Despite what he had said about politicians when at Hiram, he now had a more positive outlook. In his diary he wrote, "I have been instructed tonight on the political condition of our country, and from this time forward I shall hope to know more about its movement and interests."[15] During the spring of his last year at Williams, Garfield attended a meeting supporting the newly founded Republican Party. He also developed a growing interest in the abolitionist movement, in part as a result of antislavery preaching and lectures by Henry Ward Beecher. Garfield was also aware of the voices arguing for women's rights and penned in his diary that he believed that "women [were] wronged socially and intellectually by the usages of society."[16]

Fighting the Confederates

When the American Civil War erupted following the bombardment of Fort Sumter in April 1861, Garfield was excited about the prospect of finally being able to punish the seceding states of the South. Although he suspected that the war would be bloody, he believed that it would be short. It is possible that his level of enthusiasm would have been lower had he known that the fight would last for four long years and result in the highest numbers of dead in the annals of American wars, both in absolute numbers (750,000) and as a percentage of the population (2.39%). (The number of casualties in the Civil War was higher than the combined numbers of dead in the American Revolutionary War, World War I, World War II, the Korean War, and the Vietnam War and by far exceeded the deaths as a percentage of the population in any American military conflict.)

Garfield was eager to get involved in the war, and in the absence of previous personal military experience, he promptly got to work studying the narratives of historical war heroes, including Napoleon Bonaparte and the Duke of Wellington. Although there is no doubt that Garfield's strong antislavery sentiment and disgust over the efforts by the South to break up the Union were leading factors in his engagement, there was at least one additional motive. Garfield realized that several of the country's presidents, including George Washington, James Monroe, and Andrew Jackson, had gained political prominence because they had been successful military leaders, and Garfield thought that might be an important queue to follow. Indeed, Garfield was subjected to the scorn by some of his anti–Republican enemies who suggested that he was driven by a political ambition "to leap from the walks of a private citizen to the position of a military chieftain."[17]

Thanks to his hard work raising funds for volunteer regiments in Ohio and to his political connections, Garfield was appointed colonel of the 42nd Ohio Infantry Regiment. In December 1861, he was ordered to bring the 42nd to Louisville in Kentucky to help stave off Confederate troops who had infiltrated the eastern parts of the state. In those efforts, Garfield saw action in the Sandy Valley campaign. At the Battle of Middle Creek on January 9, 1862, Garfield led Union forces in their defeat of the rebels. The victory made Garfield a hero in Ohio, and in March he was promoted to brigadier general. The following month, Garfield again saw action, this time at the bloody Battle of Shiloh.

In the summer of 1862, Garfield was struck by dysentery and hepatitis-induced jaundice and had to return to Ohio for recuperation.[18] Back in Ohio, he was persuaded by his friends to run for Congress, and in November he defeated his Democratic opponent with a decisive two-to-one margin. Although Garfield still felt that his place was in the Union Army as long as the war was dragging on, the fact that the new Congress would not be assembled until December 1863 led him to believe that he would have ample time to see the conclusion of the war before he would take his seat in the House of Representatives.

After regaining his health, Garfield was ordered to go to Washington for instructions as to where to go next in the war. He used his time in the capital to make connections with members of the administration and other leaders of the Republican Party. In particular, he rekindled his friendship with the former governor of Ohio, Salmon Chase, now in Lincoln's administration as secretary of the treasury. Chase generously invited Garfield to spend several weeks at his Washington home, and they shared many hours discussing politics and the state of the war. They also had time for their mutual love of the game of chess.[19] Chase remained a close friend and important mentor to Garfield for many years. Garfield had a lot of admiration for Chase and at one point commented that "Chase is by far the strongest man in the administration," adding that Chase "seems to be thoroughly imbued with a moral and religious sense of the duties of the government in relation to the war."[20]

In early 1863 Garfield was ordered to join Major General William S. Rosecrans, who at the time was with his troops at Murfreesboro in Tennessee. Garfield was appointed by "Old Rosy" to be his chief of staff. Although they expressed mutual respect and even admiration for each other, Garfield grew increasingly frustrated by what he perceived as Rosecrans's inaction and passive approach to the war. In July, Garfield wrote a letter to Chase expressing his disappointment with Rosecrans. Garfield complained that "thus far, the General has been singularly disinclined to grasp the situation with a strong hand.... I beg you to know that this delay is against my judgment and my every wish."[21]

Garfield's disappointment with Rosecrans's leadership came to a point with Garfield's legendary "ride" at the Battle of Chickamauga on September 19 and 20. When the Union forces' line was broken by the Confederates, Rosecrans considered the battle lost and wanted his troops to fall back on Chattanooga. Garfield, however, did not agree with Rosecrans's pessimistic view and wanted to see with his own eyes what the situation was like. Garfield undertook a daring ride through enemy lines to be able to better survey the conditions on the field and found that the troops were holding their positions better than expected. Ultimately, however, the Confederates were victorious, and Rosecrans withdrew to Chattanooga. Garfield's brave ride was reported in newspapers all over the country, and his enterprise became part of his political legend.

With the Union forces held down at Chattanooga by the surrounding rebels, Garfield sent a telegram to Washington pleading with Secretary of War Edwin M. Stanton to send reinforcements. In just a little more than a week, 20,000 Union soldiers arrived at Chattanooga by train to strengthen Rosecrans's beleaguered troops. In light of the outcome at Chickamauga and Garfield's communications with Chase and Stanton, it did not take Abraham Lincoln long to relieve Rosecrans of his command.

In late October, Garfield returned to Washington to give a report on the conduct of the military operations in Tennessee. The time for the new Congress to assemble was fast approaching, and Garfield was struggling with the dilemma of whether to go back to the Union Army or take his seat in the House that he had won about a year earlier. He decided to seek Lincoln's advice. When Garfield met with the president, Lincoln recommended that Garfield take his House seat because, he explained, there was an excess of generals but a shortage of congressmen with military experience and in support of the administration. In a letter to his previous mentor, the president of Williams College, Mark Hopkins, Garfield wrote that "the President told me he dared not risk a single vote in the House" and explained that "I did not feel it right to consult my own preference in such a case."[22] Garfield resigned from the army and took his seat and began what would become a more than seventeen-year career in the House of Representatives.

Congressman

Garfield took his seat in the House of Representatives on March 3, 1863, and would remain a congressman until November 8, 1880, when he was elected president. During his time in the House he kept growing in prominence, initially mainly because of his involvement in the fiscal issues of the country. His political influence peaked during the first half of the 1870s, when he was the chairman of the powerful House Appropriations Committee (1871–1875). As further evidence of Garfield's influence on policies of monetary issues, he was a member of the Ways and Means Committee and chairman of the Committee on Banking and Currency.[23]

Many financial debates in Congress during the early years after the Civil War were centered on the question of how to pay off the huge budget deficits incurred during the war and how to pay for the reconstruction of the South. Garfield was in strong favor of the gold standard and was an opponent of the reliance on paper money, the greenbacks, that the Treasury had started to print to support the war efforts and later to pay back the debt.

During his years in Congress, Garfield would reevaluate some of his colleagues and personal friends. Even Abraham Lincoln did not escape a reassessment in Garfield's eyes. In early 1861 when Lincoln was visiting Ohio as the president-elect on his way to the capital, Garfield was optimistic about the future with the new president (despite his lack of refined social skills) and commented in a letter to a friend that "he clearly shows his want of culture and marks of western life" but still added that Lincoln's "remarkable good sense, simple and condensed style of expression, and evident marks of indomitable will, give me great hopes for the country."[24] Among the more radical Republicans there were other opinions, with accusations that Lincoln was a "dictator with the sole interest of personal gain."[25]

It did not take long before Garfield began to be openly critical of the president. In 1864, Garfield refused to support Lincoln's reelection hopes within the Republican Party, and although understanding that "he will probably be the man," Garfield felt that "we could do better."[26] When Lincoln issued the Emancipation Proclamation in January 1863, Garfield voiced criticism and thought it was a "strange phenomenon in the world's history when a second-rate Illinois lawyer is the instrument to utter words which shall form an epoch memorable in all future ages."[27] One important reason why Garfield was critical of Lincoln was that he felt that the President was weak in his war efforts and that his plan for the South, once the war would be over, was too conciliatory. Garfield agreed with the more radical Republicans that the Confederates ought to be punished and that all legal rights should be taken away from them.

When Garfield explained to his constituency in Ohio that "Lincoln was not his first choice for the presidency,"[28] the voters were upset. Garfield, however, did not change his mind and declared that "I hold it to be my privilege under the Constitution and as a man to criticize any acts of the President of the United States." He concluded by declaring that "I cannot go to Congress as your representative with my liberty restricted in this respect in any degree. If I go to Congress I must go as a free man." His speech was convincing, and "those present rose to their feet and broke into resounding cheers."[29] Despite the critical view of Lincoln, Garfield expressed deep sorrow when the president was assassinated. In a letter to his wife, he wrote, "I am sick at heart and feel it to be almost like sacrilege to talk of money or business now."[30]

Another person for whom Garfield's feelings changed over time was his old friend and mentor, Salmon Chase. When Andrew Johnson, Lincoln's successor, was impeached, Garfield wanted to see him found guilty. The impeachment trial was presided over by Chase, who was now the Supreme Court chief justice. When the impeachment failed by one vote in the Senate, Garfield was outraged and called the outcome of the trial a "great betrayal" and thought that a "great wrong was consummated."[31] Garfield felt that the outcome was Chase's fault and accused him of favoring the defense. In a letter to a friend, Garfield wrote, "It is the hardest thing I ever have to do, to withdraw confidence and love from a man to whom I have once given them, but the conduct of Mr. Chase has been outrageous." Garfield then added the accusation that "I have no doubt that he is trying to break the Republican party and make himself president."[32]

Although Garfield had risen in political power and influence during the early 1870s, this was also a period when he was challenged by political scandals. In the summer of 1872, Garfield was accused of being involved in the Crédit Mobilier scandal. The fraudulent scheme involved money that had been appropriated by Congress to the Union Pacific Railroad for building the Transcontinental Railroad and was siphoned off to a fictitious company called Crédit Mobilier of America. Union Pacific executives swindled the U.S. government of more than $44 million. Almost a quarter of that money was used to bribe congressmen for additional funding and for regulation rulings favorable to the Union Pacific Railroad. Some of the bribes of the Washington politicians were in the form of Crédit Mobilier stocks. Garfield was accused of lying to the House investigating committee when denying that he had received Crédit Mobilier stocks and dividends. He was sharply criticized in the press for his less than truthful testimony but was relieved when a House vote to censure him failed. Even if he had weathered the storm for now, he understood that the ordeal could hurt his future political career. In his diary he wrote that although he had done nothing wrong, he feared "that the shadow of the cursed thing would cling to my name for many years."[33] And sure enough, the scandal would resurface eight years later during his presidential campaign.

It would be only one year after the Crédit Mobilier scandal when Garfield again found himself in hot water. In what became known as the "Salary Grab of 1873," the members of Congress had voted themselves a 50 percent pay increase (from $5,000 to $7,500 per year) and decided it would include retroactive compensation from the start of the session, two years earlier. The press and the public were enraged, in particular since this happened in the wake of the Crédit Mobilier scandal and gave additional fuel to the view that the Washington politicians were corrupt. Garfield was a major target for the anger, being the chairman of the House Appropriations Committee.

Garfield was shaken by the disdain expressed by people and found the salary grab to be even tougher to deal with than the Crédit Mobilier scandal. In a letter to his wife, Lucretia (Crete), he wrote that he was surprised to find "that just now there is more agitation in regard to my vote on the increase of salaries of members of Congress than there is in regard to Crédit Mobilier."[34]

The situation looked grim, but Garfield decided to fight back. He promised his wife "to meet manfully whatever comes to my lot."[35] He communicated with his voter base in Ohio and explained his actions. "It was not a crime, and we have no right to say that those who advocated it were thieves and robbers."[36] Somehow he managed to survive this crisis as well, but there was one more lurking.

Like many other congressmen in those days, Garfield opted to practice law on the side of his job in Congress. In 1873, he was retained to represent the DeGolyer-McClelland Company that was bidding for a contract with the District of Columbia's Board of Public Works to install a patented system of wooden sidewalks. Being chairman of the House Appropriations Committee put Garfield in a position of conflict of interest when DeGolyer-McClelland's bid was reviewed. When the contract was secured, Garfield was given a reward of $5,000 from the company, something that angered the press and resulted in Garfield being accused of corruption. Garfield, however, was defiant and angrily stated, "I prepare to stand on my rights as an American citizen," adding that "there is nothing either of law or morals to prohibit a member of Congress from practicing his profession."[37] After all, he was a licensed attorney. Although looking threatening, the DeGolyer-McClelland incident did not take away the support of the voters. In the election of 1874, Garfield won the reelection to his House seat with a comfortable margin.

As if the political scandals were not enough of a threat, Garfield also had issues in his personal life that could become a problem. His womanizing was a ticking time bomb ready to explode and ruin his political career. Even though the press and political opponents seemed less eager to exploit this type of private questions than we see now, there were rumors about "Garfield's persistent philandering" already during the first decade of the marriage.[38] Lucretia, of course, was not happy about her husband's behavior and pleaded with him "to let the fire of such lawless passion burn itself out, unfed and unnoticed."[39] Lucretia's comment was prompted by an affair her husband had had with "a young and attractive reporter for the *New York Times*" whom he had met when she interviewed him in New York City.[40] When Garfield confessed the tryst to Crete, he admitted that the young reporter "excites in me the fire of lawless passion."[41] Luckily enough for James, Lucretia forgave him and saved their marriage.

When Garfield was in Congress and living separated from his wife and family, additional strains were put on the marriage. To help salvage their relationship, James and Lucretia built a home in Washington in 1869 where they could be together when Congress was in session. Based on comments by Lucretia at the time their home in Washington was being constructed, one gets the impression that she had concerns about her husband's commitment and was ready to forgive his missteps as long as that would save the marriage. She told him, "I am sure if our home should be really finished and you permitted to take me into it, I shall feel more than ever before that I am your wedded wife taken to your hearth and heart."[42]

Despite the frictions, the bonds between husband and wife survived and even improved over the years. One of Garfield's biographers commented that despite the ups and downs in their relationship, "the middle and later years of the Garfields' marriage were marked by a strong sense of togetherness and familial bonding."[43] Their affection for each other would be ultimately tested and found to be strong during the last seventy-nine days of Garfield's life.

In 1880, the political landscape in the country had changed. President Rutherford B. Hayes had announced that he would not seek a second term. Garfield had been elected to an open seat in the U.S. Senate. Garfield's name had even started to be mentioned as a "dark horse candidate to replace the retiring Hayes."[44]

Running for President in 1880

When President Hayes declared that he would not seek a second term, the race was on for the Republicans to nominate their presidential candidate. When the party convention assembled in Chicago, the top contenders were Ulysses Grant, James Blaine, and John Sherman. Although Garfield was now a highly regarded member of Congress, soon to become a senator, with a national reputation and thought about as a potential presidential candidate in some circles, he distanced himself from the idea and publicly declared that he was not and would not be a candidate. In a letter to a friend, he wrote that "I long ago made a resolution that I would never permit myself to let the Presidential fever get any lodgment in my brain" and emphasized his feelings by adding, "I think it is the one office in this nation that for his own peace no man ought to set his heart upon."[45]

The convention in Chicago exposed a fractured Republican Party full of bitterness and angry infighting. Grant, a Stalwart with strong conservative opinions, was supported by Senator Roscoe Conkling of New York. Conkling was an outspoken troublemaker who would continue to stir the pot long after Chicago. Garfield was sympathetic to the more moderate Half-Breeds, represented by the retiring President Hayes as well as Blaine and Sherman, and became a strong supporter of and spokesman for Sherman.

After several days of heated debates and multiple ballots, none of the candidates had managed to gather a winning majority. Following long nightly deal-making sessions, the deadlock was finally broken. Garfield had emerged as the dark horse and had won the nomination on the thirty-sixth ballot. The Stalwarts, Conkling in particular, were unhappy with the outcome. In order to appease the conservatives, the delegates chose Chester Alan Arthur, a Conkling confidant and considered a true Stalwart, as their vice presidential candidate.

In the presidential campaign, Garfield faced the Democratic candidate Winfield Hancock in a "hard-fought contest, full of personal attacks and bitter recriminations."[46] When the final outcome of the fight was announced, Garfield had won with fewer than two thousand votes of the more than nine million ballots that had been cast. The electoral vote gave Garfield a clearer majority, 214 to 155.

The months after the election were hectic and saw continued fractions and infighting among Republicans seeking positions in Garfield's administration. There were also continued political tensions in the nation with the threat of violence. Some were even concerned about the safety of the president-elect and feared that Garfield could become the target of an assassination attempt. Garfield shrugged off those sentiments, stating that "assassination can be no more guarded against than death by lightning; and it is best not to worry about either."[47]

When inauguration day finally arrived on March 4, 1881, Garfield was exhausted from dealing with bickering fellow Republicans fiercely fighting for positions in the government. As Garfield stepped out to deliver his address, he looked tired. His speech, thirty-five minutes long, was described as "entirely unworthy of the high reputation that Garfield had justly earned as one of the most effective American orators."[48] His voice was hoarse, and he was lacking his typical "dramatic and exuberant body language, which he had used so effectively throughout his career."[49]

The pressure on Garfield did not end on inauguration day. If anything it grew worse, with throngs of office seekers demanding the attention and favors of the president. In those days, job seekers had free access to the White House and were often aggressive in their job-chasing pursuits. Garfield was weary and distracted by "the indurated office seeker who pursues his prey with the grip of death."[50] One office seeker who was particularly demanding was Charles Julius Guiteau.

When Garfield appointed several individuals to New York patronage positions, all of them turned out to have ties to Conkling. This outraged Blaine, who rushed to the White House and talked Garfield into appointing William H. Robertson, an enemy of Conkling, to the most coveted appointment, the collector of customs at the Port of New York City. The result was an even more deepening fissure between Garfield and Conkling. Their constant feuds started to make daily headlines in the press.

Guiteau was one of the most persistent office seekers. When he realized that he would not be rewarded with the consulship in Paris or the mission in Vienna for what he considered was his essential help to get Garfield elected president, he turned against the president. During the spring and early summer of 1881, Guiteau sent several letters to Garfield criticizing him for appointing Robertson collector of customs in New York and demanding that a Stalwart should instead be chosen. Guiteau felt that Garfield was a weak president betraying the ideas of the Republican Party and decided that Garfield needed to be removed and replaced by a Stalwart president to prevent another civil war from breaking out.

From now on, Guiteau was obsessed with finding a way to eliminate Garfield. Guiteau bought a .44-caliber snub-nose revolver, a "British Bull Dog" known for its killing power. He went down to the Potomac River at the foot of Seventeenth Street and "planted a stick in the soft mud on the river-bank, where the tide had gone out, and deliberately practiced his arm and tested his weapon."[51] Guiteau wanted to make sure that "there should be no failure in the accomplishment of the crime for which he had been preparing." He began stalking the president and his wife and initially developed a plan to assassinate Garfield during a church service. When that scheme fell through, Guiteau planned to kill the president when he accompanied Lucretia for a train ride to New Jersey, where she was to spend time to recuperate from malaria. However, when Guiteau spotted Mr. and Mrs. Garfield at the train station and saw that "Mrs. Garfield looked so thin, and she clung so tenderly to the President's arm," he realized that "he did not have the heart to fire on him."[52]

Guiteau remained obsessed with the idea of killing Garfield and saving the country by having him replaced by a Stalwart, but the shooting would have to wait until the morning of Saturday, July 2, when Garfield was scheduled to travel by train to New York City and meet Lucretia, who now felt well enough to leave New Jersey. They were going to be joined by several cabinet members and their wives on a two-week journey through New England. Guiteau knew from the president's schedule, made public in newspapers, that Garfield was to board the train at the Baltimore and Potomac depot (the present site of the National Gallery of Art) with a departure time of 9:30 a.m.

The Shooting

Garfield was accompanied by two sons and his secretary of state, James Blaine, on the short ride from the White House to the train station on the morning of that fateful July 2. Garfield and Blaine had previously been political rivals but were now the best of friends, in particular since Blaine had been rewarded with the most prominent position of the cabinet next to the president. They had a good time of conversation and fellowship in the horse-drawn carriage bringing them to the depot. Blaine was not planning to join the president on the travels to New England but wanted to come along that morning to see Garfield off and get a chance to greet several of his colleagues in the cabinet and their wives. To get to the train, Garfield and Blaine entered the station by walking through the ladies' waiting room, which was almost empty at this time on an early weekend morning. Except for a few passengers and a female attendant, there was only one additional person in the room: a "down-and-out-looking man" who was hiding in a dark corner of the room.[53] He was initially unnoticed by Blaine and the president. Once they had passed, Guiteau stepped out from the shadow and approached the president from behind. Guiteau pulled his weapon and fired twice.

The first shot hit Garfield in his right upper arm, causing only a superficial wound. The second bullet hit the president in the back and felled him to the floor. People hearing the shots at first thought that firecrackers had gone off in honor of the president, but Blaine understood better. When he turned around, he saw Guiteau with a smoking gun in his hand. Blaine recognized Guiteau from the State Department, where he had been several times with the same demands as at the White House. At the time, Guiteau was "an easily recognized nuisance in Washington, a disgruntled office seeker, and a delusional loner who had left a trail of debts

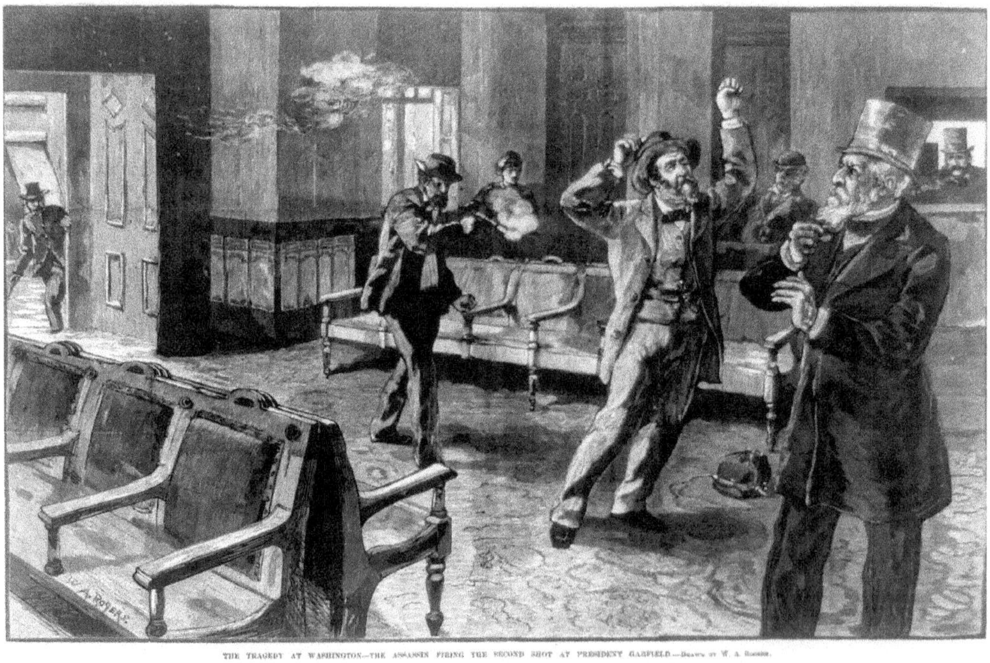
THE TRAGEDY AT WASHINGTON—THE ASSASSIN FIRING THE SECOND SHOT AT PRESIDENT GARFIELD.

Scene of the shooting of President Garfield on July 2, 1881. Charles Guiteau is seen shooting the president in the back. Secretary of State James Blaine is looking on in horror. Engraving, December 21, 1881. Library of Congress, Prints and Photographs Division, Washington, D.C.

and angry acquaintances."[54] Guiteau was immediately apprehended and led away, mumbling, "I did it and will go to jail for it. I am a Stalwart and Arthur will be president."[55]

Guiteau was "rapidly driven through the howling mob" to the police headquarters.[56] When the crowds realized Guiteau had been brought there, shouts of "Lynch him!!," "Tear down the building!," and "Hang him!" were heard. When Guiteau arrived at police headquarters, a letter was found in his pocket. The letter started "July 2, 1881. TO THE WHITE HOUSE. The President's tragic death was a sad necessity, but it will unite the Republican party and save the Republic."[57]

With the president on the floor in a pool of blood, panic erupted. A railway worker rushed out to the platform where cabinet members and their wives had gathered to board the train. When he was screaming that the president had just been shot, the waiting passengers first thought it was an inappropriate jest. The postmaster general, Thomas James, who was in the group, cried out, "What! There is no joke in a thing like that."[58]

People immediately crowded into the ladies' waiting room to see the bleeding president. Garfield was put on a mattress and carried up a flight of stairs to a second-floor room to get him away from the throngs. A frantic search for any available physician was started. Within a couple of minutes, Dr. Smith Townshend arrived. His first action was to have Garfield swallow "a half ounce of brandy and a dram of aromatic spirits of ammonia."[59] Garfield immediately complained of back pain and a "prickling sensation" in his right leg and foot,[60] and he would soon experience "numbness and pain radiating to the right groin,"[61] followed by hypersensitivity of the skin of his feet and ankles.[62] Townshend's second action was to insert one of his unwashed fingers into the wound on Garfield's back, probing for the bullet. Townshend did not find the slug, only "a small clot of blood" that he removed with his finger.[63] Townshend's finger would be followed by numerous additional dirty digits inserted into the bullet hole by surgeons called to the president's side.

Word about the shooting spread like wildfire. There were rumors about a coordinated conspiracy rather than a lone gunman, and a palpable anxiety was rapidly engulfing Washington. Federal troops took up positions throughout the capital, and the White House was closed off to the public.

The second doctor to arrive at the Baltimore and Potomac depot was Charles Purvis. He was the surgeon in chief at the Freedman's Hospital (founded in 1862 to provide care to former slaves). Doctor Willard Bliss ("Doctor" was one of his given first names) was the third physician to arrive on the scene. He had been summoned by Robert Todd Lincoln, President Lincoln's son and Garfield's secretary of war and was among the cabinet members scheduled to accompany Garfield on the journey to New England. Robert Todd Lincoln had met Bliss when he was attending the dying President Lincoln. Bliss was considered an expert in gunshot wounds after serving as a surgeon in the Civil War and was considered by some as "one of the best surgeons in the army."[64] Lincoln's son also knew that Bliss was a good friend of Garfield since their childhood in Ohio. Bliss reported that he had known the president "as an earnest, industrious boy, a little younger than I, whose ambitions were evidently far above his apparent advantages."[65]

Although admired by many, Bliss certainly also had his detractors. He had been accused of poor care of injured soldiers at the Battle of Bull Run in 1863. He had previously been arrested for government fraud and for taking bribes. In 1853, he had been expelled from the Washington D.C. Medical Society for selling the bark of a South American vine, claiming it was a "wonderful remedy for cancer, syphilis, scrofula, ulcer ... and all other chronic blood diseases."[66] Bliss was also looked down upon by some doctors for being a homeopath with less than desirable education. It is interesting that despite being a homeopath by training and in much of his practice, some of his adversaries did not feel that he was homeopathic enough.

Bliss had a domineering personality and was quick to take control of Garfield's medical care when he arrived at the train depot. Despite rushing to the site of the shooting on horseback and not washing his hands before examining the president, he used his little finger, "passed to its full extent into the wound,"[67] to search for the bullet. When probing the wound, Bliss could feel a fractured rib but not the bullet. When his finger was not enough, he used a Nelaton probe and a silver probe, both unwashed, again to no avail. By following what he believed was the track of the ball, he convinced himself that the slug had ended up in the president's liver.

The Care of the President

Within an hour after the shooting, almost a dozen doctors had gathered around the president. He was complaining of pain in his legs and requested to be moved to the White House. He was carried out on the mattress to a waiting horse-drawn ambulance and rushed to the Executive Mansion. Washington was now a city in panic; "five thousand sympathizing friends—men, women, children, of all ages, black and white—followed the ambulance on the run until it reached the White House."[68] Once Garfield had reached the White House it was sealed off, and the area was secured by military. The members of the cabinet were instructed to come to the White House without delay and remain there until the situation became clearer. Blaine sent telegrams with updates to Vice President Arthur, who was in his home at New York City. When Arthur was informed that Garfield had been subjected to an assassination attempt, he promptly consulted with his mentor, Conkling. When receiving a second telegram in the evening stating that "the President is no better, and we fear sinking,"[69] Arthur decided to take a midnight train and arrived at Washington on the morning of Sunday, July 3.

Meanwhile, Lucretia, who had not yet left Elberon in New Jersey, was informed about the shooting. At around lunchtime, she was on board a special Pullman car racing to Washington at the astonishing speed of sixty miles per hour. To Lucretia's horror, the train engine broke down just outside Baltimore. After being stranded for several hours, she finally reached Washington at around seven o'clock in the evening.

With the president now back in the White House, news about the shooting spread quickly through the country, with "bulletins flashed over newly strung telegraph wires to every frontier town all the way to the Gulf Coast and the Pacific

Ocean."[70] People were shocked by the news, and unrest and riots erupted in many cities. When the foreign-sounding name of the perpetrator became known, immigrants became targets of hatred.

Not until five o'clock in the afternoon of Saturday, seven and a half hours after the shooting, were the president's clothes removed, allowing for a more thorough examination of the patient. One hour later, "a catheterization of the bladder" had to be performed.[71] Against all odds, the president was still alive the following morning. By now, a multitude of doctors had gathered at the White House. Tension had started to develop between the physicians, mainly because of different opinions of what should be done next but also because of a power struggle between some of the colleagues. Bliss felt that he was the most qualified surgeon in the group and deserved to be in charge. On Sunday morning, he assembled his fellow physicians and claimed that the president and his wife had requested that he should have the authority to lead the president's medical care. He appointed Drs. Robert Reyburn (professor of anatomy and surgery at Howard University), Joseph Barnes (surgeon general of the U.S. Army), and Joseph Woodward (newly appointed president of the American Medical Association and more a researcher than a clinician) as his permanent staff and then bluntly explained that most of the other doctors' service was no longer needed and ordered them to leave the White House.

Although Bliss and his team and some of the other surgeons consulted during the course of Garfield's treatment were prominent doctors, they have been described as "arrogant physicians who did not accept the new theory of antisepsis."[72] As the days went on, Bliss became increasingly authoritative. He kept the president isolated behind screens, blocking access to the patient. Blaine was not able to see the president for several weeks after the shooting. Even the first lady and other family members had only limited access to Garfield.

Not surprisingly, several of the doctors who had been dismissed from the White House started to voice their critique of Bliss. He was accused of egomania and of allowing dirty fingers to cause harm. One physician was reported as saying "I am afraid Bliss will probe the wound, and if he does inflammation will set in and the President will die."[73] Other colleagues complained that Bliss did not include homeopathic medicines in Garfield's treatment. Bliss, of course, did not let the critique dwarf his self-assurance: "If I can't save him, no one can."[74]

Bliss's control of the president's medical management (and of his own authority) resulted in an almost absurd situation on the afternoon of July 3. Only a couple of hours after Bliss had dismissed most of his colleagues from the White House, Dr. Jedediah Baxter arrived, requesting to see the president. Baxter, who had served during the Civil War, had been appointed chief medical purveyor of the U.S. Army in 1872 with the rank of lieutenant colonel. He was promoted to colonel in 1874. As chief medical purveyor, one of Baxter's duties was to serve as personal physician to the president of the United States, a duty that often extended to include the president's family.

When Baxter arrived, Bliss denied him access to Garfield. Naturally, this made Baxter furious. After all, he was not only the official physician to the president but had also recently treated the first lady for malaria and had been Garfield's physician for several years. As Baxter explained, "He is my patient. I have prescribed for him for the past five years and insist on seeing him."[75] Baxter did not take no for an answer and "lunged toward the door of Garfield's room," trying to force his way to the president's bedside. Bliss engaged his own son to push away Baxter, who was screaming and shouting in protest. The brawl ended up with Baxter being escorted out of the White House by armed guards. The incident provided material for newspaper headlines all over the country.

Realizing that the controversies may end up hounding him, in particular if the president would die, Bliss decided to find coverage for his actions. He asked two of the country's most respected surgeons to come and see the patient: David Hayes Agnew, professor of surgery at the University of Pennsylvania School of Medicine in Philadelphia, and Frank Hamilton, professor of surgery at Bellevue Hospital Medical College in New York City. Bliss wanted his colleagues to give an assessment of his care of the president and how to proceed from there.

Agnew and Hamilton arrived early on July 4. They found a patient with high fever but otherwise seemingly not in critical condition. They repeated what Bliss had already done, inserting unclean fingers and instruments into the wound feeling for the ball. Like Bliss, they could not locate the bullet. When describing the actions taken by Agnew and Hamilton, Bliss wrote that "they individually examined the wound with great care" and then added that "these examinations consisted in the introduction in different directions of probes."[76] In contrast to Bliss, Agnew and Hamilton did not believe that the president's liver had been injured. Bliss was relieved to see a public bulletin released by Agnew and Hamilton at the end of the day "stating their satisfaction with all that had been done."[77] When returning to New York, Hamilton told a *New York Times* reporter, "When I left Washington at 3 o'clock this afternoon, President Garfield was no worse than he was at 6:30 o'clock this morning when I arrived there." And he added, "There was no evidence that he was sinking—nothing to lead to a suspicion that he was."[78]

Despite these optimistic proclamations, Garfield would have another seventy-six days of suffering before finally succumbing to the injuries caused by Guiteau's shooting.

The unfortunate fight between Bliss and several of his colleagues partly reflected Bliss's personality. There were reasons why he was accused of egomania, "arrogance and hubris"[79] and why he considered himself "godlike."[80] In addition, Bliss's abrasive attitude toward other physicians also reflected differences in education and practice between different groups of doctors. Although most doctors were allopaths (regular or orthodox), a substantial number (including Bliss) were homeopaths (irregular or sectarian). Allopaths often prescribed harsh remedies (following centuries-old traditions) such as bleeding and purging using high doses of toxic substances, frequently making patients suffer more from the treatments than the disease. In contrast, the homeopaths used much milder treatments, using several times lower doses of medications. Their philosophy was that the effectiveness of drugs was improved by pronounced dilution.

Allopaths often looked down on their homeopathic colleagues, whom they considered less well educated and knowledgeable. Homeopaths were not allowed to practice at some hospitals for the same reasons. The friction between groups of physicians was no secret. One commentator wrote, "The quarrels of physicians are proverbially frequent and bitter, and their hatred, in intensity and duration, seems to exceed that of other men."[81] Some allopaths even refused to provide treatment if a homeopath was involved in the care of the patient.

Although the Garfields were strong believers in homeopathic medicine, when Bliss claimed that he had been asked by Garfield to be in charge of his medical care, it is questionable whether he was truthful. Indeed, after Garfield's death, a handwritten note by Dr. Silas Boynton indicated that Garfield and his wife had never asked Bliss to take charge of the president's care after the shooting but that they considered Baxter to fill that position. This was confirmed by Lucretia, who attached her own handwritten note stating that "I have read the statement [that Garfield considered Baxter, not Bliss, to be his doctor] … and will say that it is entirely correct."[82]

In addition to Baxter, James and Lucretia Garfield regarded two homeopaths, Susan Edson and Silas Boynton, as their family doctors. Edson and Boynton had graduated from the same homeopathic medical school in Cleveland, Ohio. Edson was a personal friend of Garfield and had taken care of both James and Lucretia as well as their son Neddie when he had fallen ill with whooping cough during the early years of Garfield's career as a congressman. Edson and the Garfield family became particularly close after Neddie's death, not yet two years old. Edson had also cared for Lucretia in May 1881 when she suffered from malaria; she visited the White House frequently and was at Garfield's bedside after his shooting.

Silas Boynton was a first cousin to Garfield and was also close to the family. Like Edson, Boynton was a frequent visitor to the White House and was consulted several times by the president and his wife during Garfield's short presidency.

Despite the close ties of Edson and Boynton to the president, Bliss did not allow them to make any medical decisions regarding Garfield after the shooting. Bliss was disdainful and called them nurses rather than doctors. Whereas Edson was able to keep her mouth shut, Boynton did not stay quiet. On several occasions, he voiced his anger with Bliss's attitude and treatment of the president. Arguments between Bliss and Boynton were frequent and heated and became fodder for newspaper headlines.[83]

Despite being a homeopath, Bliss prescribed generous amounts of morphine to the president, resulting not only in pain relief but side effects as well. Garfield received "heroic" doses three to four times daily, resulting in nausea and vomiting and constipation. Edson and Boynton, as Garfield's family physicians, were well aware of the president's long-standing problems with stomach pain and indigestion, something Bliss was unaware of.

Boynton's critical view of Bliss's care of Garfield continued and escalated. Three weeks after the shooting, Garfield started to show signs of "blood poisoning" (sepsis in today's language), with clinical manifestations including "rigors" (shaking chills), high fevers (up to 104 degrees Fahrenheit), and a heart rate of 120 beats per minute. The wound on Garfield's back kept draining large amounts of pus, now also containing pieces of the president's cotton shirt and fragments of wool from his coat brought deep into his tissues with the bullet. An abscess on Garfield's back kept enlarging. Seeing what was happening, Boynton feared for the president's life and could not keep quiet any longer. He went public with a report of Garfield's condition and gave a scathing critique of the care Bliss provided. On July 23, Boynton told reporters that the president was dying and gave details: "Pus had through carelessness and neglect been allowed to be in the wound till it rotted and pyemia had done its perfect work."[84]

On the other side of the Atlantic, the surgeon Joseph Lister had already in the 1860s discovered the role of germs in the development of infections following surgery. He had introduced antiseptic systems, mainly using carbolic acid in the wound during operations, and showed the importance of clean hands and surgical instruments. Whereas his ideas and recommendations had gained acceptance in Europe, in particular in England and Germany, American surgeons were harder to convince. Even after giving a keynote lecture and demonstrating how to use carbolic acid in the operating theater to an audience of almost five hundred doctors attending the International Medical Congress in Philadelphia 1876 (held as part of the Centennial Anniversary of the Declaration of Independence), surgeons in the United States remained skeptical. Bliss and other physicians involved in the care of Garfield were aware of Lister and his antiseptic system but were not ready to forget the old teaching of the "laudable pus."

Seventy-Nine Long and Painful Days

It would be seventy-nine days, including the day of the shooting, of pain and suffering before Garfield died. The summers in Washington, D.C., are hot and humid, and the weather in July 1881 was no exception. With temperatures in the upper 90s, the president felt like he was melting away. The problem of the soaring heat and humidity in the sickroom was "brilliantly solved" by a group of engineers who, together with the scientist and astronomer Simon Newcomb, "invented and installed what may well have been the world's first air-conditioner."[85] The device had a blower forcing air over six tons of ice whereafter the cool air passed through a cast-iron box filled with cotton screens, drying the air. The cool and dry air was delivered through the sickroom's heat vent, resulting in a reduction of the temperature by about twenty degrees.

The wounded president was cared for by multiple physicians, including surgeons deemed the best in the country. Unfortunately, some of the doctors cared more about their own reputation than the life of their patient and were even willing to use deception to reach their goal. In light of today's knowledge, most observers would agree that the president died because of the physicians' malpractice, but even at the time, several colleagues pointed out the recklessness and incompetence of Garfield's care. A central point in their critique was that the massive infection that finally felled the president was caused by the surgeons and could have been avoided and indeed would have been avoided if only the surgeons had bothered to apply knowledge that was actually available at the time.

The fact that arrogance, jealousy, and rivalry among the doctors played important roles in the tragic outcome of the July 2, 1881, event adds to the frustration. That the surgeon, appointed by himself to be in charge of the president's care, was a principle culprit in the death of Garfield does not make the verdict by history less serious.

As we have seen, the mismanagement of Garfield started almost immediately after the shooting when Dr. Townshend put one of his unclean fingers into the president's bullet hole. The number of dirty fingers and unwashed surgical probes that would subsequently be inserted into the wound were too many to be counted. Not only did this cause a fatal infection, but the search for the slug was not even warranted; lessons learned during the Civil War had clearly shown that many soldiers recovered with the bullet left in place.[86]

The efforts by surgeons to find bullets in battlefield wounds had been the subject of interest and research for a long time and generated writings that, at least in retrospect, are fascinating. Ten years before Garfield's assassination, Thomas Longmore, a renowned military surgeon in England, had published a review of different methods to "detect bullets in gun-shot wounds."[87] In the paper, various "bullet explorers," including a "probe-nipper" and instruments using electricity to find the bullet, were described. Amazingly, an endoscope had been developed to visualize the bullet and pieces of cloth in the wound. Wisely, the author pointed out that if all efforts had failed to find the ball, "there must be a limit to search … especially if the patient … [was] suffering pain or [was] in an exhausted condition … [in which case] … the exploration should be at once discontinued."[88] Longmore concluded that "the wound may heal favourably, not withstanding its [the bullet's] presence, the foreign body … remaining lodged without causing either pain or mischief for many years afterwards."[89] If Bliss and his colleagues had adopted these recommendations, Garfield would have had a good chance to survive his injury.

The obsession to find the bullet fascinated Alexander Graham Bell, the inventor of the telephone. He developed a device that he hoped would help save the president's life. The "Induction Balance" was invented in Bell's Volta Laboratory only a couple of blocks from the White House. It was designed to track metallic objects in the body and had been tested in several veterans who had bullets left behind since the Civil War. Based on the results in those tests, Bell was convinced that he would be able to locate Garfield's ball. To his great disappointment, the search for the president's bullet failed, and he had to leave Garfield's sickroom feeling ashamed and upset. Bell would later blame interference from metal springs in Garfield's mattress. Bell was aware of this potential problem and had therefore instructed Bliss to "move the President to a bed without metal box springs" before he used the induction balance. Bliss had ignored this request.

The days, turning into weeks and months, that followed the shooting, continued to take Garfield through enormous anguish. The president suffered not only physically but also mentally. At one point Garfield, an otherwise jovial and outgoing individual, was prohibited from talking by his doctors. One historian described how on one occasion

> Dr. Woodward stepped to the bedside and forbade General Garfield to talk any more. "Mr. President, you are feeling very much refreshed now after all the sleep you have had, but if you keep on talking you will injure yourself, and may undo all the work we have done." He then

> explained to the President that when talking he moved the diaphragm, and this moved the liver, and was liable to injure the prospect for recovery. "But I move the diaphragm every time I breathe." The doctor explained again that in breathing the movement of the diaphragm was very gentle, while in talking it was violent. The President then promised that he would talk no more except by permission of his doctors and he ... kept his word since.[90]

During the last several weeks of his life, Garfield had periods of high fevers, chills, and other signs of sepsis. The repeated probing of his wound caused tremendous pain. Some of the medications prescribed at high doses by Bliss and some of his colleagues induced constipation, nausea, and vomiting. Partly because of that but also because of the infections, Garfield lost all appetite; he stopped longing "for the foods of his childhood, squirrel soup and Minerva Austin's hard bisquits."[91] He became malnourished and was "rotting from the inside out."[92] At the time of his death, Garfield had lost almost one hundred pounds in weight. Already in August the weight loss was obvious, as commented on by Dr. Robert Reyburn: "In spite of all efforts to nourish the President he is emaciating so rapidly that it is distressing to look at him. His weight when he was wounded was 210 pounds, and his weight now is probably not more than 130 or 135 pounds."[93]

Efforts were made to provide Garfield with nutrition by administering calories via the rectum, but despite containing beef bouillon, egg yolk, milk, and whiskey, these "nutritive enemas" did not prevent Garfield's weight loss and continuous decline.

Although the insertion of dirty fingers into Garfield's bullet hole was performed by surgeons, the procedures did not always involve the use of a knife and therefore were not what we typically think of as surgeries. A scalpel, however, was used on several other occasions. The abscess on Garfield's back close to the bullet entrance wound was growing in size and kept draining pus but not enough for the infection to heal. On Sunday, July 24, the star surgeon Agnew, assisted by Hamilton, opened the abscess by performing a surgical incision and drained purulent matter. Despite being "two inches in length and an inch and a half in depth,"[94] the incision was not big enough, and a second operation was needed just two days later to more completely drain the abscess. Even though the procedures were performed by two of the country's top surgeons, the operations were considered "an exercise in surgical incompetence" by a recent surgical historian.[95] Despite excruciating pain during the operations (done without anesthesia), "the President displayed his usual courage" and "neither flinched nor moved."[96]

The infection of the bullet tract kept spreading in the body, with abscesses popping up in different locations. Over the next several weeks, Garfield had to suffer "numerous surgical drainages of abscesses," and "one was so extensive it required general (ether) anesthesia."[97] Ironically, Bliss cut one of his own fingers and developed an infection when incising one of the president's many abscesses.[98] The surgeon, however, was luckier than his patient, and his finger healed by itself.

In late August, the doctors, to their dismay, discovered a swelling on Garfield's right cheek and diagnosed it as an abscess of the right parotid gland. They believed that it was yet another manifestation of Garfield's infected bullet tract and began cutting into the area. They had to repeat the operation several times, but despite multiple incisions, the abscess was not effectively drained. Instead, after several days the abscess drained spontaneously, with matter emptying into Garfield's right ear canal and into the inside of his mouth.[99]

A Frustrated Garfield Finally Demands to Be Moved to Elberon

With the miseries growing worse, Garfield finally was losing his patience and requested to be moved from the White House to Elberon, the resort area along the coast of New Jersey where Lucretia not long ago had recovered from a bout of malaria fevers. Garfield was also getting tired and sick of Bliss who, with his arrogant and dictatorial demeanor, continued to create frictions in the Executive Mansion. When Garfield sensed that Bliss was not going along with his request, he raised his voice and stood his ground, telling Bliss, "No, no, I don't want any more delay."[100]

At six o'clock on the morning of September 6, the president was carried out to a waiting train. A track had been laid from the station to the White House, and "people on Pennsylvania Avenue early Tuesday were surprised to see a train with three cars in the middle of the street."[101] When Garfield waived goodbye to the staff, they were horrified to see their president for the first time in two months; although "he was fully conscious [he] looked like a ghost."[102] The president's car had been equipped with an extra-thick mattress to reduce the impact of bumps along the track. Drs. Bliss and Agnew were on the train to monitor the president's condition. Dr. Hamilton had left ahead of Garfield and his entourage and was waiting for the president in New Jersey.

When the train arrived at Elberon shortly after lunchtime, word of Garfield's expected coming had spread, and the president was greeted by throngs of people standing "silently, with uncovered heads, hats in their hands, and tears in their eyes."[103] Railroad workers had been laboring through the night laying a temporary track connecting the train station with the Francklyn Cottage, a "comfortable and roomy dwelling" at the seaside and owned by Charles G. Francklyn, a wealthy New York financier.[104] The president was given an upstairs large chamber, fifteen by twenty-five feet, overlooking the ocean. Garfield loved his new view, so different from the enclosed sickroom at the White House. "From the bed, the occupant could look out a window to the left toward the ocean or over the foot of the bed to the south, ... [and] James Garfield could hear the waves breaking on the shore."[105]

This was where Garfield would spend the last two weeks of his life.

Despite the beautiful place, the fevers, pain, and misery continued. Garfield even had to put up with having Bliss remaining in charge of his care. In all his sufferings, Garfield remained stoic. He won the admiration of Susan Edson, who commented that the president was a "wonderfully patient sufferer."[106]

Bliss continued to deceive the public about the president's condition and fired some of his colleagues when he felt they were no longer needed due to the president's "improved condition."[107] Bliss even got Dr. Hamilton to buy into the false belief that Garfield was getting better. Hamilton was reported to have told a colleague surgeon that "he had the strongest hope of recovery."[108]

Susan Edson was so outraged by Bliss's continued deceptions that she left Elberon. Silas Boynton stayed but kept contradicting Bliss's optimistic announcements on a daily basis. The president's condition continued to deteriorate despite Bliss's pronouncements. Eleven days after Garfield's arrival at the New Jersey sea shore, his condition was "critical."[109] He was delirious and had high fevers, severe chills, and a violent cough. On the evening of September 19, Garfield woke up at ten o'clock with severe chest pain and complained of "this terrible pain," pointing to his heart. Finally, reality caught up with Bliss who, when he saw Garfield's agony, cried out "My God ... he is dying!"[110]

Garfield died at 10:35 p.m. on Monday, September 19, 1881. Even Bliss now had to admit that things were not looking good and whispered, "It is over."[111] Vice President Arthur was informed at his residence in New York. He was sworn in by a New York Supreme Court judge as the twenty-first president of the United States at 2:15 a.m. on September 20, 1881. The new president then left for Elberon to escort Garfield's body to Washington.

The Autopsy

Garfield's body underwent an autopsy in the afternoon the day after his death. The necropsy was performed in the bedroom where Garfield had died only eighteen hours prior. The room was crowded by several of the president's surgeons, including Agnew, Hamilton, Bliss, Barnes, Reyburn, and Woodward. The body had already been embalmed when the procedure began. The dissection was carried out by Daniel S. Lamb from the Army Medical Museum in Washington, D.C. Of course, the major attention was focused on finding the bullet.

The bullet had fractured the right eleventh and twelfth ribs and injured the twelfth thoracic and first and second lumbar vertebrae but had miraculously spared the spinal cord.[112] Several medical historians have reported that at the autopsy, the bullet was found behind and below the lower edge of the pancreas, where it was "encysted."[113] In contrast, when Bliss was cross-examined during the trial and asked where the bullet had been found during the autopsy, he replied that "all the viscera had been taken out and placed in a bowl, and in that bowl the ball was found in its cyst."[114] The official government stenographer and court reporter confirmed this by again stating that "according to the testimony of Dr Bliss the bullet was found in a basin at the time of the autopsy."[115] If this was the only way by which the slug was localized, its exact relationship to the pancreas and other organs and structures must have been difficult (if not impossible) to establish.

These observations may explain why another medical historian described the location of the bullet as "among the viscera."[116] The observations may also explain why one of the physicians who was present as an observer during the autopsy refused to sign the autopsy report and dismissed Lamb (who had performed the dissection) as "merely a medical student" who had "haphazardly removed and thrown the abdominal viscera off to the side."[117]

The predominant finding of the postmortem examination of Garfield's body was that of widespread infections with abscesses located at multiple sites in the abdomen, in the retroperitoneal space, and at distant locations, including in the right parotid gland. A remarkable finding was a pseudoaneurysm (a pseudoaneurysm is a saclike widening of an artery not caused by an original intrinsic weakness of the arterial wall but instead by an extrinsic factor causing the weakness of the artery, such as an infection close to the artery or an injury to the blood vessel) of the splenic artery, "nearly as large as a man's fist."[118] The pseudoaneurysm was filled with clotted blood, and there was evidence of a recent rupture of the blood vessel. Although the tear of the artery was described as being the result of direct injury by the bullet, it seems likely that the pseudoaneurysm of the splenic artery was caused by infection, which also caused weakness of the vessel wall. The rupture of the splenic artery with the ensuing bleeding was considered the immediate cause of death by the doctors who performed the autopsy.[119]

Despite the overwhelming evidence of the role of infection in the president's death, Bliss still had a hard time acknowledging the damage caused by his and the other surgeons' dirty fingers and instead ascribed the death to a "broken backbone."[120] It is remarkable that the potential role of the surgeons' unclean hands was not brought up during Guiteau's trial by the prisoner himself or his defense counselors, despite Guiteau's forceful and repeated claim that Garfield's death was caused by the physicians and not by him.

The medical and surgical treatment of President Garfield attracted an immense amount of both national and international interest and criticism. In Germany, Professor Friedrich Esmarch, a world-renowned military surgeon, was particularly critical in a lecture given to the Physiological Society of Kiel in February 1882. The speech was reprinted in the *Boston Medical and Surgical Journal* the same year.[121] In his lecture, Esmarch lambasted his American colleagues for not understanding the risks of the unnecessary digging for the bullet with unclean fingers and instruments. He criticized the American surgeons for the error of doing too much rather than too little and declared that if "no search had been made for the ball … the unfortunate patient would be alive now."[122] This view certainly supported the claim that Guiteau made at his trial: "I simply shot him, [but] it was the doctors that killed him."[123]

Also in this country, voices of harsh criticism of the president's surgeons were raised. Some even suggested that the doctors had committed malpractice.[124] Bliss, of course, continued to defend the treatment Garfield had received, but his views were strongly contradicted by others, causing additional controversies.[125]

Although most historians, including medical historians, have attributed Garfield's death to the incompetent management by his surgeons, in particular their disregard of aseptic systems and repeated probing of the president's back wound with dirty fingers, a different opinion was offered recently. In a paper published in 2013, Pappas and Joharifard, two academic surgeons and medical historians, proposed that most of the infection suffered by Garfield was caused not by contaminated fingers of the surgeons but instead by an abscess caused by the rupture of an inflamed gallbladder.[126] The basis of this claim was a thorough reevaluation of the autopsy report, which described "an abscess cavity between the undersurface of the liver, the transverse colon, and the transverse [mesocolon] which involved the gallbladder …

[and] ... contained about two ounces of greenish yellow fluid—a mixture of pus and biliary matter."[127] Because there was no mentioning of gallstones, the authors suggested that the president's sepsis was caused by a ruptured "acalculous cholecystitis" (acute inflammation of the gallbladder without the presence of gallstones), a condition that can be seen in patients with other severe conditions, such as severe injury.

It may be argued that even if Garfield's surgeons had suspected that the president's fevers and declining condition were caused by an abscess originating from a ruptured gallbladder, nothing else would have been done, and the outcome would have been the same. (Removal of an inflamed gallbladder was not yet part of the surgeons' armamentarium.) The observation, however, would shift the blame away from the doctors' alleged mistreatment of their patient to the assassin who caused the president's injury and condition ultimately causing a ruptured gallbladder. In their report, Pappas and Johariard concluded that "first, President Garfield died of a ruptured pseudoaneurysm of the splenic artery, a complication of the initial gunshot wound. Second, the President's clinical course ... was not caused by an infected bullet tract but was more likely secondary to complications of an undiagnosed and unmanaged course of cholecystitis."[128]

Guiteau's Trial

Guiteau had an unhappy and less than honorable life. In his youth, he inherited $1,000 from his grandfather (more than $30,000 in today's money) and promised to use the money for his education. He went to Ann Arbor hoping to attend the University of Michigan. Instead of studying hard and preparing for the university application, Guiteau got involved with the Oneida Community and neglected his studies for the admission tests, which he flunked.[129] The experience and the lost money upset Guiteau's father, who kept sending letters to his son asking about the progress of his studies.

Having failed in Michigan, Guiteau moved to Chicago. He found a job as a clerk in a law firm and somehow managed to pass a cursory examination to be admitted to the bar. He did not achieve any successes as a lawyer; reportedly, he argued only one case in court. His legal work was relegated to collecting bills. The temptation to put some of the collected dollars in his own pocket became too big, and soon he had to look over his shoulder for angry clients. Guiteau's fraudulent life continued after he moved to New York, where his activities eventually resulted in jail time.

In 1869 Guiteau married Annie Bunn, an "attractive young librarian."[130] That endeavor also failed; after five years, his wife filed for divorce for adultery and abuse. Annie "did not like the way he would drag her out of bed in the middle of the night and lock her in a hall storage closet."[131] She also despised her husband for his "shameful method of bill collecting."[132]

Guiteau's life would continue to spiral out of control. He became involved in extreme religious groups and traveled around the country to preach "a new Gospel." His father did not like what he saw and at one point even felt that his son was "possessed by the devil."[133]

Guiteau's interests started to turn to politics, and we have already seen the ultimate disastrous result. During the early months of 1881, Guiteau lived in Washington, D.C. He went from one boarding house to another, typically checking out without paying his bills. He was often "sleeping in the public park ... and was seen to go out with a small parcel under his arm and change his linen behind a tree in the public grounds."[134] He kept pestering both the White House and the State Department, demanding either the consular appointment in Paris or a position in Vienna. When Guiteau realized he would not be successful, he developed hatred toward Garfield and decided it was time to "remove" the president.

The trial of Guiteau began on Monday, November 14, 1881, and would turn out to be the spectacle of the year. The press followed the legal proceedings obsessively, and the fact that Guiteau was an odd fellow, behaving in a bizarre manner (in addition to being the assassin of a beloved president), helped create a tremendous amount of interest in the case. The crowds watching were huge from day one. The official government stenographer and court reporter described the chaotic scene: "As soon as the main door opened there was a general rush for seats, men climbing and pulling over chairs in their haste to get a good position whence they could hear the proceedings and better observe the actors."[135] The courtroom was filled to capacity from day one by four hundred persons, with many of the spectators "standing on chairs in order to get a view of Guiteau."[136]

It was not only the general public that crowded the courtroom during the trial. Other people cramming the court included "foreign ministers and attachés, prominent officials of various departments of the Government [and] White House attendants."[137] Women dressed up for the event, and "a bevy of female beauty and fashion occupied a considerable portion of the court-room and contributed by their unusual presence to a remarkable scene."[138] There was no doubt that Guiteau enjoyed the attention. "From the way he addressed the crowd it was evident his overweening vanity was flattered by their presence."[139]

Guiteau was arrested and jailed immediately after the shooting, initially charged with attempted murder of the president. When informed that the president had died, Guiteau understood the implications of the upgraded charge and that he would now stand trial for murder. On the news of Garfield's death, Guiteau immediately broke down but soon found his footing. Already the day after Garfield's passing, Guiteau wrote a letter to the new president, Arthur. In the letter, Guiteau described Garfield as a "good man but a weak politician." He also reminded Arthur that his salary had risen from $8,000 to $50,000 a year thanks to the death of Garfield.

The defense planned to base its case on two points: first, the insanity of the defendant, which his legal counsels hoped would "be a good reason for sending Guiteau to the asylum for the insane instead of the gallows."[140] This line of defense was adamantly opposed by Guiteau, something that created frictions between himself and his legal team. The second defense point was that the wound was not mortal and that the president died from the surgeons' failures. Guiteau reasoned that because Garfield's physicians soon after the shooting had "officially decided he would recover," the president's death two months later proved that Garfield died "from malpractice." Guiteau added that the surgeons "ought to be indicted for murdering James A. Garfield, and not me."[141] Repeatedly, Guiteau pleaded with the judge, "I admit the shooting, but deny the killing."[142]

Guiteau spent time in his cell reading and writing. He was fantasizing on being acquitted and even voiced plans to run for president in 1884. He wrote an autobiography with the title page declaring that he was a "Lawyer, Theologian, and Politician."[143] In the introduction, he tried to explain his crime and wrote, "I have not used the words 'assassination' or 'assassin' in this work. These words grate on the mind and produce a bad feeling."[144] Instead, he continued, "I think of General Garfield's condition as a removal and not as an assassination. My idea simply stated was to remove as easily as possible Mr. James A. Garfield, a quiet and good-natured citizen of Ohio, who temporarily occupied the position of President of the United States, and substitute in his place Mr. Chester A. Arthur, of New York, a distinguished and highly estimable gentleman."[145] To emphasize his reasoning, Guiteau added, "Mr. Garfield I intended to quietly remove to Paradise (which is a great improvement on this world), while Mr. Arthur saved the Republic."

After this and many additional twisted ideas, Guiteau ended his writing with "two matters strictly personal." First, he explained that he was "looking for a wife," and he wanted her to be an "elegant Christian lady of wealth, under thirty, belonging to a first-class family."[146] Second, he wrote that "for twenty years I have had an idea that I should be President," and he went on to declare, "If I were President I should give the nation a first-class administration in every respect."[147]

It is no wonder that Guiteau's defense lawyers were hoping that insanity would be a way to save the prisoner's life.

During the time leading up to the trial and during the trial itself, many Americans developed a deep hatred toward Guiteau. When he was led out of his cell and brought to the van that transported him to the court, crowds gathered and shouted, "There he goes, the villain!"[148] It was obvious that Guiteau was universally detested. On several occasions, plans were plotted to kill him. At one time, a guard at the Old Capitol Prison fired at Guiteau but missed. On another occasion, Guiteau was shot at by "a red-faced man on a sorrel horse who followed along in the rear" while Guiteau was being transported in the van from the courthouse back to the jail after the end of the day's proceedings.[149] Due to fears of lynching, Guiteau was moved to a cell with thick brick walls and only a small opening in the bullet-proof door. From now on, the prisoner demanded better protection and requested "not less than six or eight mounted policemen to guard the van from the jail to the Court, and in going from the Court back to the jail in the afternoon."[150]

The jury to serve during the trial was selected from a pool of 159 persons. Some candidates were easy to exclude after expressing biased statements such as "nothing save the rope should be used" and "no amount of torture is too great for the prisoner."[151] The trial commenced about four and a half months after the shooting and would last for almost ten weeks. On January 25, 1882, it took less than thirty minutes for the jury to reach a verdict: "Guilty as indicted." The assassin was executed by hanging on June 30, 1882, two days before the first anniversary of the shooting.

The entire trial was characterized by Guiteau's bizarre behavior. He was constantly interrupting witnesses, cursing and yelling at them. When guards tried to restrain the prisoner and prevent him from interrupting the proceedings, he shouted, "You mind your business, you confounded fools! You ain't got no sense."[152] Not even the judge and the jury members were spared Guiteau's screaming and disdainful comments. His lead defense counselor, George Scoville, a lawyer from Chicago and Guiteau's brother-in-law whom the accused had requested as counselor, was particularly badly treated in front of spectators, witnesses, and everybody else present in the courtroom. On several occasions, Guiteau did not spare his invectives when scolding Scoville. Heated verbal exchanges between Guiteau and his counselor illustrated Guiteau's strange behavior. For example, when a witness was cross-examined by Scoville about Guiteau's potential insanity, the prisoner interrupted and yelled at his counselor: "You are about as stupid as you can be, Scoville, on this subject. You have no more sense than a baby on the insanity business." Scoville pretended he did not hear Guiteau and continued the cross-examination. Guiteau again interrupted and told his defense lawyer, "You are as stupid as you can be, Scoville."[153]

On another occasion, Guiteau "in a rage" interrupted Scoville and declared, "You are stupid, Scoville, as the witness is. You are just compromising my case every time on cross-examination."[154] Again, Scoville was able to brush off Guiteau's outrage and calmly continued his interview of the witness. Finally, however, Scoville ran out of patience and stood up to Guiteau. When Guiteau again interrupted a witness, the following exchange took place:

> Mr Scoville (angrily)—Now, shut up.
> The Prisoner—I won't, I will go on.
> Mr Scoville—Then go on and I will get off the case.
> The Prisoner—We will have a new man to-morrow. This is your last day, Scoville.[155]

Luckily enough for Guiteau, tempers cooled off, and Scoville was at the prisoner's side the next day and would remain there until the end of the trial.

Although Guiteau was difficult to control and had outbursts of anger, throwing tantrums most of the days during the trial, on some days he appeared subdued, having "the same restless, furtive expression as of a hunted wolf."[156]

The last time Guiteau had a chance to scold somebody in the courtroom was when he directed his anger toward the jury that had just found him guilty of murdering the president. Despite attempts by his defense team to have Guiteau shut up, he screamed at the jury members, "My blood will be upon the heads of [the] jury. Don't forget it!" Then the verdict sank in, and Guiteau "dropped completely his air of flippant arrogance and sat with rigid features and compressed lips," but even so he could not totally restrain himself and "called out in tones of desperation 'God will avenge this outrage.'"[157]

Guiteau's weirdness would continue to the bitter end. He was reported to have "danced his way to the gallows," smiling and waving at the crowds and shaking hands with his executioner. He had been writing a poem, "I am going to the Lordy," toward the end of his time in the cell and had requested that an orchestra be allowed to play while he sang the poem on the gallows. The request for music and singing was denied, and instead Guiteau read the poem. He kept smiling as a black hood was placed over his head. The trapdoor opened, the rope immediately broke his neck, and gone was one of the most bizarre political murderers this country has seen.

Consequences of Garfield's Assassination

The shooting of Garfield had many consequences. Garfield, of course, died. Guiteau was hanged. A Stalwart was sworn in as president (one of Guiteau's objectives), but to the surprise of many, Chester Arthur became less of a Stalwart as president than expected. He distanced himself from Conkling, his mentor, and did not even appoint him to the cabinet.

A scandal around bills submitted by the surgeons erupted when it became known that Bliss and Hamilton had requested that the federal government to compensate each of them with $25,000 (almost $710,000 each in today's money). Congress balked, and after public hearings in which Bliss and other doctors were harshly criticized, it was decided to offer Bliss $6,500 (still a whopping $184,000 in today's dollars), an offer that Bliss refused to accept, and Hamilton "only" $5,000.[158] Considering the mismanagement of Garfield's injury, which was now openly discussed in newspapers and even echoed by Garfield's young daughter Mollie, who commented that "the surgeons didn't know anything about the wound,"[159] the surgeons' bills were not looked upon favorably by the public. The spectacle certainly did not boost the reputation of surgeons.

Because it was obvious that the omission of antiseptic principles had resulted in severe infection of Garfield's gunshot wound and caused the president's death, Lister's discoveries and recommendations started to get a foothold even among American surgeons, particularly among younger surgeons. As one medical historian explained, "The controversies surrounding Garfield's death became a dividing line between the new and the old in American medicine."[160]

Another aspect of the critique directed at Garfield's medical team was that Bliss did not recruit qualified nurses to assist in the care of the president. Nursing schools had started to be established in the 1870s, and by the time of Garfield's assassination several schools were in full swing, training nurses throughout the country. People had a hard time understanding why experienced nurses had not been called in to help care for the wounded president. A comment in a surgical journal did not mince words: "The absence of trained and experienced nurses from the patient's bedside has unquestionably excited comment upon the part of many."[161]

Although Bliss and some of his colleagues were criticized, it may be argued that they were working hard during the months following the shooting of the president and for the most part were adhering to principles that were observed by many surgeons at the time. They were in the spotlight in a stressful environment and were constantly feeling the pressure from the media. The experience and the critique Bliss was subjected to took its toll. He tried to defend himself and wrote in a medical journal asking "whether the conditions could have been improved or mitigated, or his [the president's] life preserved longer by any other line of treatment."[162]

Even though Bliss tried to be optimistic in his comments to the press and wanted to give the impression that he had everything under control (something that was criticized by others as attempts to deceive the public and his colleagues about the president's condition), he seemed to have suffered mental stress from the experience. Some of his supporters claimed that "his health was broken from the pressures of treating Garfield."[163] When Bliss died eight years later from heart failure, he was an "embittered and lonely man."[164] In recent writing, Bliss has been called "the inept doctor who killed President Garfield."[165] And another article had the title, "Ignorance Is Bliss."[166]

When Bliss asked Dr. Joseph Woodward to serve as his second-in-command and take responsibility for the daily bulletins provided to the press, many raised their eyebrows. Notwithstanding that Woodward was the president of the American Medical Association, he was considered a researcher with little or no clinical experience. One of the doctors taking care of Garfield sarcastically commented that Woodward "knew nothing about gunshot wounds, practically, but that he had looked up the matter in the books and found that the way to treat gunshot wounds of the abdomen was the following—reading off the notes."[167] The stressful experience of taking care of Garfield had even greater impact on Woodward's life than Bliss's. When the truthfulness of Woodward's bulletins started to be questioned after Garfield's death, Woodward was quite disturbed and "went into a state of severe mental and physical depression."[168] Three years after Garfield's death, Woodward committed suicide after having spent those years in and out of mental institutions.

Dr. Reyburn, who was also criticized for his management of the president, defended himself by stating, "I know that I speak only the truth when I say that no wounded man ever received more tender, loving, and devoted service, not only form his surgeons, but also from the faithful friends who nursed him through his long and weary illness. We gave him this cheerfully and would have killed even our lives for him, if by so doing we could have saved his."[169] Dr. J. Marion Sims, a prominent surgeon and gynecologist at the time, gave further support to the surgeons treating Garfield, commenting that "the President's surgeons did all that men could do, all that the present state of science would permit.... He had not the least chance of recovery under any circumstances or any treatment."[170]

Two of the most prominent surgeons involved in the treatment of Garfield did better. Agnew continued his remarkable career, impacting the practice of surgery in this country as well as internationally. Thomas Eakins's painting *The Agnew Clinic* remains an important part of the annals of surgery. Maybe one reason why Agnew's reputation was not negatively affected by his participation in Garfield's care (despite the fact that he, like Bliss, kept probing the gunshot wound with unclean fingers and dirty surgical instruments) is that he managed to come across as less greedy than some of his colleagues. When a delegation arrived to give Agnew payment for the help he had provided, Agnew nobly refused the money: "Gentlemen, I present no bill for my attendance to President Garfield. I gave my services freely and gratuitously." This was a less than a truthful statement, since he had initially submitted a bill for $14,700 ($421,250 in today's money).

Dr. Frank Hamilton, like Agnew, did not experience a setback of his reputation or career after Garfield's death. Hamilton was more candid than Bliss and admitted his errors in Garfield's care but, at the same time, surprisingly and against most witnesses, claimed that "throughout the whole course of the treatment, contrary to what has been publicly said repeatedly, so far as it was possible to apply the system of antiseptic surgery advocated by Mr. Lister to a wound of this character, it was rigorously employed."[171] Agnew died five years after Garfield's assassination, "having taught many medical students, having founded medical schools and departments and leaving a chapter in American history."[172]

Chapter Four

Grover Cleveland

The President with a Rough Spot on the Roof of His Mouth

The Twenty-Second President

March 4, 1885–March 4, 1889

The Twenty-Fourth President

March 4, 1893–March 4, 1897

Even though most of the events detailed in this chapter took place during Grover Cleveland's second term as president, it may be worthwhile to consider some aspects of his earlier life as well.

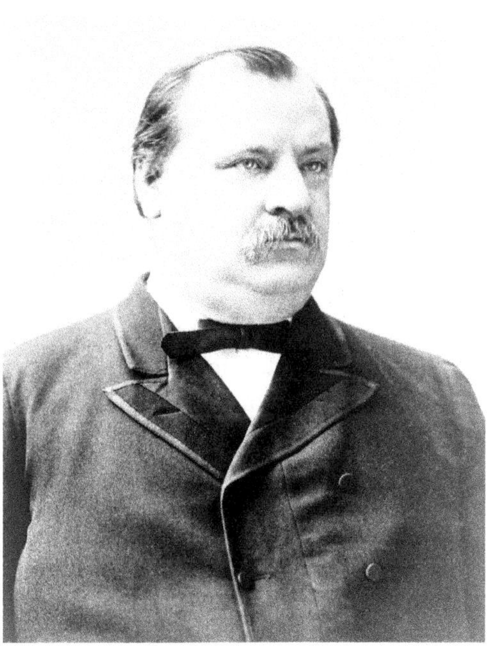

Portrait of Grover Cleveland. Library of Congress, Prints and Photographs Division, Washington, D.C.

Lifelong Struggle with Obesity

Grover Cleveland was born on March 18, 1837, in Caldwell, New Jersey. His father, Richard, was a Presbyterian minister from Connecticut who had married Cleveland's mother, Ann, "the pretty daughter of a bookseller," in Baltimore in 1829.[1] Cleveland was christened Stephen Grover after his father's predecessor in the congregation and was known to most people as Steve (sometimes nicknamed Big Steve) until his early twenties, when he started to use Grover as his first name, convinced that would sound "more sonorous and distinctive."[2]

Grover was blessed with a good appetite and was known to be eating too much his entire life. Already as a boy, he was described as "chubby and large for his age."[3] In his mid-thirties, he earned the nickname "Uncle Jumbo" and became the "butt of a great many jokes about his obesity."[4] Not only did he enjoy big (and frequent) portions at the table, but he also consumed a lot of liquid calories. One of his favorite drinks was lager beer; no wonder he developed "a huge beer belly."[5] At the time of his second presidency, Cleveland was described as "an overweight cigar smoker who savored beer and heavy foods"[6] and was what we today would call morbidly obese. His body constitution made him an extremely high-risk patient when he underwent a surgical procedure in 1893, an operation that would be risky even in a fit and normal-weight person.

Cleveland grew up being "full of fun and inclined to play pranks."[7] He liked outdoor activities and sports. His favorite was fishing, for which he was passionate. He developed his love for fishing early in life, an affection that would stay with him as long as his physical condition allowed. Cleveland's ardor for fishing was well known and would come in handy when the public was deceived after his surgery for cancer and after his delayed arrival at Buzzards Bay in Massachusetts in July 1893.

Early in his first presidential term, Cleveland was afflicted by ankle gout. He was at high risk for the disease, having "obesity, large intake of alcoholic beverages, and lack of exercise."[8] The joint pain would remain with Cleveland for years and would have political consequences; it would make it difficult for him to carry out his campaign for a second term in 1892.[9] In 1901 at William McKinley's funeral, Cleveland was seen limping severely, with his right foot in bandages. Obviously, carrying around an overweight body was not helpful when suffering arthritis in the ankle joint.

Practicing Law and Getting into Politics

In 1855, Grover, eighteen at the time, moved to Buffalo, New York. An uncle took care of young Cleveland and offered him a job (paying ten dollars a month) and lodging. Buffalo was a young city with somewhat of a Wild West mentality. The place was booming, with an economy thriving on its strategic location at the Erie Canal, completed only three decades prior to Cleveland's arrival. Buffalo was in the midst of a breathtaking expansion, with its population growing from eight thousand to eighty thousand between 1830 and 1860.

Not surprisingly, Buffalo was considered a "pretty wild place" filled with temptations and dangers. It was reported that "sixty percent of the buildings on both sides of Canal Street from Erie Street to Commercial were houses of prostitution, thirty percent were saloons, and ten percent grocery stores, etc."[10] Disease and crime were widespread, and the murder rates were high. After killings, the victims were often thrown into the canal. "When the canal was dredged every spring, it wasn't unusual for eight or more human bodies to be discovered."[11]

Through his uncle, Cleveland was introduced to a prominent lawyer, Henry W. Rogers, and was offered a position as an office clerk in Rogers's law firm. It paid enough to allow Cleveland to rent a small room in the center of the city, where he would spend hours "reading law." After studying hard for three and a half years, Cleveland was admitted to the bar by the New York Supreme Court in May 1859.

In 1862, Cleveland was offered the position of assistant district attorney for Erie County, and three years later he won the Democratic nomination for election to the district attorney office. He lost the election to his Republican opponent and went back to private practice but had by now been bitten by the political bug.

When Cleveland returned to the law firm, one of his best friends, Oscar Folsom, was a new partner. They were of the same age, had similar interests and temperament, and were very close both at work and outside the office. In 1864 Folsom and his wife had a daughter, Frances. Cleveland was happy to see the baby and "bought her a baby carriage and doted on her as if she were his own."[12] Not in his wildest dreams could Cleveland imagine the little girl would one day be his bride.

Cleveland would remain in Buffalo for almost three decades before ending up in Albany as governor of New York state. His time in Buffalo spanned the American Civil War era, and he saw some of the unrest that plagued many American communities during that time. The Conscription Act of 1863 spawned violence and riots in Buffalo. It was an intriguing coincidence that John Wilkes Booth was in town the week of the worst riots performing on the stage of the Metropolitan Theatre.

When Cleveland went back to his law practice after losing the election for Erie County district attorney, he found more time to participate in "Buffalo's boisterous nightlife."[13] He was seen several nights every week visiting Buffalo's many saloons, enjoying his cigars and plenty of lager beer. Although Buffalo's saloons offered many opportunities to find female company, Cleveland "was discreet about his romantic interests and kept his distance from the city's belles."[14] However, when Cleveland later reminisced about his years in Buffalo, he admitted that he "had not been a saint."[15]

In 1870, only five years after Cleveland lost the election for district attorney, the temptation to get back into politics became irresistible. He ran for the position as Erie County sheriff and won the election. Despite being successful and respected for honesty and integrity, he was not happy and decided not to run for reelection in 1873. Instead, he again went back to practice law.

The next several years propelled Cleveland's political career at a speed that took even Cleveland himself with surprise. As one of his biographers explained, "the stars were with him."[16] In January 1882, Cleveland was elected mayor of Buffalo. Already in November he quit the position of mayor and threw himself into the campaign for governorship of New York state. He won the election, and on January 1, 1883, he was sworn in as the twenty-eighth governor of New York.

Soon, Cleveland would be pulled away for an even higher office. After a bitter campaign against James G. Blaine, a former Republican senator from Maine and a seasoned politician, Cleveland won the election in 1884. The campaign saw a lot of mudslinging from both sides. Cleveland was accused of having raped a woman, Maria Halpin, several years earlier and being the illegitimate father of her son, Oscar Folsom Cleveland.[17]

Cleveland was inaugurated as the twenty-second president of the United States on March 4, 1885. Four years later he lost his reelection campaign to Benjamin Harrison, a former Republican senator from Indiana, but after four additional years, Cleveland made a comeback to become the first president serving two nonconsecutive terms.

When the Cleveland's left the White House in 1889, the president's wife, Frances, told one of the staff members, "I want you to take good care of all the furniture and ornaments in the house, for I want to find everything just as it is now, when we come back again." When asked when that would take place, she replied, "We are coming back four years from today."[18] And that is what happened.

In the meantime, Mr. and Mrs. Cleveland headed to a more private life in New York City where the former president joined a private law firm but could also spend more time at the couple's summerhouse at Buzzards Bay in Massachusetts. Finally, Grover Cleveland could go fishing as much as he wanted to and stay away from politics, which is what he did, at least initially.

Seeing President Harrison pushing for policies that supported protectionism, such as the McKinley Tariff, and that favored silver rather than gold as currency standard, in particular the Sherman Silver Purchase Act (requiring the government to purchase 4.5 million ounces of silver every month to mint coins), Cleveland became increasingly frustrated. He finally lost his patience and broke his silence. In 1891, he wrote an open letter to a political meeting in New York expressing his objections.[19] The letter became known as the "silver letter" and put Cleveland back in the center of the nation's political debate. He was jumping into the hotbed just in time for the 1892 election. His actions helped set the stage for a rematch with Harrison, and this time Cleveland was the winner.

Cleveland's Second Inauguration

On March 4, 1893, Cleveland was sworn in for his second term as president.

The weather on the day of Cleveland's repeat inauguration was miserable, described by one congressman to be "as bad as mortal man ever endured, windy, stormy, sleety, icy."[20] It was dramatically different from the weather at Cleveland's first swearing in eight years earlier. At that ceremony "the day was one of the perfect ones that finally gained, from the new President, the distinctive name of Cleveland weather," meaning beautiful weather.[21] When Cleveland stepped out to take the oath for the second time on the platform constructed at the steps of the Capitol, the weather was cold and drizzly. The newly reelected president looked out on an audience of about ten thousand but did not see all their faces. Many were huddling under umbrellas, freezing and shivering.

It was not only the weather that was nasty when Cleveland was sworn in. The political and economic climate in the country was miserable as well. In 1892, Cleveland had won a disgruntled fight against Adlai Stevenson (the grandfather of his namesake who ran for president in 1952 and 1956) for the Democratic presidential nomination. In an effort to unite the divided Democratic Party, the party leaders

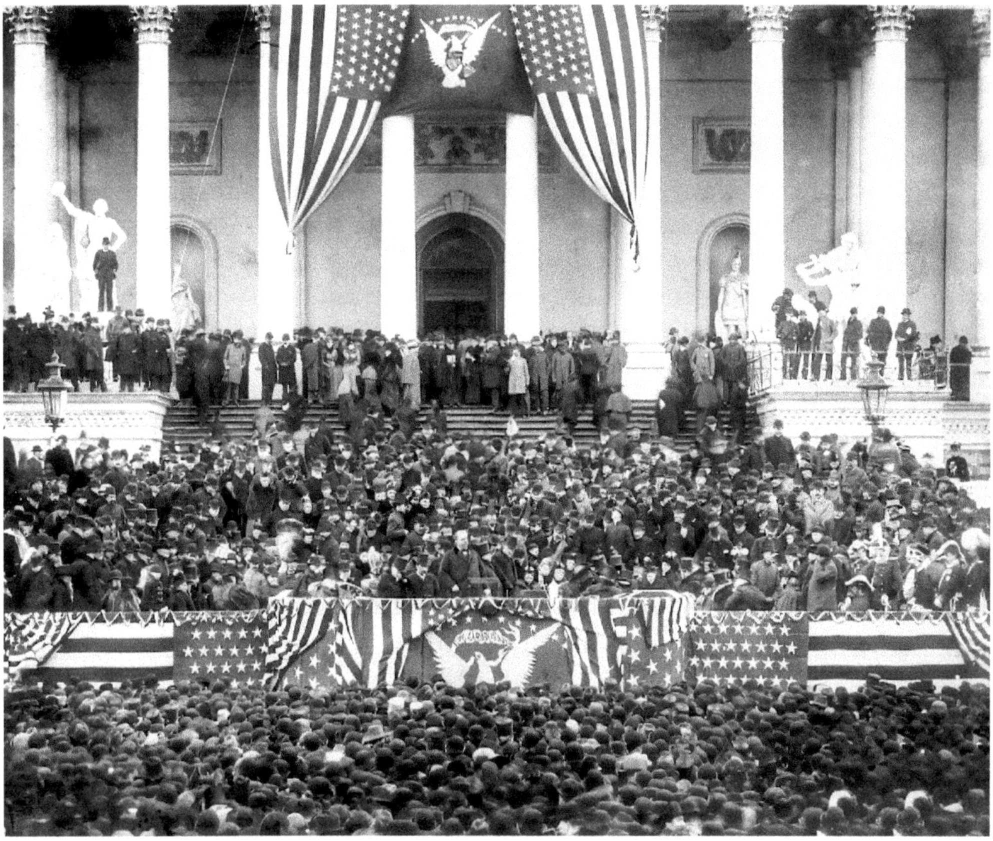

Grover Cleveland's second inauguration, March 4, 1893. Getty Images. Credit: New York Daily News Archives.

had picked Stevenson as Cleveland's running mate, resulting in a ticket with two individuals who were at each other's throat and held radically different views on fiscal policies. (It was not until the 1940s that the candidate for vice president would be chosen by the man on the top of the ticket rather than by the party.) As opposed to Stevenson, Cleveland was a conservative "sound money man" or "goldbug"[22] who favored the gold standard and despised "the waste of public money."[23] He was hoping to gain support for his programs and win over Stevenson's supporters, the Silverites, once back in power.

The stakes were high, with the nation facing the worst economic situation since its founding. The crisis was called "the most deep-seated storm in the history of our country." Others wrote that "Mr. Cleveland is about all that stands between the country and absolute disaster."[24]

The Panic of 1893 was already under way when Cleveland took office. The bankruptcy of the iconic Reading Railroad in late February had been one of the igniting events. Hungry citizens out of work were roaming the streets of American cities, and trust in the federal gold reserve was quickly evaporating. When the National Cordage Company went belly-up on May 4, the markets collapsed. The next day, the *New York Times* described the floor of the Wall Street stock exchange as "a morning at Bedlam."[25]

Cleveland understood that he needed to provide strong and unquestioned leadership to defeat Stevenson's supporters and push his fiscal programs through Congress. More than ever before, the country needed a powerful and healthy leader, and any question about the president's vigor could make the political and economic situation worse.

Things got complicated when in early May, only two months into his second term as president, Cleveland felt a "rough spot" on the roof of his mouth. Although initially not too concerned, when realizing that the swelling was growing bigger, he became increasingly alarmed not only because of the potential political fallout if he was found to be sick but also because he was scared about cancer. He was well aware of Ulysses Grant's diagnosis of oral cancer only eight years prior and had followed the extensive press coverage of Grant's struggle with a tumor that prevented him from swallowing food and ultimately choked him to death. Like Grant, who reportedly could go through twenty cigars in a day, Cleveland was an ardent cigar smoker (and chewer). He also loved his whiskey and his lager beer. The president realized that these habits may put him at risk for something bad going on in his mouth.

The Workup of Cleveland's Oral Tumor

When Cleveland initially felt the swelling in his mouth, he had more important things to worry about. In addition to the political divisiveness and disastrous economic situation in the country, the time-consuming and tiring interviews of a multitude of jobseekers looking for employment in the new administration weighed heavy on the president's shoulders. In addition, his wife, Frances, twenty-seven years younger than the president, was pregnant. The thought of anything dangerous going on in his mouth was initially brushed aside; Cleveland believed that the swelling could be caused by irritation from his teeth. As time went on, however, and the rough spot grew bigger, the president started to get anxious and began to fear a fate similar to that of Grant.

Toward mid–June, Cleveland asked his White House physician, Dr. Robert M. O'Reilly, to take a look. O'Reilly was an army doctor with the rank of major who had been assigned to take care of health issues among government officials. When the doctor looked in the president's mouth, he was not sure what he saw but agreed with Cleveland's initial suspicion that the lesion may be caused by bad teeth. The next day, however, a dentist called to the White House concluded that "the president's teeth were not the cause of the irritation."[26] With better light available, O'Reilly reexamined the president and was now able to see "an ulcerative surface nearly as large as a quarter with cauliflower granulations and crater edges."[27]

What O'Reilly saw made him uneasy. He scraped some tissue off the lesion and sent it for microscopic testing. Pathologists at the Army Medical Museum (later called the Armed Forces Institute of Pathology), uninformed about the patient's identity, reported that it was probable that "the specimens are from a case of epithelioma."[28] In other words, the lesion "presumably could be cancerous."[29]

It was now time to call in the experts. O'Reilly consulted Dr. Joseph Bryant, a famous surgeon at Bellevue Hospital in New York and a good friend of Cleveland and his wife. In a letter to Bryant, O'Reilly wrote, "Foreseeing the [diagnosis of epithelioma] and believing that an operation would be required I had yesterday told Mr. C that the bone was a little rough and the possibility some dead matter would have to be removed and advised him to accompany Mrs. C. to New York and see you because if you were at Gray Gables [the president's summer home at Buzzards Bay] nothing would be known, whereas here it would be difficult to keep it a secret."[30]

At this stage, the first lady had been alerted to the president's condition. She was about to leave for Gray Gables for the summer visit and wrote a letter to Bryant asking for a meeting with him during a stop at the railroad depot in Jersey City, New Jersey. She wrote, "I wish very much to speak to you, especially about something that the President has on the roof of his mouth." When they met, Bryant listened to Frances's description of the lesion in the president's mouth and decided to travel to Washington to examine Cleveland firsthand. Bryant was not only a renowned surgeon and a good friend of the Cleveland family but was also considered an expert on oral tumors.

The day after his arrival in Washington, Bryant performed a detailed examination of Cleveland's oral cavity. What he saw, "an ulcerated surface with an oval outline about the size of a quarter of a dollar,"[31] convinced him that the president had a malignant tumor in his mouth and would need surgery. Cleveland, who probably sensed that Bryant was concerned, asked, "What do you think it is, Doctor?" The surgeon replied, "It is a bad looking tenant. Were it in my mouth I would have it removed at once."[32]

First, however, Bryant wanted the character of the tumor better defined. He scraped some additional samples from the lesion and sent them to Dr. William Henry Welch at Johns Hopkins University in Baltimore. Welch was considered an "unquestioned authority in these matters," and in addition to being a professor of pathology, he was also an internationally recognized bacteriologist. This was particularly important, since one of the differential diagnoses of the malignant-looking tumor in the president's mouth was a syphilitic lesion. Syphilis, more common in those days, could mimic many other conditions, including tumors.

Bryant, however, felt so convinced about the diagnosis of cancer that he informed the president that surgery would be necessary and started making preparations for the procedure even before Welch's report was back. The surgeon leaned on his clinical experience: "To one familiar with the macroscopical appearance of epithelial growths, no reasonable doubt could exist in his mind regarding the certainty of the malignant nature of this."[33] Only two days before the surgery, Bryant received "an elaborate and detailed report" from Welch. The report has been lost for history, and it remains a mystery whether Welch had confirmed the cancer diagnosis. This uncertainty has fed into conspiracy theories surrounding Cleveland's tumor, his surgery, and his surgeons.

When Cleveland realized what Bryant had found and that he would need surgery, he panicked not only for having a disease that could kill him but also for the political ramifications if his condition and upcoming surgery would become known to the public. He swore his doctors and a few additional individuals in his inner circle to secrecy. He was adamant that the procedure must take place out of the view of the press. Nothing could be noticed on the president revealing that something had happened to him. No visible scars would be tolerated, and the mustache needed to stay![34]

The political stakes were extremely high. Cleveland had called for a special session of Congress for the first week of August. He planned to deliver a message addressing the economic crisis in the country. His ultimate goal was to have Congress repeal the Silver Act. The president needed to look healthy and robust when the message was delivered.

So, here we were: a fifty-six-year-old patient, obese (weighing 250–300 pounds) with a neck so thick that people jokingly said that "he could take off his shirt without unbuttoning the collar,"[35] a heavy smoker and drinker, and overworked and tired from a stressful political situation ("just the build and age for a brain stroke," as one of Cleveland's surgeons, Dr. William W. Keen, expressed it),[36] about to undergo major and dangerous surgery in the saloon of a yacht under sail.

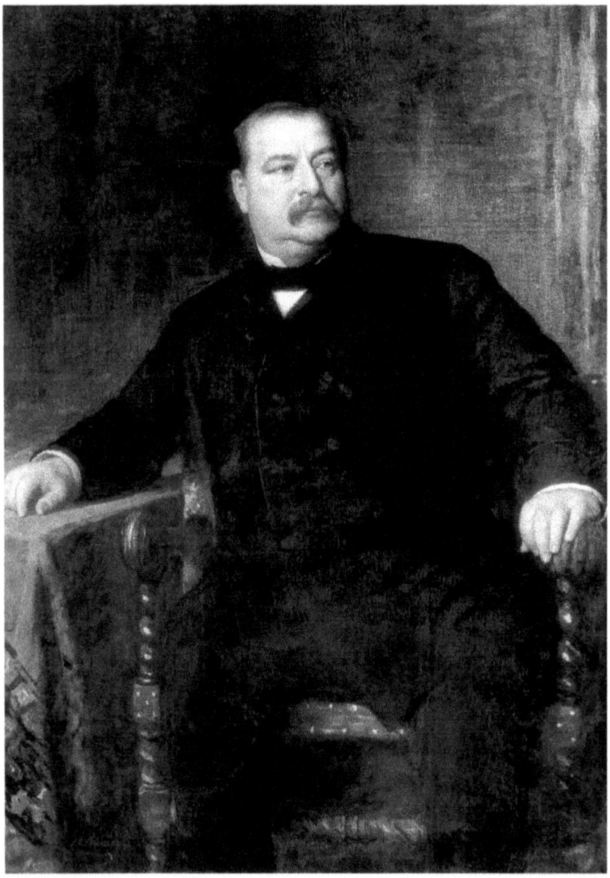

Official portrait of President Cleveland by Eastman Johnson (1824–1906) in 1891. The image shows a morbidly obese Cleveland, who was weighing close to 300 pounds and would undergo major and risky surgery about two years later. Alamy Stock Photo. Credit: NMUIM.

Although the saloon where the surgery would take place had been emptied of furniture, cleaned, and disinfected and the surgical instruments had been sterilized by boiling them in water, the space was far from an operating room with lighting and sterile environment and the ability to have vital signs safely watched during and after the procedure. A chair had been tied to the mast in the middle of the saloon, and this was where Cleveland would be sitting during the operation rather than lying on an operating table. The only light would come from a single bulb powered by a portable battery.

One medical historian described the whole situation as "bizarre" and added, "It is almost beyond comprehension that either patient or doctors would be so foolhardy as to place themselves in such a position."[37] To perform major surgery under suboptimal conditions in a "56-year-old obese, sedentary president who drank too much, smoked too much, and ate too much" was reckless, to say the least. No wonder the surgical team was nervous. One of the doctors commented, "If the president dies during surgery, I hope the yacht sinks and we all drown!"[38] The only person who seemed to be calm at this point was the president. He reportedly slept well the night before surgery even without getting any sedative, "lulled by the gentle rocking of the yacht."[39]

With today's standard, Cleveland's surgery would probably be considered a clear case of malpractice, and even with the norms of the late 1800s, the procedure and the circumstances under which it was performed would be considered dangerously risky.

Preparing for Secret Surgery

In addition to keeping the surgery hidden, it was also a matter of finding a secret place for the operation and how to get there without being detected. Despite all efforts to keep the affair secret, Cleveland understood that it would not be easy to keep his condition and upcoming surgery out of sight of probing journalists. Already during his first term, the president had experienced the intrusiveness of the press and its less than truthful reporting. He had been outraged by the "keyhole correspondents" and their probing. In a letter to the *New York Evening Post*, he had expressed his frustration with the reporters: "They have used the enormous power of the modern newspaper to perpetuate and disseminate a colossal impertinence, ... as professional gossips and tattlers."[40] In another letter, he had complained about how the "falsehoods daily spread before the people in our newspapers."

Elias Cornelius Benedict (one of the possible namesakes of eggs Benedict) was a wealthy banker and industrialist in New York City who was one of Cleveland's close friends and supporters. Benedict also happened to be a devoted yachtsman and the owner of a luxurious steam yacht, the *Oneida*. The vessel was usually anchored in New York when not under sail. Because it was not uncommon for Cleveland to visit Benedict and join him on the *Oneida* for fishing expeditions and socializing, it would not raise too much of suspicion if Cleveland were to be seen paying another visit to Benedict. Of course, having a team of surgeons onboard waiting for the president would be more difficult to explain.

The plot was to fake a fishing trip along the East Coast up to Cleveland's summer residence at Buzzards Bay. The surgery was planned to take place on July 1 in the yacht's saloon, which was converted into an "operating room."

Cleveland arrived in New York the day before surgery and boarded the vessel on the evening of June 30. Even the travel to New York was veiled in secrecy. The president's good friend Daniel Lamont, who had previously been Cleveland's private secretary but was now part of the cabinet as secretary of war, traveled with the president from Washington to Newark, New Jersey, in a private railroad car. Lamont had brought his wife and daughter along to make the travel look innocent in case they were spotted.[41]

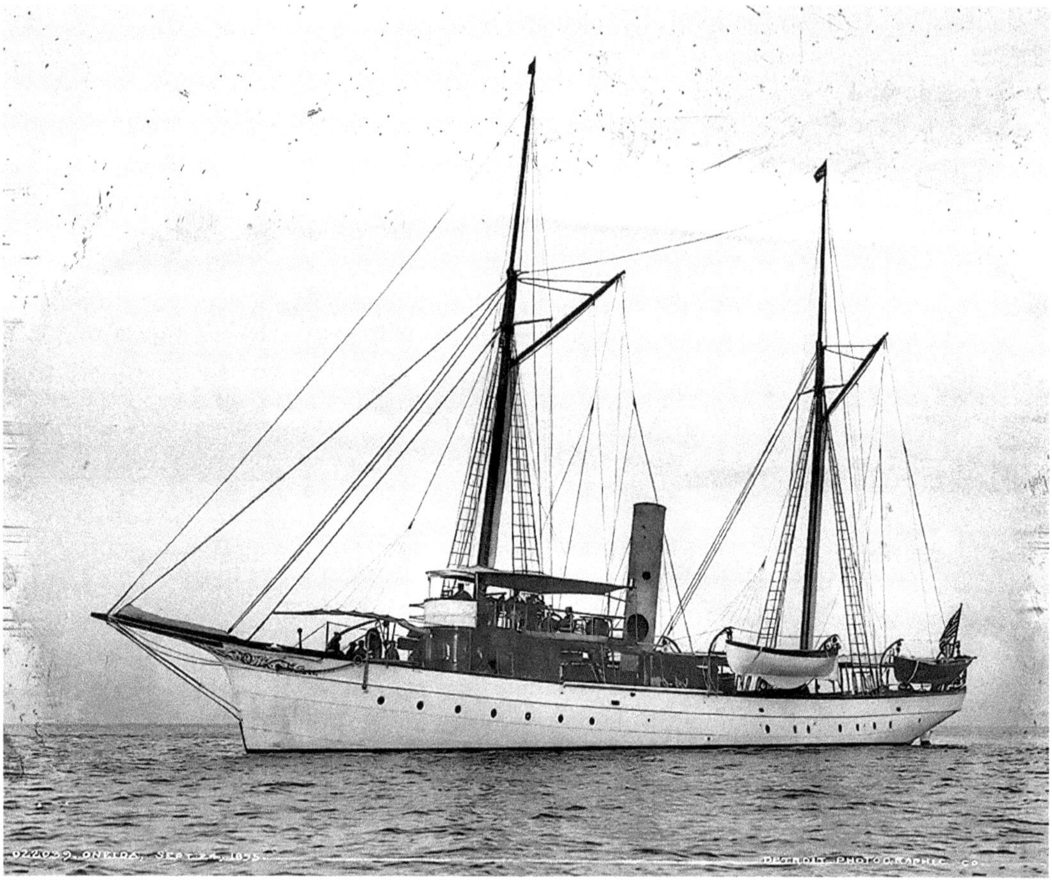

Cleveland's surgery took place on the yacht *Oneida* on July 1, 1893. The *Oneida* was one of the most spectacular yachts of the Gilded Age. It was fast and luxurious. Library of Congress, Prints and Photographs Division, Washington, D.C.

On the ferry crossing from New Jersey to New York, Cleveland was noted by a journalist from the *New York Times*. When asked what he was up to, the president evadingly answered, "It is a fact that I have … nothing to say for publication, except that I am going to Buzzards Bay for a rest."[42] This, of course, was the truth but not the whole truth.

When Cleveland boarded the *Oneida*, the team of doctors was hiding below deck. The ship crew had been told that the surgical team, also holding one dentist, had been assembled to work on an infected tooth in the president's mouth. When sailing out of New York Harbor, the yacht passed by Bellevue Hospital. This was a problem, because by now Cleveland was sitting on the deck enjoying his cigar and in conversation with the surgeons, some of whom actually worked at Bellevue. They had to quickly hide below deck in order not to be detected by colleagues looking out from the hospital.

Being safely out of the harbor and out of sight, Cleveland was brought to the "operating room" around noontime on Saturday, July 1. The *Oneida* was now proceeding through the calm waters of Long Island Sound. The team of doctors was ready and nervously awaiting the prominent patient.

The Medical Team

The group of six doctors assembled on the *Oneida* to operate on the president was impressive. The leader of the team, Dr. Joseph Bryant, the renowned surgeon from New York, had impressive credentials as an expert on oral cancers. Only three years prior, he had published an article in the prestigious *Annals of Surgery* titled "On Excision of the Superior Maxilla: A Study of Two Hundred and Fifty Cases."[43] The article described patients needing partial removal of the upper jaw because of cancer in the mouth. Two of the cases described by Bryant were his own patients. Bryant was indeed qualified to tackle the surgery that his president—and friend—needed.

The journal that Bryant had chosen for publication of his article is one of the oldest and most prestigious surgical journals in America. In his report, which had initially been read before the New York State Medical Society in February 1890, Bryant described 230 cases of removal of part of the maxilla (upper jaw) and 24 cases where parts of both the maxilla and mandible (lower jaw) had been removed. Bryant found it "proper to state" that the "two hundred and fifty cases"[44] indicated in the title of the paper were less than the 254 cases actually described in the article, but he did not explain why he had not given the correct account in the title (maybe he liked round figures).

Bryant had great respect for the procedure and commented that the removal of the superior maxilla put the surgery among the group of "formidable operations."[45] In addition to facial deformity and recurrence of the disease (if malignant), Bryant mentioned that "profuse" and "dangerous haemorrhage"[46] was among the immediate threats of the operation. He described various ways to prevent or stop hemorrhage, including local pressure, packing with "stryptic compresses,"[47] and ligation of the external—and even common—carotid artery. He felt that ligating the common carotid artery was too risky (he did not mention how many of the patients in whom it was done suffered a stroke) and referred to a quote by Professor Samuel Gross (famous surgeon in Philadelphia) who had stated, "I have never found it necessary in any of my operations upon the upper or lower jaws to secure the carotid artery as means of preventing haemorrhage. Indeed, one can be but surprised that such a procedure should ever have been recommended, much less employed by any sensible surgeon."[48]

Despite reporting a mortality rate of 14 percent after "removal of a single jaw" and despite classifying the procedure as a "formidable" operation, Bryant concluded at the end of his paper that removal of the superior maxilla "is not a dangerous operation." He even added that "excision of both superior maxillae is not a specially dangerous procedure." Bryant also explained that "ligature of one or both external carotids is a safe and commendable procedure when dangerous haemorrhage is apprehended as the result of operations" but repeated that "ligature of the *common* carotid ... is unwise, unsurgical and unwarrantable."[49]

Certainly, Bryant was well aware of the risks involved in the procedure he was planning for Cleveland and was prepared to ligate the president's external carotid if needed.

Dr. William Williams Keen of Philadelphia was another well-known and accomplished surgeon who contributed important expertise to the team. Keen was one of the most respected surgeons in the United States at the time and one of the pioneers in the field of neurosurgery. He had studied medicine at Jefferson Medical College in Philadelphia and remained faithful to his hometown throughout his professional life. Earlier, he had participated as a surgeon in the American Civil War and had coauthored a publication, "Gunshot Wounds and Other Injuries to Nerves." After having learned about the importance of antiseptic surgical techniques and listened to Joseph Lister, the "father" of antiseptic surgery, give a talk in Philadelphia in 1876, Keen had become one of the American forerunners of Lister's antiseptic practices. Important for the task that was awaiting him on the *Oneida,* Keen was also a leader in the field of cauterization of blood vessels with an electric device, a technique that was essential in neurosurgery but also became helpful during Cleveland's operation performed in a very vascular area of the body.

Anticipating the need to remove some of Cleveland's teeth to facilitate access to the tumor, Bryant had recruited a New York dentist, Dr. Ferdinand Hasbrouck, to participate. Importantly, Hasbrouck was also experienced in the use of nitrous oxide (laughing gas) during tooth extractions and other painful procedures. He understood that the nitrous oxide may not be sufficient to keep the president pain-free throughout the entire procedure, but he was prepared to use it at least during the initial phase of the surgery. Hasbrouck would become the source of the leak to the press that Cleveland had had surgery aboard the *Oneida.*

Dr. John Erdmann was the youngest surgeon on the team, only twenty-nine years old. He was brought aboard to assist Bryant. Erdmann was Bryant's favorite assistant in the operating rooms of Bellevue Hospital and would later become a renowned surgeon in his own right.

Dr. Edward Janeway was an additional accomplished New York physician and one of the most respected internists in the country. Like Bryant, Janeway was a professor at Bellevue. His main task was to monitor Cleveland's vital signs and general condition during and after the surgery.

We have already met Dr. Robert O'Reilly, Cleveland's White House physician who had been the first to investigate the president's tumor. O'Reilly was invited by Bryant to join the team of surgeons and would become important in administering ether anesthesia if Hasbrouck's nitrous oxide would be insufficient at keeping the president pain-free and still in the operating chair.

The Operation

Shortly after noon on July 1 Cleveland emerged from his cabin, where he had undressed down to his underwear. He made his way to the operating room, where he was positioned for surgery. At 12:32 p.m., Hasbrouck placed a mask across the president's face and began to administer nitrous oxide. When the patient appeared to be anesthetized enough, Hasbrouck grabbed his dental pliers and extracted two of the president's teeth from the left upper jaw. The bleeding that ensued was stopped by applying local pressure and cautery. O'Reilly reported that the pulse "remained first rate" and that the president appeared to have "no pain."[50]

At 12:47 p.m., cocaine was injected around the tumor as a local anesthetic but also to reduce blood flow to the area. More nitrous oxide was also administered. Bryant made an incision around the tumor to prepare for its removal. In order to achieve a radical removal of the cancer, surrounding tissue that was involved by the tumor, including parts of the hard palate and some of the upper jaw (maxilla), and three additional teeth had to be removed. This was when the operation entered "the more severe and bloody part," as Keen explained it.[51] Bryant understood that the nitrous oxide would not be sufficient to keep Cleveland pain-free and ordered O'Reilly to switch to ether for the duration of the operation.

At 1:14 p.m., Bryant started the actual removal of the tumor together with the nearby portions of the hard palate and a segment of the left maxilla with the three additional teeth. To accomplish this, the surgeon used "a surgical hammer, chisel, and bone-cutting instruments."[52] With the removal of a major part of the hard palate, the nasal cavity and maxillary sinus were entered. What Bryant saw at that point made him concerned; the presence of "a gelatinous mass" that he had to scoop out with a small spoon indicated that the president's tumor could be a myxosarcoma, a more aggressive type of cancer.

The surgery resulted in a large hole in the roof of the mouth that was packed with iodoform gauze to prevent infection.[53] The packing also helped stop the bleeding. The defect in the hard palate measured two and a half inches in length and almost one inch in width and resulted in a communication with the nasal cavity resembling what Keen described as "the worst imaginable case of cleft palate."

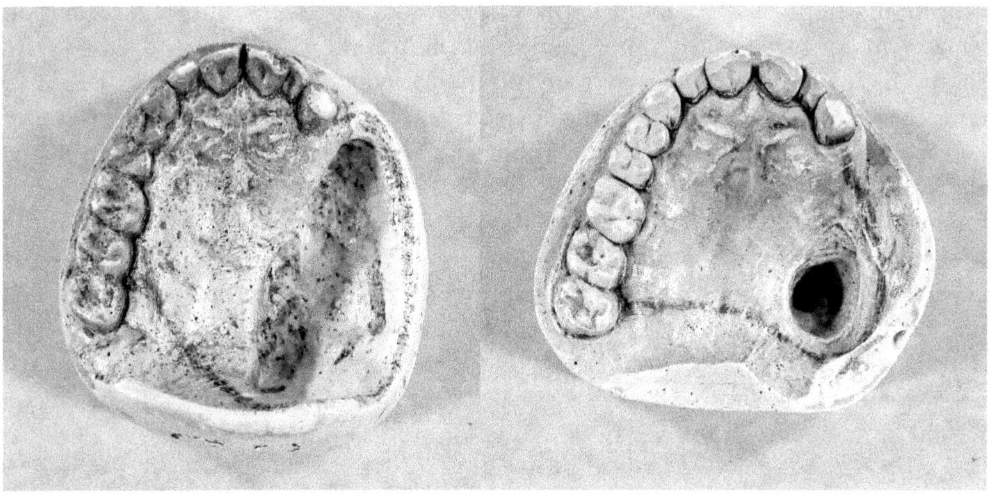

Casts of Cleveland's mouth used to make a rubber prosthesis to cover the defect in the roof of the mouth created by his surgery. The two casts were made with four years interval (1893 and 1897), and the picture illustrates the remarkable healing of the initial defect that measured 2.5 inch (6.35 cm) in length and 13⁄16 inch (2.06 cm) in width shortly after the surgery in 1893 (left panel) and 11⁄16 by 7⁄16 inch (1.75 by 1.11 cm) in 1897 (right panel). Courtesy New York Academy of Medicine Library.

At 1:55 p.m., almost an hour and a half after Hasbrouck had started to administer nitrous oxide, the surgery was over. By now, the surgeons had removed the tumor with a significant part of the hard palate and left upper jaw and a total of five teeth. At the end of the procedure, the patient's temperature was recorded at 100.8°F. The president had lost not more than six ounces of blood. All of this had been done without leaving any visible scars and with the president's mustache still in place!

Although similar surgeries had been performed many times before, as reported by Bryant already in 1890, the overwhelming seriousness of performing such a procedure under suboptimal conditions on the president of the United States and the potential consequences for the country, the president and his family and the surgeons and their future careers if something would go wrong weighed heavily on the doctors' shoulders. Keen would comment later in life that he had never felt "such a deep, almost overwhelming sense of responsibility as during that operation." He added that although the surgery "in itself was nothing as compared with many others I have done of greater difficulty and danger, but in its possible consequences for good or evil, none I ever was involved in could compare with it." He also commented, "What a sigh of intense relief we surgeons breathed when the patient was once more safe in bed can hardly be imagined."[54]

No wonder that the surgeons, when realizing the president had survived, went up on the deck for a meal and finished the evening with whiskey and cigars.[55]

After waking up from the ether anesthesia, Cleveland was carried back to his cabin for recovery. He was out of bed in the evening the following day, and on Monday he was "up and about," walking about the yacht.[56] Indeed a remarkable bouncing back after the major procedure in this high-risk patient!

A couple of weeks after the initial surgery, Bryant became concerned when he examined the president's mouth. The surgeon noticed that a "suspicious looking growth ... appeared at the inner margin of the wound which it was deemed wise should be removed for the sake of giving the patient the benefit of every doubt."[57] On July 17, Bryant reassembled the surgical team—with the notable exception of Hasbrouck—on the *Oneida*. It is possible that Hasbrouck was not included in the team this time because Bryant did not trust the dentist to be able to keep a secret after he had been suspected of being the person behind the leak resulting in the report by United Press on July 5. It is also possible that Hasbrouck was not invited because Bryant did not think nitrous oxide or removal of additional teeth would be needed. Although it is not exactly known what was done at the second surgery, Bryant removed "the suspicious appearing tissue and re-cauterized the entire surface of the wound with galvino-cautery."[58] Keen would later comment that "all suspicious tissue was removed."[59]

The Aftermath: Continued Secrecy

After the surgeries, the secrecy and deceptions continued, both short- and long-term.

To have the surgeons avoid detection, not only was the initial boarding of the

Oneida concealed, but getting off the ship also needed to be kept out of sight. To achieve that, the surgeons did not leave the vessel together as one group after the operation. On the day after the surgery, Hasbrouck disembarked early in the morning at New London, Connecticut, and not until the evening of July 4 did the remaining surgeons, with the exception of Bryant, get off at Sag Harbor, Long Island. Dr. Bryant stayed aboard the *Oneida,* accompanying the president to Buzzards Bay.

The reason Hasbrouck left the ship first may not only have been the need for secrecy. An additional rationale, perhaps even more important, was the fact that the dentist, who was in high demand, was scheduled to participate in a surgery in Greenwich on the day after Cleveland's procedure. Despite the planning, Hasbrouck was unable to make it back to the appointment in time. When he finally arrived, one day late, he was met by a surgeon "in a very angry frame of mind" who had been forced to cancel the procedure and send the patient home when Hasbrouck did not show up to administer anesthesia as planned.[60] When Hasbrouck was pressured by the surgeon to provide an explanation about why he had been delayed, he felt compelled to come up with a reason. What better excuse could he give than he had been on a ship pulling teeth out of the mouth of the president of the United States and providing laughing gas to the same illustrious patient undergoing surgery for cancer. Hasbrouck was hoping that the surgeon would be able to keep the secret, but the astounding information was soon leaked to other doctors. One of the doctors was a good friend of a newspaper man, Elisha Jay Edwards, and the stage was set for a sensational news leak.

The *Oneida* arrived at Buzzards Bay on the evening of July 5 and the late hour made it possible for Cleveland to get to his summerhouse without being spotted by the journalists who had started to assemble in the area to welcome him. The members of the press, most of them lodging at Walker's Hotel just a few minutes down the road from Gray Gables, had started to become suspicious about why it had taken Cleveland five days to reach Buzzards Bay from New York when about fifteen hours should have been enough. Lamont lied to the reporters and explained that the delay had happened because Cleveland and his company had "found good fishing grounds" on the way up from New York and that the president's health was "excellent except that he was suffering from a slight attack of rheumatism."[61]

Already on July 5, United Press had reported that the president had undergone surgery to remove a "malignant growth," a report that became widely spread and noticed and likely was based on Hasbrouck's failure to keep the secret.[62] On the afternoon of July 6, a journalist from United Press managed to corner Dr. Bryant to get an interview:

> United Press: Doctor, a number of conflicting stories are told concerning the illness of the president. Some of them make the matter very serious. You would confer a great favor by making some sort of official statement.
>
> Bryant: The president is all right.
>
> United Press: From what is he suffering?
>
> Bryant: He is suffering from rheumatism, just as was reported this afternoon. Those reports were correct.
>
> United Press: Then, Doctor, to report that he is suffering from a malignant or cancerous growth in the mouth and that an operation was necessary and had been performed to relieve it is not correct?

BRYANT: He is suffering from his teeth; that is all.
UNITED PRESS: Has an operation been performed?
BRYANT: That is all.[63]

The interview was reported in newspapers around the country the following day. The fact that Bryant had not fully denied that the president had undergone surgery fed speculations that the entire truth had not been spoken. Bryant stated that the news printed in the papers was false; he even denied ever having met the journalist from United Press, even less having given an interview. The disinformation from the president and his medical team managed to suppress the rumors about Cleveland's surgeries at least for the time being.

On August 29, however, the story resurfaced in a large front-page article published by the *Philadelphia Press* and authored by Elisha Jay Edwards, the *Press*'s New York correspondent. Edwards titled his piece "THE PRESIDENT A VERY SICK MAN. An Operation Performed on Him on Mr. Benedict's Yacht. PART OF THE JAW REMOVED." The newspaper correctly described the details of the operation (Edwards did not include details about the second operation, probably because he had no information about it) and listed some of the surgeons who were involved. The article, which was based on the information initially leaked by Hasbrouck to the angry surgeon in Greenwich, was considered "one of the greatest scoops in the history of American journalism."[64] It was immediately picked up by the wire services and transmitted to every major newspaper in the country and made headlines in local newspapers as well.

The piece by Edwards created not only a sensation but also bitter animosity. The facts, of course, were denied by the doctors involved (except Hasbrouck), the president, Lamont, and Benedict. The story was also vilified by the Philadelphia newspaper mogul Alexander McClure of the *Philadelphia Times*. McClure, a friend and supporter of Cleveland, did not spare his venom directed at the Philadelphia *Press* and in particular at Edwards, who was accused of being a "Panic-Monger" and messenger of "conscienceless sensationalism" and "deliberate falsity."[65]

The President's Recovery

Although Cleveland's recuperation from his surgery aboard the *Oneida* was remarkable, the recovery was not without struggle. Two weeks into the convalescence, Attorney General Richard Olney (later secretary of state) finally managed to get in to see the president. He urgently needed to discuss with Cleveland the upcoming message to the special session of Congress scheduled for early August. Olney described his encounter with the president:

> After a fortnight more or less during which I made frequent attempts to see Mr. Cleveland, I succeeded in having an interview. He had changed a great deal in appearance, lost a great deal of flesh, and his mouth was so stuffed with antiseptic wads that he could hardly articulate. The first utterance that I understood was something like this: "My God, Olney, they nearly killed me." He did not talk much, was very much depressed, and at the time acted, and I believe he felt, as if he did not expect to recover. He was very depressed about the progress he was making and complained that his mind would not work."[66]

Despite Cleveland's struggle, his condition improved gradually over the next couple of months. In August he was again able to participate in political activities, and his speech was starting to get back to almost normal with the help of the rubber prosthesis to cover the hole in the hard palate. The prosthesis was engineered by Dr. Kasson Gibson, an expert dentist and prosthodontist in New York. On September 5, Cleveland was so well recovered that he was able to give a talk at the opening of the Pan-American Medical Congress in Washington, D.C., with a voice that was "clearer and more easily understood than it had been since the surgery."[67] Two weeks later, Cleveland gave a speech at the opening of the centennial of the founding of the nation's capital. In October, Cleveland's dentist was able to replace the initial prosthesis covering the hole in the palate with a permanent prosthesis of hard rubber that Cleveland wore the rest of his life.[68]

Leaving the White House and Retiring in Princeton

Indeed, Cleveland's appearance and behavior were getting so close to normal that the story about his surgery was almost forgotten. The secrecy about what had happened aboard the *Oneida* in July 1893 was maintained for decades.

When Cleveland left the White House for the second (and final) time in 1897, he retired to his estate, Westland Mansion, in Princeton, New Jersey.[69] He finally got more time to spend with his family. He stayed active outside his home by engaging himself as a trustee at Princeton University. Always outspoken, he could not help himself from getting involved in the political debates in the country and voice his opinions, which were sometimes controversial. For example, he let people know what he thought about giving women the right to vote. In an article written for *Ladies Home Journal,* he was blunt in his opposition to the women's suffrage fight: "Sensible and responsible women do not want to vote," and he even told his readers that to deny women the right to vote was of divine origin. "The relative positions to be assumed by men and women in the working out of our civilization were assigned long ago by a higher intelligence."[70] Not surprisingly, his article created significant backlash, and numerous women canceled their subscriptions to the magazine.

In 1904, tragedy struck. Grover and France's eldest daughter, Ruth, died from diphtheria at the age of twelve. The grief was deep, and the thought of Ruth now lying cold in the ground was unbearable to Cleveland. Three days after her death, Cleveland lamented, "I had a season of great trouble of keeping out of my mind the idea that Ruth was in the cold, cheerless grave instead of in the arms of her Saviour."[71]

Toward the end of 1907, Cleveland's health started to deteriorate. He died on June 24 the following year, aged seventy-one. The cause of death was officially listed as "heart failure complicated with pulmonary thrombosis and edema."[72] With Frances at his side, the former president's last words were "I have tried so hard to do right."[73]

It would be almost a decade before the interest for Cleveland's operation aboard the *Oneida* resurfaced. The renewed interest was prompted by an article written by one of the surgeons who had participated in the operation.

Dr. Keen's Article about the Secret Surgery

On September 22, 1917, the weekly journal *Saturday Evening Post* published a three-page article titled "The Surgical Operations on President Cleveland in 1893" and credited to "W.W. Keen, M.D., LL.D., Emeritus Professor of Surgery, Jefferson Medical College, Philadelphia."[74] The article was republished later the same year as a sixty-two–page book.[75] The article described in detail what had happened during Cleveland's surgeries. At this time Keen and Erdmann were the only surviving members of the presidential surgical team, and Keen saw it as his obligation to let the nation know the details of the story before it was too late. The article also offered an opportunity to vindicate Edwards, the journalist, who had been harassed in the press and by people close to Cleveland and labeled a "Fakir," an epithet that was associated with him for years. Before submitting the article, Keen had asked for permission by Cleveland's widow to publish the piece.

The same year, Keen presented to the Mutter Museum in Philadelphia the remains of Cleveland's tumor together with surgical instruments used during the procedure. The surgical specimen had up until then been kept in a glass jar by Gibson, the dentist who designed the prostheses for Cleveland's mouth. Keen also donated a scrapbook containing his personal notes about the surgeries. Interestingly, the secrecy continued for another fifty years, and not until 1967 did the museum allow an outside expert to review Keen's notebook. That review revealed that in 1893, surgeons and pathologists had lengthy discussions about the character of Cleveland's tumor and expressed different opinions about whether it was malignant. It would be another eight years before a panel of outside expert pathologists were allowed to examine the surgical specimen from Cleveland's operation. Historians have suggested that one reason the museum and the Cleveland family were reluctant to allow pathological examination of the surgical specimen was that the investigation would end up showing that the tumor had been caused by syphilis (which turned out not to be the case).[76]

The panel, led by the pathologists Horatio Enterline and John S.J. Brooks, concluded that there was "no evidence that the lesion was carcinosarcoma, mixed tumor or cancer, nor was there anything to support Dr. Keen's interpretation of myxosarcoma," a highly malignant cancer suspected by Keen when he encountered mucinous substance in the maxillary sinus (antrum) during the president's surgery. Instead, the panel felt convinced that Cleveland's tumor was a "verrucous carcinoma."[77]

The pathological diagnosis of verrucous carcinoma had not been reported at the time of Cleveland's surgery. A detailed description of the disease was published by the pathologist Lauren V. Ackerman in 1948.[78] Although Ackerman's account is often quoted in writings about Cleveland's tumor as the original description of verrucous carcinoma of the mouth, Ackerman pointed out that almost identical findings had been published seven years earlier by Friedell and Rosenthal.[79] In both reports, tobacco chewing was considered the most important factor in the etiology of the tumor.

When Cleveland discovered the rough spot on the roof of his mouth, he was younger (fifty-six years old) than most of the thirty-one patients reported by

Ackerman. The majority of his patients were "rather aged" men with a mean age of sixty-seven, and only one patient was younger than fifty-seven.

In his report, Ackerman pointed out that verrucous carcinoma, even when extensive, has an excellent prognosis "with proper treatment." Because the tumor can quickly become attached to and invade surrounding bony structures, such as the mandible, the maxilla, and the hard palate, "radical surgery" with removal of parts of affected bones may be necessary to provide adequate treatment. In light of Ackerman's report, it is probably not fair to imply that Cleveland's surgery was "too radical," as has been suggested.[80] It may also not be justified to suggest that the president's long survival, seemingly without evidence of recurrent disease, would support the suspicion that the surgeons involved in Cleveland's operation tried to cover up a mistake of removing a benign tumor by overly aggressive surgery. As mentioned, Ackerman pointed out that the tumor had an excellent prognosis even when advanced, provided "proper treatment" was provided.

The secrecy surrounding Cleveland's surgery therefore was more likely politically motivated rather than a conspiracy among the surgeons.

CHAPTER FIVE

William McKinley

Brought to the Wrong Hospital, Got the Wrong Operation, by the Wrong Surgeon

THE TWENTY-FIFTH PRESIDENT

March 4, 1897–September 14, 1901

William McKinley was only six months into his second term as chief executive when he became the third president to be shot and killed, not a very proud record for a country that was still young. It was only thirty-six years after Abraham Lincoln's assassination, and many still remembered when their twentieth president, James Garfield, died with a bullet lodged in his body in 1881, only four months into his presidency.

William McKinley

Born in the town of Niles, Ohio, 1843, McKinley would ultimately become the fifth of seven presidents originating in the midwestern state. He grew up in a religious home of strict Methodist beliefs and remained a lifelong devout member of the Methodist Church.

Some of the groundwork of McKinley's political career was laid during the American Civil War. He joined the fight against the states in the South at the onset of the conflict.

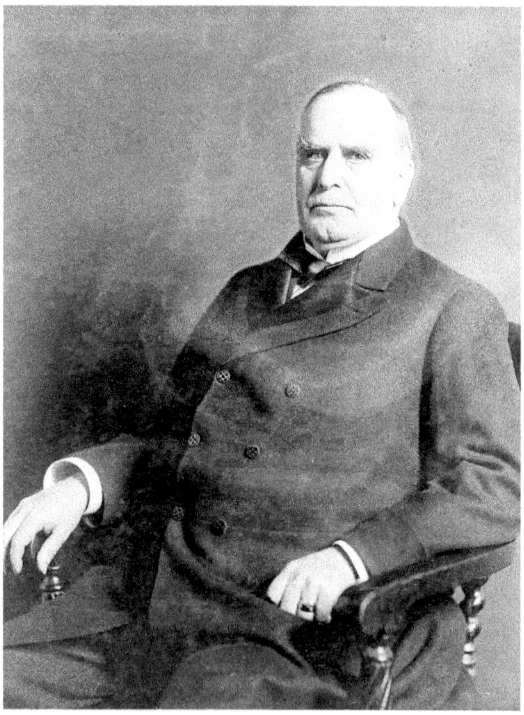

Portrait of William McKinley. Library of Congress, Prints and Photographs Division, Washington, D.C.

During the war, he became a close friend of future president Rutherford B. Hayes, a friendship that would last until Hayes's death in 1893. Before his presidency, Hayes, another Ohioan, had served as governor of his state twice.

Hayes became not only a friend of McKinley, almost twenty years younger, but also his mentor, and Hayes's support would play a big role in McKinley's political life. Like Hayes, McKinley served as governor of Ohio before ascending to president of the United States in 1897.

McKinley was a popular president. One of his biographers even thought that McKinley "died the most beloved president in history."[1] During his first term, McKinley was a strong advocate for the gold standard and for tariffs. Foreign policy was also high on the agenda. He was forced to devote much time and energy to the Spanish-American War of 1898 that erupted after the battleship USS *Maine* was blown to pieces in Havana Harbor, killing more than 260 of its crew. One of McKinley's slogans during the campaign of 1896 was "Prosperity at Home, Prestige Abroad."[2] McKinley's reelection in 1900 was an easy win, with 291 to 155 in the electorate college and about 52 percent of the popular vote.[3]

Even though McKinley's political life was successful and happy, his private life had a sorrowful side of illness and death. McKinley married Ida Saxton in January 1871. Ida was an Ohio girl from Canton, the daughter of a wealthy local banker. The McKinleys had their first child, Katherine, on Christmas day 1871. A second daughter, named Ida after her mother, was born in 1873. Sadly, little Ida died the same year. This tragedy sent Mrs. McKinley into a deep depression that would get even worse when Katherine succumbed to typhoid fever in 1875, only four years old. McKinley's wife never recovered from her children's death, and when she developed epilepsy around the same time, she became dependent on her husband's constant support and help through the remainder of their marriage.

Despite her frail condition, Ida frequently followed her husband on political tours and other travels. When, after his second inauguration on March 4, 1901, the president went on a victory lap, he was accompanied by Ida. The couple traveled mainly by train, and the journey took them through the South to the Southwest with plans to extend the travel up the coast of California and to finally go back east to arrive at the Pan-American Exposition in Buffalo on June 13.[4] Plans, however, had to be changed when Mrs. McKinley fell ill on the West Coast. The president had to cancel several public events and speeches and the visit to the Exposition had to be postponed almost three months.

It would not be until early September that the president and his wife arrived at Buffalo. After leaving Canton, Ohio, on the morning of September 4, their train pulled into the railroad terminal at the Nickel City on the evening of the same day. The arrival at Buffalo turned out to be triumphant. Large crowds had gathered to greet their president, and "factory whistles blew, brass bands played and cannons boomed."[5] Mrs. McKinley, epileptic and frail, became nervous from all the commotion, and the president decided to retire as soon as possible to their retreat at the home of their host, John Milburn, a well-known lawyer in town and the president of the Exposition.

After a night's rest, the following day, Thursday September 5, was going to be even more glorious. It was labeled the President's Day, giving McKinley an opportunity to give a speech at the fairgrounds in front of fifty thousand cheering spectators, during which he laid out the plans for his second term.[6] Much of the speech was centered around reciprocal tariffs and treaties. The address would be the president's last public oration.

Friday, September 6, was scheduled for more relaxed activities. In the morning, the president, his wife, and their entourage traveled the short distance to Niagara Falls for sightseeing. Lunch was enjoyed at the International Hotel at the falls,[7] and the return trip to Buffalo was on a special train, arriving at the exposition at 3:30 p.m. It was now only about forty minutes before McKinley would be fatally shot.

The Pan-American Exposition of 1901

The world's fair of 1901 opened on May 1 and remained open for the next six months. The Pan-American Exposition, as the world's fair was called this year, had initially been planned for Cayuga Island at Niagara Falls, but the Spanish-American War of 1898 forced a postponement of the event. When plans were reactivated, nearby Buffalo was the successful bidder.

Initially, the number of visitors to the exposition was lower than hoped for, mainly because of a rainy and cold start to the summer.[8] As time went on the audience grew, and with events such as the president's visit in early September, the numbers steadily improved. When all was said and done, a total of eight million people had visited the fairgrounds, and with a price of fifty cents for a ticket (approximately $30 in today's money),[9] the Exposition generated a revenue of about $240 million.

The Pan-American Exposition, like other world's fairs, was designed to showcase modern inventions and progress in society. When McKinley gave a speech on September 5, he began by stating that "Expositions are the timekeepers of progress. They record the world's advancement."[10] Three attractions that garnered great interest during the fair were an X-ray machine, the thousands of light bulbs that illuminated the fairgrounds, and the Temple of Music, all with relevance for the aftermath of the shooting of McKinley. A prototype "electric ambulance" and an emergency hospital constructed on the premises would also play important roles in the story told here.

Despite the fact that the X-ray machine might have become useful in the search for the bullet that killed the president, the machine was not brought into action. Doctors at the time were not yet acquainted with the use of X-ray and were not convinced of its benefits. After all, this was the same year Wilhelm Conrad Röntgen was awarded the first Nobel Prize in Physics for his discovery of X-ray, and it would be some time before the novelty became generally accepted as a tool in medicine.

The massive number of light bulbs used to illuminate the exposition was made possible by the advent of alternating current for power transmission. With the emphasis on electricity and the centerpiece of the exposition being the Electric Tower, Thomas Edison's name loomed large over the fair. Edison was also busy

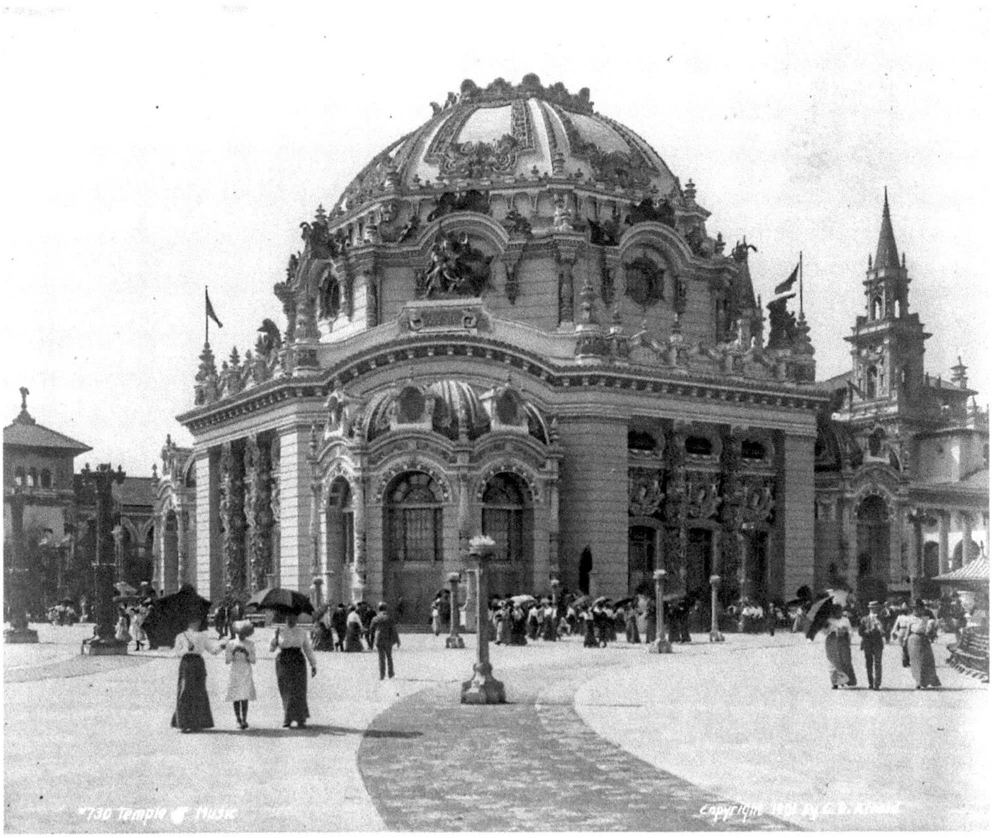

The Temple of Music was considered the most beautiful building at the Pan-American Exposition of 1901 and was the site of many live performances of various styles of music. It would become the place for President McKinley's assassination. Library of Congress, Prints and Photographs Division, Washington, D.C.

filming many of the events during the exposition, including McKinley's arrival at the Temple of Music on the fateful afternoon of September 6.

Ironically, despite the excessive number of electric lights at the exposition, no lights were available in the operating room of the emergency hospital when McKinley was brought there for surgery after being shot.

The Temple of Music hosted many live performances of various styles of music and was one of the most popular buildings of the exposition. The Temple of Music accommodated one of the largest pipe organs in the country. An audience of two thousand people could also enjoy the prominent use of interior electric lighting. Sadly, the site would also become the place for the president's assassination.

The Assassination of President McKinley

The Temple of Music was chosen as the place where McKinley would shake hands with a long line of admirers. The president's private secretary, George Cortelyou, was not happy with the location or any other site; fearing for the safety of the president, Cortelyou wanted the entire event canceled. There had been rumors about anarchist plots to kill McKinley already when King Umberto I of Italy was assassinated by an agitator in July 1900, but a warning issued at that time by New York City police lieutenant Joseph Petrosino had been ignored.[11] The jitter increased when Louis Babcock, the grand marshal of the exposition, overheard someone making a joke at lunch in a restaurant at the fair that the president might be killed during the reception at the Temple of Music.

Cortelyou pleaded several times with the president to change his schedule, but McKinley did not want to listen. "Why should I? No one would wish to hurt me."[12] Cortelyou tried to rationalize his arguments by pointing out that there may be people who would get mad because they did not reach the end of the line to shake the president's hand. But McKinley did not budge. "Well, they'll know I tried, anyhow."[13]

When getting toward the end of McKinley's excursion to Niagara Falls on September 6 and when Cortelyou realized he would not be able to stop the president from going through with his "favorite part of the job," he sent a telegram to Buffalo urging the authorities to provide extra security for the president.[14] Finally, McKinley at least agreed to cut down on the event, limiting the reception to ten minutes.

The Temple of Music was one of the most beautiful buildings of the Pan-American Exposition, considered one of the architectural features of the fair. There were additional reasons why the construction was considered ideal for the presidential reception on Friday afternoon, September 6. The hall was large, and when seats were removed from the floor, a wide aisle could be created for the line of well-wishers. The structure had doorways on all sides, making it possible to have a fast flow of people entering on one side and quickly exiting on the other side after shaking hands with the president. There was room for beautiful plants to be placed around the president, adding to the alluring sight. And of course, majestic music from that huge organ would give additional glory to the occasion.

Although the level of security would ultimately turn out to be insufficient, extra measures had indeed been taken, at least in part thanks to Cortelyou's telegram. Constables from the exposition police and officers from the Buffalo police force were protecting the doors, and detectives had been called in to guard the aisle. Louis Babcock had assigned artillerymen to be at the reception dressed up in uniforms to keep an eye on the line of people queuing to greet the president and stop anyone who might be suspicious-looking. The artillerymen, despite being impressive in their uniforms, had no police training and made no attempts to prevent the assassin-to-be, Leon Czolgosz, from getting close to the president.

When McKinley had arrived, punctually at 4 p.m., and taken up his position in the front of the hall, the pipe organ blasted out "The Star-Spangled Banner." The president signaled that the doors could be opened, and lines formed in the aisle. Cortelyou was visibly nervous and kept looking at his watch. Babcock moved toward the doors and waited for Cortelyou's order to close them.[15] The organist was now playing music by Johann Sebastian Bach, and Cortelyou couldn't wait for the time to be 4:10 p.m. and have the event concluded.

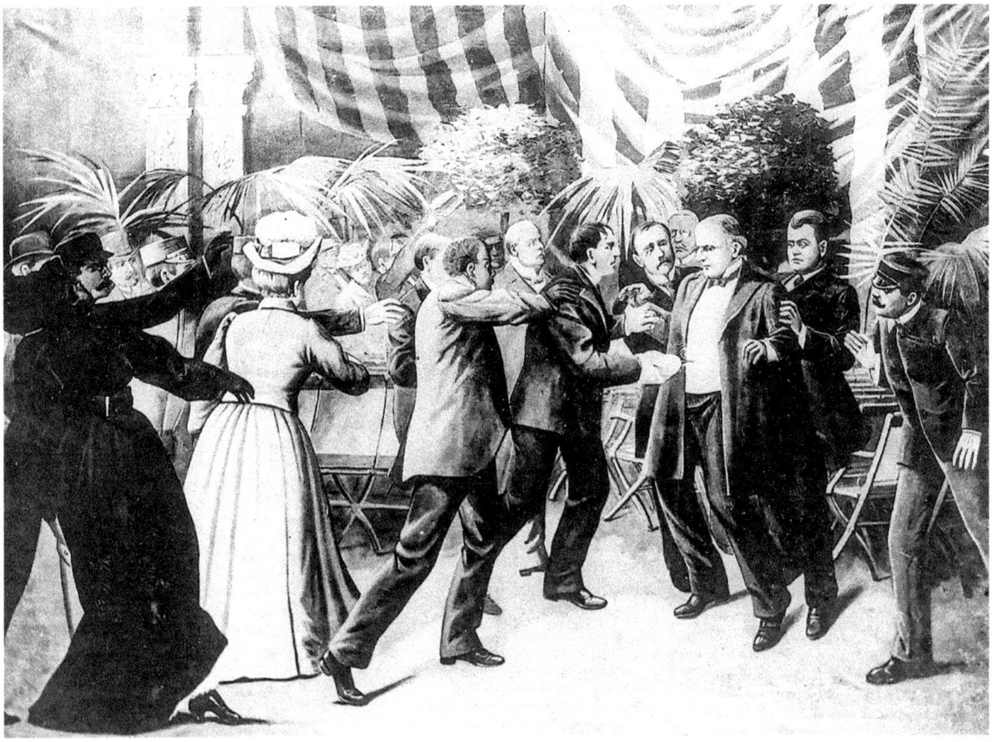

The shooting of President McKinley at the Temple of Music at 4:07 p.m. on September 6, 1901. A tabloid illustration by T. Dart Walker. Library of Congress, Prints and Photographs Division.

When Czolgosz finally reached the end of the line, only three minutes remained of the reception. Having his right hand covered by a white handkerchief did not raise suspicions. The day was hot, and people were using handkerchiefs to wipe sweat from their faces. Of course, Czolgosz's handkerchief had another purpose. The president might have thought that Czolgosz was injured and reached for his left hand. That's when two shots rang out and the music stopped.

Within seconds, people behind Czolgosz realized what had happened and threw him to the floor. He was disarmed and received heavy beatings from fists and the artillerymen's rifle butts. One of the shots had been deflected by a button in McKinley's coat and had just grazed the president's skin. The other bullet, however, had entered McKinley's abdomen. The president initially did not understand that he had been seriously injured, but when blood started to stain his white vest, he and people standing close by realized the gravity of the situation. When the president started to stagger to his right, he was caught by Cortelyou and helped to a chair. Within minutes, McKinley was carried out on a stretcher to the electric ambulance that had immediately been summoned to the Temple of Music.

On the way out, the president saw Czolgosz being attacked by angry bystanders and police. He told them, "Don't let them hurt him."[16] He also instructed Cortelyou, "My wife—be careful, Cortelyou how you tell her—oh, be careful."[17]

The president was loaded onto the prototype electricity-powered ambulance

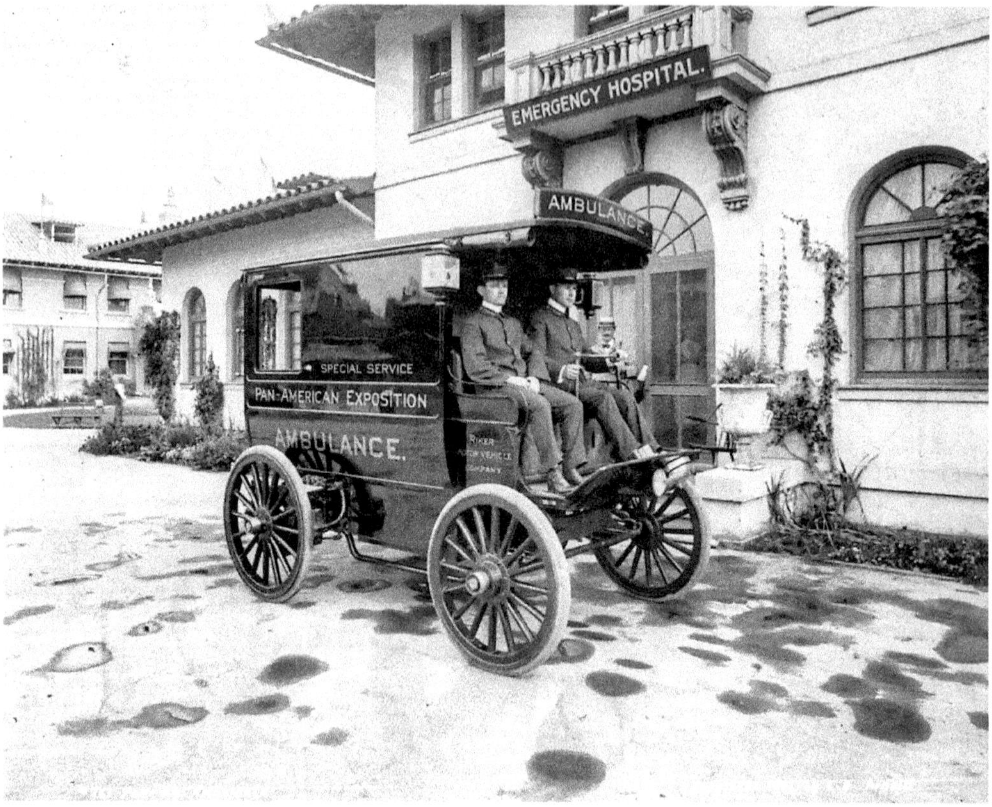

The prototype electric ambulance exhibited at the Pan-American Exposition of 1901. Library of Congress, Prints and Photographs Division, Washington, D.C.

displayed at the fair and rushed to the Exposition emergency hospital, where he arrived at 4:18 p.m. "Dr. G. McK. Hall [a local physician] and Mr. Edward C. Mann, medical student, of the house staff, were in charge of the ambulance, medical student T.F. Ellis being the driver."[18]

The Surgery

When McKinley arrived at the Exposition hospital, nurses immediately scrambled to set up the operating room and commenced a frantic search for doctors. One of the most famous physicians in Buffalo at the time was Dr. Roswell Park. He was an expert surgeon and had experience with trauma and abdominal gunshot wounds. In addition, he was the medical director of the Exposition and would have been the obvious choice if surgery would be needed. Unfortunately, however, he was out of town performing an operation in a hospital at Niagara Falls.

The first surgeon to arrive at the Exposition hospital was Dr. Herman Mynter, an experienced abdominal surgeon. Mynter, who had emigrated from his native Denmark in the 1870s, was a professor of surgery at Niagara University. When he arrived at the hospital at 4:45 p.m., he immediately examined the president, who by now had been stripped of his clothes and placed on a table in the operating room. Mynter quickly decided that an operation would be needed and promptly informed McKinley about the recommendation. The president recalled that he had briefly met with Mynter the day before and commented, "Doctor, when I met you yesterday, I did not imagine that today I should have to ask a favor of you."[19] Dr. Mynter was soon joined by several other surgeons, including Dr. John Parmenter, a general surgeon and professor of anatomy and clinical surgery at the Buffalo Medical College; Dr. Wallace Lee, a surgeon from St. Lois who happened to be visiting the exposition on the day when McKinley was shot; and Dr. Matthew Mann, an eminent gynecologist at Buffalo General Hospital and a professor of gynecology at the Buffalo Medical College. Mann was fifty-six years old at the time and was described as being "at the height of his career."[20] He was the father of one of the medical students who had transported the president to the Exposition hospital in the electric ambulance.

Although an accomplished surgeon, Mann did not have any expertise in upper abdominal surgery and had no previous experience with abdominal gunshot wounds. Despite these shortcomings, it was decided that he would be in charge of the operation, assisted by Mynter, Parmenter, and Lee. Dr. Eugene Wasdin, an abdominal surgeon with the United States Marine Hospital Service, would be in charge of the anesthesia. The surgical team was also joined by seven nurses and by McKinley's personal physician, Dr. Presley Marion Rixey, "a peppery, bushy-mustached naval surgeon from Virginia."[21]

When McKinley had his clothes removed, a bullet fell from his garments. This was the ball that had been deflected by a button and "had merely grazed the skin between the second and third ribs."[22] The second bullet, however, was more of a threat. It had caused a wound in the upper abdominal wall five centimeters to the left of the midline below the edge of the ribs; the surgeons were concerned that it may have entered the abdomen, a concern that was confirmed when the wound was probed and found to "extend deeply into the abdominal walls [*sic*]," with the direction being "somewhat downward and outward."[23]

With the president now undressed and placed on the operating table and with surgeons having been assembled, the induction of anesthesia was commenced at 5:20 p.m. The president was put to sleep by Dr. Wasdin with ether dropped on a piece of gauze placed on a mask over his nose. "President McKinley took the ether well, and was entirely under its influence in 9 minutes after the beginning of the anesthetization,"[24]

The surgeons prepared their hands and arms by scrubbing them with soap and water and immersing them in a solution of mercury bichloride. Rubber gloves were not routinely used by surgeons at the time, and the operation would be performed with bare hands. While the surgeons were scrubbing, the patient's abdomen was shaved and cleaned with green soap followed by alcohol, ether, and mercury bichloride.

At 5:29 p.m., one hour and twenty-two minutes after the president was shot, Dr. Mann began the operation by making an approximately ten-centimeter vertical incision in the abdominal wall, starting at the edge of the ribs and extending downward just past the bullet wound. When the skin was opened, a small piece of clothing, most likely from the president's coat, was found in the tract created by the slug. After the layers of the abdominal wall had been cut through, it was confirmed that the bullet had indeed penetrated the peritoneum and entered the abdominal cavity. The incision was extended to allow for a more thorough exploration. This revealed that the ball had perforated the anterior (front) wall of the stomach and traversed the stomach to exit through the posterior (back) wall, creating a hole there as well. Both wounds were closed with double layers of fine black silk sutures.

In an attempt to find the bullet, Mann then explored (using his fingers to feel around) the space behind the stomach, an area where the pancreas is located. A bullet could not be easily identified, and when the surgeon continued the exploration by introducing "his arm so as to palpate carefully all the deep structures behind the stomach, ... no trace of the bullet ... could be found."[25] Digging deeper had "a bad influence on the President's pulse,"[26] so the surgical team decided to end the operation. After irrigating the abdomen with warm saline solution and debriding (removing with the knife) injured tissue surrounding the bullet track, the layers of the abdominal wall were closed with sutures. Before the skin was closed, the wound was irrigated with hydrogen dioxide and covered with antiseptic powder to reduce the risk of wound infection.[27]

At the end of the operation, the surgeons discussed whether the area behind the stomach should be "drained" by inserting a device that could lead contaminated fluids out of the abdomen, thereby reducing the risk for infection. Dr. Mynter argued for the placement of a drain but was overruled by the other surgeons. Even Dr. Park, who had now arrived from Niagara Falls, did not advocate a drain. The omission of a drain would become an important point when the surgeons' performance was later criticized. Some of the doctors, including Dr. Park, would regret the decision not to use a drain.[28]

The operation lasted "one hour and 31 minutes."[29] The surgeons concluded that "the President bore the operation very well." After he had been awakened from anesthesia, the president was brought to the Milburn home and was carried in from the ambulance on a stretcher to "a room in the northwest corner of the house, where a hospital bed had been prepared for him."[30]

The surgeons were disappointed that they had not been able to find the bullet and speculated that it may have traveled deeper than they could feel and had been lodged close to one of the back muscles. The operation had been made difficult by a number of adverse circumstances, one of them being the president's body habitus. He was not only a big person but was also obese; when Mann later commented on the surgery, he mentioned that "the greatest difficulty was the great size of President McKinley's abdomen,"[31] with thick layers of fat in both the abdominal wall and inside the abdomen. "The omentum (a structure containing fatty tissue and covering the intestines) was enormously thickened with fat and very rigid." Mann also reported that he had found "the stout President's abdomen so protuberant that he was operating at the darkened end 'of a big hole.'"[32]

Another circumstance that made the operation challenging was the lack of adequate surgical instruments, in particular retractors. At the time, it was common that surgeons brought their own instruments to the operating room. On that fateful day of September 6, 1901, Park had left his private set of surgical instruments in an anteroom at the Exposition hospital before taking off to Niagara Falls but had forgotten to inform nurses and medical students staffing the hospital. When Mann recalled the events, he complained that he had not been informed what he was "wanted for" and therefore had arrived at the emergency hospital "entirely unprepared."[33] He was grateful that Dr. Mynter had his large pocket case with him, "the contents of which were of great use."[34]

The lack of sufficient lighting in the operating room was a big problem. Although a multitude of electrical lights had been installed all over the Exposition, none had been placed at the hospital. When the sun started to set, this problem grew even worse. Dr. Rixey "gave very efficient service by guiding the rays of the sun to the seat of the operation by aid of a hand-mirror and later by arranging an electric light."[35] Later, people asked why the president had not been brought to the newly built Buffalo General Hospital, where a larger and better-equipped surgical amphitheater was available. Although Park had earlier performed a successful appendectomy in the operating room of the exposition hospital,[36] McKinley might have been better served by having his surgery in a bigger operating room with efficient lighting and other equipment.

Finally, the unavailability of Dr. Park, arguably the most qualified surgeon to take care of the wounded president, was a factor that may have contributed to the unfortunate outcome of the event. The multiple problems associated with McKinley's surgery have led some writers to comment that "the President was brought to the wrong hospital, got the wrong operation, by the wrong surgeon."[37]

The Postoperative Course

Even though the Milburn family probably felt honored to host the president in their home after the operation, it would not take long before they realized that doing so turned into a spectacle. The Milburn home was immediately surrounded by a horde of journalists, and a special tent was erected nearby where the reporters could write their stories. The house was encircled by throngs of well-wishing (and gawking) people who eagerly awaited the daily briefings given by the president's doctors on the steps of the Milburn house. In order to give the patient some peace and quiet, nearby streets were cordoned off, and soldiers were stationed across the street to prevent disturbances. The home was wired, connecting it with the White House, and there was a steady stream of cabinet members and other dignitaries who had rushed to Buffalo when they heard about the shots fired at the president. McKinley's chef and house servants, who had served the president and his wife when traveling to the Exposition, were brought from the private Pullman car parked at the railroad station to help provide food for the visitors.

In the first encounter with the press, McKinley's doctors painted an optimistic picture and let the reporters know that "the condition at present justifies recovery."[38] However, they also wanted to be cautious and added, "The result cannot be foretold." The first several days after the shooting and operation seemed to support the initial upbeat view, with the physicians letting people know that the president was recovering at a favorable pace. The doctors, however, were worried about a persistently increased heart rate and elevated temperature, and on Tuesday the week after the event, the superficial part of the wound had to be opened and drained of an infection. "In the evening the dressings were examined, and as there was considerable staining from the discharge, it was thought best to remove 4 stitches and separate the edges of the wound."[39]

The local surgeons wanted to get reassurance from outside expertise and asked Dr. Charles McBurney of New York to come and see the patient. McBurney was a world-renowned surgeon who is best remembered for his work on the diagnosis and treatment of acute appendicitis. He identified an area in the right lower quadrant of the abdominal wall that is particularly tender in patients with this disease. The tenderness at "McBurney's point" remains well known by medical students and surgeons all over the world as an important finding in patients with appendicitis.

When McBurney came to see the president, he felt that the patient was doing very well and had nothing but praise for his colleagues in Buffalo. McBurney called the operation a showcase of "the epoch of the century in surgery."[40] He even predicted that McKinley would be able to return to the White House in a couple of days. Feeling reassured by McBurney's positive assessment, Vice President Theodore Roosevelt, who had hurried to the president's side after the shooting, decided to board a train and leave for vacation in the Adirondack Mountains.

During the first several postoperative days, fluids and calories were provided to the president by "nutritive" enemas consisting of saline solutions, whiskey, and eggs.[41] He also received small doses of morphine for pain relief and digitalis for his heart. A couple of days after the surgery, the patient also started to take fluids by mouth and seemed to tolerate that well. When the president was allowed chicken broth, a small piece of toast, and a cup of coffee,[42] he was happy and called the meal a "luxurious luncheon."[43]

Oh the morning of Thursday, September 12, the sixth postoperative day, McKinley looked and felt quite good, and his doctors commented that "the President now seemed at his best and his condition to warrant the favorable prognosis given out."[44] To emphasize how optimistic they felt, they added, "The time for peritonitis and sepsis had passed.... His spirits were good and his mind clear." McBurney also felt happy with the president's condition and did not feel that he was needed any longer. He left Buffalo in the morning, "having arranged to return at once if his presence was desired."[45]

Sadly, the rosy picture was about to change dramatically. It was only a couple of hours after McBurney left that "it was noticed that the character of the pulse was not quite so good."[46] The fever returned and kept rising, and McKinley could no longer tolerate fluids by mouth. In the early morning hours of Friday, September 13, a new bulletin was issued by the doctors: "The President's condition is very serious, and gives rise to the gravest apprehension," and it was noticed that his "pulse [was] growing weaker."[47] McKinley became increasingly drowsy and restless. By 6:30 p.m. that day, a bulletin was issued stating that "the President's condition is most serious in spite of vigorous stimulation," and a couple of hours later it was commented that "the President continued to sink, becoming weaker and weaker."[48] The bulletin ended by ominously adding that "the end is only a question of time."[49] Even McKinley himself understood that he was going to die, and at some point during the evening he whispered, "It is useless, gentlemen. I think we ought to have a prayer."[50] Ida sobbed over her husband: "I want to go, too. I want to go, too."[51]

The president died in the wee hours of Saturday, September 14, eight days after being shot.

The Postmortem

An autopsy was performed the morning after McKinley's death by Dr. Harvey R. Gaylord, "pathologist to the New York State Pathological Laboratory."[52] The room used for the procedure was small and crowded, with at least ten people present.[53] In addition to the pathologist, several surgeons, including Dr. Wasdin, who had participated in the operation, and Dr. Park, were present.

During the autopsy, the damages caused by the bullet were documented. The main finding was the result of the injury to the pancreas with "the apparent pancreatic necrosis being the most significant pathologic finding contributing to the death."[54] The pathologist pointed out in his report that although "the extensive necrosis of the pancreas would seem to be an important factor in the cause of death ... it has never been definitively shown how much destruction of this organ is necessary to produce death."[55] Other injuries along the tract of the bullet were also noticed, including injuries to the upper portion of the left kidney and the adrenal gland.[56] When the bullet tract was followed, it ended blindly behind the left part of the colon at one of the back muscles. Although this suggested that the bullet might have been lodged in or close to the muscle, it could not be found despite vigorous attempts. The president's obesity made the search for the slug "extremely difficult."[57] Because of the difficulties, "the autopsy continued for a longer period than was anticipated by those who had charge of the President's body, and we were requested to desist seeking for the bullet and terminate the autopsy."[58] When the autopsy was stopped, the doctors had to give up their attempts to find the bullet and argued "that nothing could be gained by locating the bullet," and the "search for it was discontinued."[59] If the procedure would have been allowed to continue longer, it is possible that the X-ray machine that was displayed at the Exposition could have been helpful. This may have diverted some of the criticism the doctors were subjected to for not finding the bullet even at the autopsy.[60]

To the relief of the surgeons present during the autopsy, both holes in the stomach repaired during the operation had remained closed; the wound on the anterior wall was "held intact by silk sutures," and the same was true for the wound on the posterior wall of the stomach.[61] Despite that, however, the tissue surrounding the gastric wounds showed "complete necrosis."[62] The autopsy findings were summarized as follows: "Anatomic Diagnosis.—Gunshot wound of both walls of the stomach and the superior aspect of the left kidney; extensive necrosis of the substance of the pancreas; necrosis of the gastric wall in the neighborhood of both wounds."[63]

The physicians involved in the surgical care of McKinley had remained united in their comments when critique of their management of the president had started to surface, in particular related to the omission of placing a drain when ending the operation. After the president's death, however, differences in opinion started to surface. Park at one point commented that the decision not to drain was "probably unfortunate,"[64] despite the fact that at the time of surgery he had not been pushing for it. Some disagreements regarding the findings at the autopsy also emerged. For example, Wasdin voiced the opinion that only a "poison-tipped bullet" could have resulted in the "massive necrosis" found at the postmortem.[65] At the time, it was not unheard of that anarchists used poison in their murderous attacks, but no evidence was found that Czolgosz's bullets had been poisoned.

How People Reacted to the Assassination

News about the attack on President McKinley spread quickly in the afternoon of the shooting, and it did not take long before most visitors to the Exposition had heard about the event. When people realized that the injured president had been brought to the Exposition hospital, they rushed there to try to find out what was happening. As the afternoon turned into evening, the crowds kept growing. The public was in shock over the event and succumbed to quiet and nervous waiting. When they finally saw the president being transported away in the electric ambulance, still alive, the masses slowly started to dissipate.

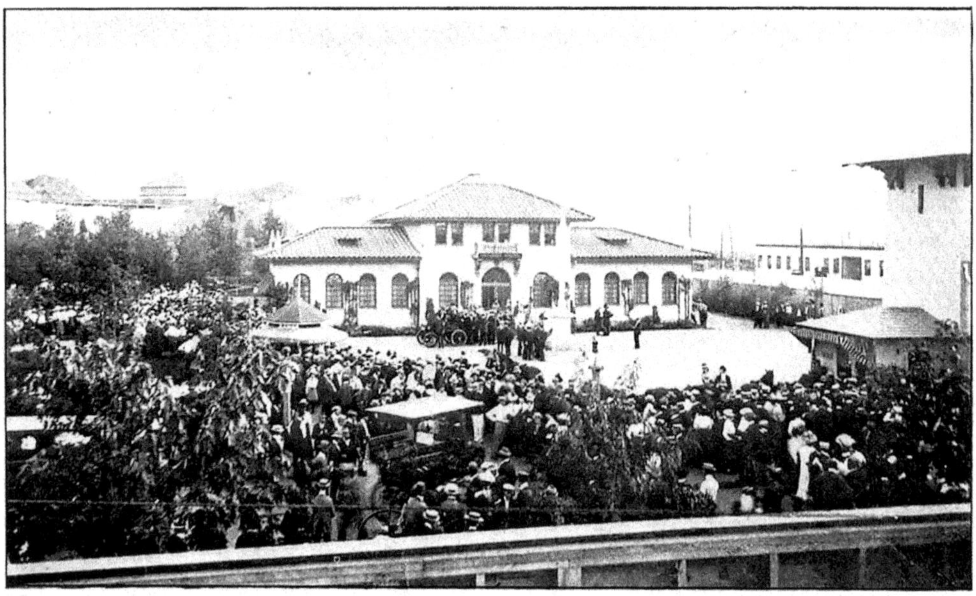

THE EMERGENCY HOSPITAL AT THE PAN-AMERICAN EXPOSITION
MULTITUDE WAITING IN SUSPENSE DURING THE SURGICAL OPERATION JUST AFTER THE FATAL SHOOTING.

Crowds gathering at the emergency hospital when President McKinley underwent surgery after he was shot on September 6, 1901. The Buffalo Pan-American Exposition of 1901 website. Collection: Pan-American Exposition of 1901/Emergency Hospital.

PRESIDENT M'KINLEY IS SHOT TWICE, BUT HIS LIFE MAY BE SAVED

Bright Hopes For His Recovery Lighten The Gloom Of An Awful Tragedy At The Buffalo Exposition.

THE ASSAILANT WAS LEON CZOLGOSZ, AN ANARCHIST

A Murderous Attack While The Chief Executive Was Holding A Reception In Temple Of Music---One Bullet Produced A Light Wound, But Other Passed Through Stomach And Has Not Been Extracted.

The news about the president's shooting spread like wildfire across the country. Depicted here is a headline from the *Baltimore Sun*, Saturday, September 7, 1901.

Not surprisingly, the news about the shooting of McKinley quickly spread beyond the Exposition in the media. On Saturday morning, big headlines were on the front pages of newspapers all over the country. The name of the perpetrator was known immediately, and the fact that he was an anarchist was trumpeted out. Despite having received two shots, the initial reporting on McKinley's condition was hopeful. The developments over the next week were widely covered by the press, and when the president's condition worsened, everybody was pausing. The ultimate outcome was mourned by the whole nation.

The Doctors Wanted to Be Paid

The surgeons taking care of McKinley after the shooting showed some less agreeable character after the events. Mann, in particular, lost some of the public respect when he became greedy. He argued that government officials, rather than members of the McKinley family, had retained the surgeons to perform the operation. The government, of course, would be able to pay higher fees than the president's rather modest estate. In his requests for payment, Mann added that "the dignity of the medical profession demands that Congress pay their bill, and that the services should be handsomely rewarded."[66] Although the surgeons were accused of being avaricious, Congress agreed to allocate enough money to pay Mann $10,000 (equivalent to $330,762 in 2022), Mynter $6,000, and Park and McBurney $5,000 each.

Who Was Leon Czolgosz?

Leon Czolgosz was born in 1873 into a family of immigrants from Eastern Europe. He grew up in Michigan but moved to Pennsylvania for work in a glass factory when he was in his midteens. At age seventeen he moved to Cleveland, Ohio, for a new job at the Cleveland Rolling Mill Company.

The economic crash of 1893 resulted in unrest in both the labor market and society as a whole. The crash created a fertile ground for socialism and, in its extreme, anarchism. When the Rolling Mill Company closed and later tried to reopen with reduced wages, a strike broke out and became violent. Czolgosz was convinced that there was something wrong in society and blamed the economic and social turmoil on inequality, allowing the wealthy to get rich on the backs of the poor. He joined socialist clubs and organizations.

When Czolgosz heard about the assassination of King Umberto I of Italy by the anarchist Gaetano Bresci in July 1900, he was intrigued by the tumultuous events and wanted to get involved in the anarchism movement. He was inspired by the American anarchist Emma Goldman when he heard her give a lecture in Cleveland in May 1901. After the speech, Czolgosz asked Goldman for reading suggestions. A couple of months later he again met Goldman, this time in Chicago in the home of Abraham Isaak, publisher of the liberal newspaper *Free Society.* Goldman introduced Czolgosz to several of her anarchist friends,[67] but because of Czolgosz's odd social behavior and his expressed curiosity about secret societies around Isaak and his friends, suspicions started to grow about Czolgosz.

After some time, there was outright fear among the anarchists that Czolgosz was a spy infiltrating the movement. In early September 1901, an article in *Free Society* warned the readers about Czolgosz:

> ATTENTION! The attention of the comrades is called to another spy. He is well dressed, of medium height, rather narrow shoulders, blond and about 25 years of age. Up to the present he has made his appearance in Chicago and Cleveland. In the former place he remained but a short time, while in Cleveland he disappeared when the comrades had confirmed themselves of his identity and were of the point of exposing him. His demeanor is of the usual sort, pretending to be greatly interested in the cause, asking for names or soliciting aid for acts of contemplated violence. If this same individual makes his appearance elsewhere the comrades are warned in advance, and can act accordingly.[68]

When Czolgosz heard about McKinley's plans to visit the Pan-American Exposition in early September 1901, he decided it was time to act. Czolgosz traveled to Buffalo on August 31 and purchased a .32-caliber Iver Johnson revolver.[69] On September 6, he joined the line approaching McKinley in the Temple of Music, not to shake the president's hand as the others where there do to but instead to kill him.

Caught in the act, Czolgosz was wrestled to the floor by angry spectators and police and was immediately arrested. He was ultimately brought to a cell at Auburn

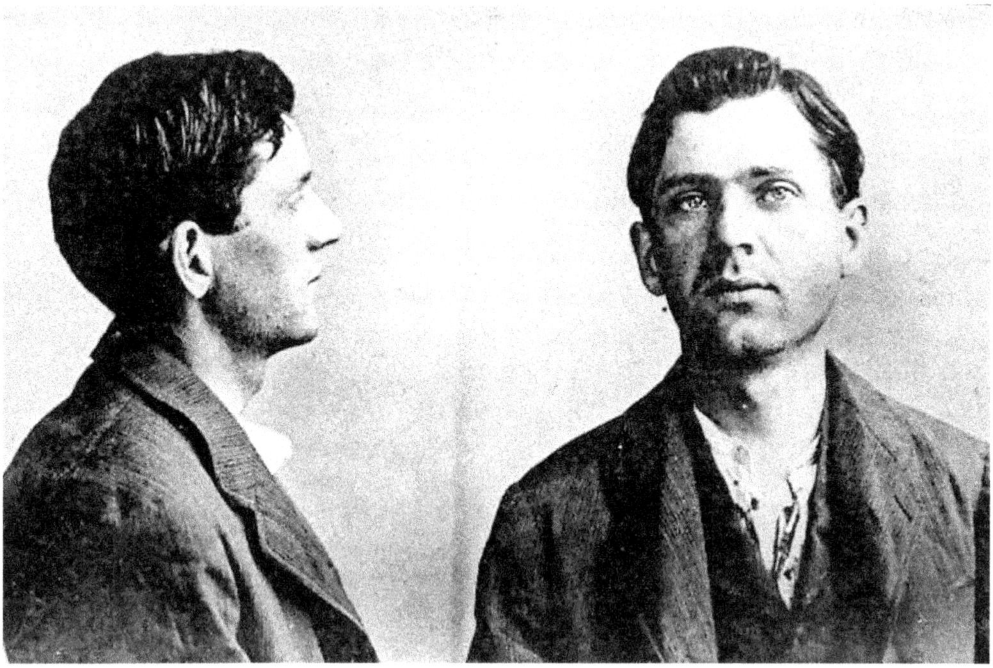

A mug shot of President McKinley's assassin, Leon Czolgosz. Alamy Stock Photo/History and Art Collection.

Prison and indicted with one count of first-degree murder. After Czolgosz's killing of McKinley, whom Goldman described as the "president of the money kings and trust magnates," she remained steadfast in her belief in Czolgosz and even compared him to Marcus Brutus, the hero assassin of Julius Caesar.[70]

During the entire pretrial period, Czolgosz refused to cooperate with the public defenders appointed to assist him. The trial began nine days after McKinley died, with the proceedings taking place at the state courthouse in Buffalo. At the trial, which was described as "quick, swift, and fair,"[71] Czolgosz was found guilty and condemned to execution in the electric chair.

Even after receiving his death sentence, Czolgosz remained combative. On the night before the execution, he was visited by two clergymen but refused to talk with them and sent them away. Later in the evening, Czolgosz's brother came to visit and asked, "Who got you into this scrape?" Czolgosz's answer was "No one. Nobody had anything to do with it but me." The brother and a brother-in-law kept pleading with Czolgosz and asked if they should call back the priests, to which Czolgosz replied, "No, fuck them; don't send them here again I don't want them." And then he added, "Don't you have any praying over me when I'm dead, I don't want it. I don't want none of their damn religion."[72] Czolgosz remained unrepentant until the bitter end. His last words before being electrocuted were "I killed the President because he was the enemy of the good people—the good working people. I am not sorry for my crime."[73]

Czolgosz died in the electric chair at Auburn Prison on the morning of October 29, 1901. In order to prevent fellow anarchists from making a hero and martyr of him, his body was completely disfigured by sulfuric acid poured into his coffin, and his clothes and other possessions were burned in the prison incinerator.

Anarchism, Gaetano Bresci, and Emma Goldman

Because Czolgosz saw himself as an anarchist and admired members of the movement, some of the features of anarchism, in particular the global involvement of anarchists at the time of McKinley, are briefly reviewed here.

The word "anarchism" originates from the ancient Greek term *anarkhia*, meaning "without a ruler," and is composed of the prefix *an-* ("without") and the word *arkhos* ("leader" or "ruler").[74] The term "anarchism" commonly describes the antiauthoritarian wing of socialism emerging from Far Left politics.[75] The movement has often been violent and has played important roles in revolutions, including the Russian Revolution and the Spanish Civil War. During the French Revolution, political opponents accused the revolutionaries of creating a society characterized by "laws that are not carried into effect, authorities without force and despised, crime unpunished, property attacked, the safety of the individual violated, the morality of the people corrupted, no constitution, no government, no justice, there are features of *anarchy*."[76]

Anarchism has had a strong foothold in Europe for centuries. The movement early developed different flavors in different countries. In the mid–1600s, the English activist Gerrard Winstanley propagated a philosophy that became important among anarchists: power corrupts, property is incompatible with freedom, and only in a society without rulers can men be free and happy.

Modern anarchism had its roots in the Enlightenment and in national uprisings taking place from the 1700s to the mid–1800s. Anarchism grew strong and was influenced by activists such as Pierre-Joseph Proudhon in France, Mikhail Bakunin and Peter Kropotkin in Russia, and Giuseppe Fanelli and Errico Malatesta in Italy. Although there were differences among the anarchists in different countries, they all subscribed to the rejection of government and political authority. Some were more violent than others and wanted terrorism to sweep away all existing institutions.

From the mid–1800s to the early decades of the 1900s, "classical anarchism" saw a shift toward more militant behavior by its members, with sabotage and terrorism becoming threats to society. During this era, political assassinations became part of the tactics. Between 1890 and 1901 several rulers lost their lives in such attacks, including the Spanish prime minister Antonio Cánovas, President Sadi Carnot of France, Empress Elizabeth of Austria, and (as we have seen) King Umberto I of Italy and President McKinley of the United States. No wonder anarchists were viewed by many as "mindless destroyer(s)."[77]

There were two people in particular who stimulated Czolgosz's fascination with anarchism. Like Czolgosz, both had European roots, one in Italy and the other in Lithuania, part of Russia at the time.

Gaetano Bresci was born in Prato, Tuscany, Italy, in 1869. As a young man, he worked as a weaver and became sympathetic to the anarchism movement because of the poverty and social injustices he saw around him. Bresci immigrated to America in 1897 and ultimately settled in New Jersey. There, he became involved in the local trade unions and started to attend meetings held by Italian immigrant anarchists.

In 1898, widespread demonstrations took place in Italy because of food shortage and exploding prices of grain. In May of that year Milan saw violent riots, with mobs roaming the streets in protest of the government's policies. The riots were struck down by the military under the command of General Fiorenzo Bava Beccaris. The military response to the riots was brutal, resulting in the death of at least eighty (and perhaps as many as three hundred to four hundred) demonstrators and scores of wounded. The streets of Milan were filled with blood from dying and wounded angry rioters. The event soon became known as the Bava Beccaris Massacre, and news about the bloodshed spread rapidly around the world. The overreaction by the armed forces resulted in bitter hatred of the Italian government, the military, and King Umberto I.

When Bresci heard about the massacre, he was outraged and swore revenge against the "murderer king."[78] Bresci bought a .38-caliber revolver and a one-way ticket to Italy and told his wife that he was returning to Italy to "take care of family business."[79] He was back in his hometown of Prato in June 1900 and the next month found his way to the town of Monza, where the king was scheduled to attend a sports event to hand out medals to athletes. However, on the day of the king's engagement, July 29, Umberto did not make it to the stadium where the sportsmen were to be celebrated. On his way there, throngs of people lined the streets to cheer on the king. Bresci was in the crowd and managed to get close to the monarch. He pulled out his revolver and shot the king dead at point-blank range.

Bresci was promptly arrested, convicted of murder, and sentenced to life in prison.[80] Less than a year later, the assassin was found hanging by the neck in his cell. Although the circumstances around Bresci's death seemed suspicious to some, his death most likely was the result of suicide.

The other anarchist who would influence the life of Czolgosz was Emma Goldman, one of the most well-known anarchists in American history. Not only was Czolgosz influenced by Goldman, but her life would be affected by Czolgosz as well.

Emma Goldman was born on June 27, 1869, in Kovno, Lithuania (part of the Russian Empire at the time).[81] Her family and upbringing were Orthodox Jewish. Emma had a rough and unhappy childhood, with a father who often used corporal punishment of his children when they dared to disobey. He did not hesitate to use a whip on the most obstinate of the youngsters, Emma.

Emma had two half sisters, Helena, born in 1860, and Lena, born in 1862. Their mother, Taube Bienowitch, had remarried when her first husband died from tuberculosis. Her second husband, Abraham Goldman, fathered four children with Taube. Emma was the first to arrive in the new family, followed by three brothers. When Abraham brought out the whip, Emma received little solace from her mother. Instead, her oldest half sister was the comforter and became the only true source of love and happiness when Emma was growing up. When Emma later reflected on her childhood, she commented that Helena provided "whatever joy it had."[82]

Emma's father was not only physically abusive but psychologically cruel as well.

When the family moved to St. Petersburg they lived through tough economic times, in part caused by Abraham's failed business adventures. The children had to quit school and work to help out with the finances. Emma ended up working in a corset shop. When she asked her father for permission to return to school, he became angry and threw her French textbook into the fire and yelled at her: "Girls do not have to learn much! All a Jewish daughter needs to know is how to prepare gefilte fish, cut noodles fine, and give the man plenty of children."[83] This mean streak of Abraham came through again when Emma asked to be allowed to accompany Helena to America to live with Lena and her husband in Rochester, New York. Abraham refused, and even when Helena offered to pay for Emma's ticket, he did not budge. Not until Emma threatened to throw herself into the Neva River did her father finally give his permission.

Helena and Emma arrived at New York City on December 29, 1885. They traveled to Rochester and moved in with Lena and her husband. This was the beginning of Emma's thirty-four tumultuous years in America, in the middle of which her life would be touched by Czolgosz and his assassination of President McKinley.

In Rochester, Emma found employment as a seamstress. She was paid two and a half dollars a week, and when she asked for a raise, her employer refused. Emma left in anger and found another job nearby. The experience rekindled her feelings against the injustice she felt workers were being subjected to, something she had also lived through in Russia.

After two years in the Flour City, she married a coworker with whom she shared interests in books, dancing, and traveling but not much else. The marriage did not turn out to be a success; he was a jealous and suspicious character, and the fact that on their wedding night Emma found out that he was impotent did not help. The couple were divorced after less than a year.

Emma's family did not approve on her divorce and considered her a "loose" woman. They shut the door and did not let her back in their home. As the independent and resolute woman she was, she took her sewing machine in one hand and a bag containing five dollars in the other and headed south to New York City.[84]

It did not take long for Emma to make connections with radicals in New York. Soon after her arrival she met with Alexander Berkman, a prominent anarchist. They developed a relationship that would last for decades. Their alliance was not only built around anarchism but included romance as well. Tragedy would also enter their lives, and Emma's love would eventually be betrayed.

Political activism would lead Goldman and Berkman to get involved in the Homestead Strike of 1892 at a steel plant in Pennsylvania. The plant was owned by Andrew Carnegie and managed by Henry Clay Frick. When negotiations between the Carnegie Steel Company and the labor union broke down, the plant was closed, and the workers were locked out. The workers went on strike, and when violence erupted between steel union workers and company guards, a twelve-hour gunfight resulted in the death of seven guards and nine strikers.

Frick hated the union and became a target for the Left's outrage after the violent events at Homestead. Goldman and Berkman decided to kill Frick to "strike terror into the soul of his class" and "bring the teachings of Anarchism before the world."[85]

Berkman was to perform "the deed," while Emma was charged with preparing the propaganda defending their act.

On July 23, Berkman, carrying a gun and a knife, managed to force his way into Frick's office. He shot Frick three times and sliced his leg with the knife. Frick somehow survived his injuries, and far from Goldman's and Berkman's predictions that they would be joined by angry workers, a group of workers got hold of Berkman and beat him up. Berkman was arrested, convicted of attempted murder, and sentenced to twenty-two years in prison (he was released after fourteen years).

The years that Berkman spent in jail were long and lonely for Goldman. She missed him and at times suffered depression. During the Panic of 1893, she became involved in hunger demonstrations that sometimes turned into riots. Her activities landed her in jail for a year. During this time Goldman decided to study midwifery, and once out of jail, she spent several years dividing her time between giving political lectures and delivering babies.

In 1901, Goldman met Czolgosz on at least two occasions. We have already learned about her brief encounter with him after a talk she gave in Cleveland and when he tracked her down to Isaak's house in Chicago.

After McKinley's assassination, the police had strong suspicions that Goldman and other anarchists had been involved in the plot. The authorities were looking for Goldman and found her at the Isaak house in Chicago. She was arrested together with Isaak and several other anarchists, but no evidence was found that Goldman had been involved in McKinley's murder, and she was released after two weeks of interrogations. After the shooting of McKinley, Goldman even offered to provide nursing care to the president, an offer that was turned down. Commenting on the mortally injured president, she mentioned that he is "merely a human being."[86]

Anarchism was at a low point in people's eyes in the aftermath of McKinley's murder. Czolgosz was hated and vilified by most Americans, even anarchists. In contrast, Goldman remained a steadfast supporter of Czolgosz up to the time of his execution. She was disappointed with many of her fellow anarchists and felt that they had abandoned a "supersensitive being."[87] Because of her support of the president's killer, Goldman became the object of hatred in the press, where, among other things, she was labeled the "high priestess of anarchy."[88]

The execution of Czolgosz weighed heavy on Goldman. She withdrew from public life and from many of her friends. For a decade, she lived an isolated life in an apartment in New York. She continued to be held in contempt by fellow anarchists was harassed in the newspapers, and she was missing Berkman. In her memoirs, she lamented this period of her life and wrote, "It was bitter and hard to face."[89] She was depressed, added another name (Smith) to her real name, and supported herself with various jobs as a private nurse.

Berkman was released from jail eight years ahead of the twenty-two years he had been sentenced to. When Goldman, with roses in hand, met him after his release in May 1906, she was shocked to find how much he had changed during his time in prison. He had lost weight and was pale and looked distraught. She later commented that she was "seized by terror and pity" when she saw him.[90]

Berkman felt lost when reentering the world outside the prison walls. He was so distressed that he contemplated taking his own life; he even bought a gun for that purpose but did not follow through. Instead, he regained his footing and together with Goldman started to plan for renewed anarchist activities.

Only one year after Berkman's release from prison, Goldman was hit by a painful experience. Her lover betrayed her with a fifteen-year-old fellow anarchist named Becky Edelsohn (who later created headlines as a hunger striker). Despite this event, Goldman continued to work with Berkman in the anarchism movement for another decade (although the romance was now gone). In 1917, with the United States engaged in World War I, Goldman and Berkman were again in trouble with the law; they were arrested for inducing people to resist military conscription and were sentenced to two years in prison.

Soon after their release, they were again arrested. Based on the Anarchist Exclusion Act, they were sentenced to deportation from the United States. On December 21, 1919, Goldman and more than 240 additional activists (including Berkman) were deported to the Soviet Union aboard USS *Buford*, nicknamed in the press "the Soviet Ark." The deportation took place almost to the day thirty-four years after Goldman's arrival at New York from St. Petersburg.

It did not take long before Goldman found herself disillusioned by the Soviet regime. In December 1921 she left the Soviet Union and spent the rest of her remaining nineteen years in Europe and Canada. She died on May 14, 1940, at the age of seventy after having suffered a major stoke in February of the same year.

Although Czolgosz committed the murder of President McKinley without the involvement of anybody else, there is no doubt that his thinking was influenced by two of the most influential anarchists of the time.

Theodore Roosevelt and the Assassination of McKinley

One person who was especially affected by the shooting of President McKinley was his vice president. When Theodore Roosevelt heard about the assault, he had a hard time believing it. His initial reaction was "stunned amazement," and when lamenting the event to his fellow Republican Henry Cabot Lodge, he said that the report seemed "literally incredible."[91] Roosevelt developed his thoughts further and commented to Lodge, "You and I have lived too long … to be astounded at ordinary folly or ordinary wickedness." He then went on to say that "it did not seem possible that just at this time in just this country, and in the case of this particular president, any human being could be so infamous a scoundrel, so crazy a fool as to attempt to assassinate him."[92]

Initially Roosevelt reflected on the sensitivity of the situation, being next in line if McKinley died, and pondered the options of not going to Buffalo immediately, risking to appear "callous and indifferent" or "to fly there too fast" and risk giving "the impression of unseemly ambition."[93] However, he did not hesitate long before doing what he judged to be the "natural thing." He swiftly commandeered a train and rushed to the president's bedside.

When the vice president arrived, McKinley had already undergone surgery, and although the bullet had not been found, his condition looked favorable. When McKinley's condition continued to improve and the doctors were pleased with the situation, Roosevelt decided on September 10 to leave Buffalo and did so "with a light heart."[94] He headed north to join his wife, Edith, and their children for vacation in the Adirondacks.

The weather was rainy and misty, but true to his character, that would not stop Roosevelt from enjoying his outdoors vacation in the mountains. On September 12 Roosevelt, accompanied by Edith and the children, set out on a hike aiming for the top of Mount Marcy at an elevation of 5,300 feet. The climb was difficult and was slowed by the rain and muddy trails. The party spent the night in cabins beside a small lake below the mountain peak. When they woke up the next morning, the rain kept pouring down. This, of course, would not discourage Roosevelt, but Edith and the children had had enough and decided to call it quits and returned down the slopes to the base camp at the Tahawus Club. Roosevelt and the rest of the party resumed the climb. They reached the top of the mountain at midday. Although the sun was now breaking through, they were freezing and wet from rain and sweat and decided to head down the mountain to break for lunch. While they were eating they suddenly saw a man coming out of the woods; he was bringing a telegram from McKinley's secretary, Cortelyou. The message was "The President's condition has changed for the worse."[95]

Roosevelt and his group at once headed down to the Tahawus Club to rejoin Edith and the children. When they reached the camp around six o'clock in the evening, no further messages had arrived from Buffalo. This made Roosevelt feel somewhat more relaxed, and he sat down for dinner with the family. Within a couple of hours, however, bad news arrived; the president's condition was getting worse and was now critical. In the middle of the night Roosevelt took off, heading for the nearest railroad station at North Creek. The morning sun was just about to rise when he reached the train station, where a special train had arrived to pick him up. He was informed that McKinley had died early in the morning.

Roosevelt's daughter Alice was seventeen years old when the family was camping in the Adirondacks. When she understood that McKinley had died and her father was about to be president, she was asked by journalists how she felt about it. She was proud and happy for her father but did not admit it publicly; to honor McKinley she "put on a sorrowful face," but as soon as the reporters had left, she "performed a joyous jig."[96]

Racing through the morning hours, Roosevelt reached Buffalo at 1:30 p.m. on September 14. McKinley had now been dead for almost twelve hours. Roosevelt took the oath of office from a local judge to become the twenty-sixth president of the United States.

Chapter Six

Franklin D. Roosevelt

Did He Have Surgery for Malignant Melanoma?

The Thirty-Second President

March 4, 1933–April 12, 1945

It has been said about Franklin Delano Roosevelt that "in spite of his splendid physical appearance, he was always getting sick."[1] Many of his early health problems, however, were mild and easily overcome. This would all change in the late summer of 1921.

Roosevelt's Paralytic Illness: Disability and Deception

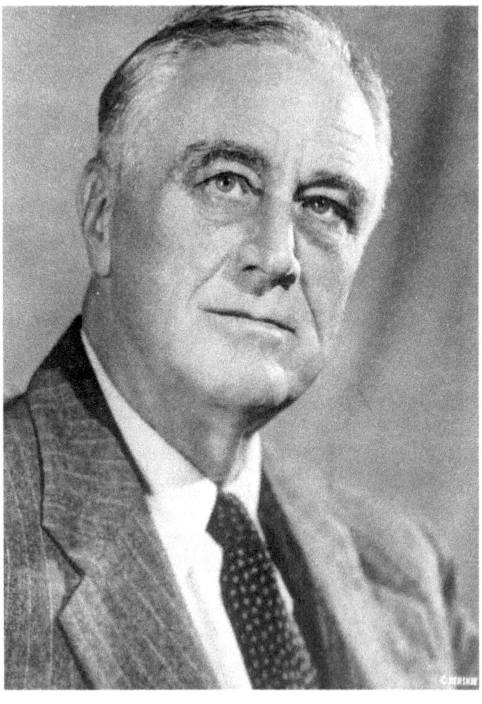

Franklin D. Roosevelt. Collection: FDR Photos, Franklin D. Roosevelt Library Photographs.

In August 1921 Roosevelt arrived at Campobello, a beautiful Canadian island off the coast of Maine, to join his family at their vacation home. Waiting for him were his wife Eleanor and their children. They had also been joined by Roosevelt's confidant, Louis Howe, and his family. Roosevelt had recently been implicated in a political scandal that had occurred during his time as assistant secretary of the navy, and when he arrived for his vacation, he was exhausted after giving testimony to a Senate committee. It was also going to be his first real time away from work at the Navy Department in more than eight years.

About ten days before going to Campobello, Roosevelt had spent time at Lake Kanowahks to visit the New York Boy Scout camp. Historians have speculated that it was during his visit with the boy Scouts that Roosevelt was exposed to the polio virus.[2]

Shortly after arriving at their summerhouse, Roosevelt and his family spent a day of outdoor activities that included picnicking, sailing, and fishing. On the way back to their cottage, the Roosevelts helped neighbors fight a wildfire. To remove the soot, they took a swim in the waters of Lake Glen Severn and an additional dip in the ice-cold waters of the Bay of Fundy. When returning home, Roosevelt complained of chills, nausea, and back pain. He skipped supper and went to bed. When waking up the following morning, August 11, Roosevelt still was feeling sick and had fever and chills. He experienced weakness of his left leg, and by the end of the day it was paralyzed.[3] In addition, the other leg had started to become weak. Dr. Eben Bennet, a good friend and family doctor living nearby, made the diagnosis of "a heavy cold."[4]

Soon, however, Roosevelt and his family would realize that this was not just a cold. Roosevelt's symptoms worsened rapidly. The next day both of Roosevelt's legs were paralyzed; his temperature was 102°F (39°C); and he had pain in his feet, legs, and back. Dr. Bennet understood that his diagnosis had underestimated the seriousness of the situation and recommended that Dr. William Keen be consulted. We have already met Dr. Keen, a famous neurosurgeon from Philadelphia who participated in President Grover Cleveland's surgery aboard the *Oneida* in 1893. At the time Roosevelt fell ill, Keen, now retired, was vacationing in the neighborhood.

When he came to see Roosevelt, Keen gave him "a most careful, thorough examination."[5] Roosevelt's condition had deteriorated further, and he was now paralyzed from the chest down. His hands, arms, and shoulders were getting weak, and he had difficulties moving his bowels. In addition, he needed a catheter, a "thin glass tube,"[6] to empty his bladder. Keen, like Bennet, misdiagnosed the condition. Keen thought that a blood clot had formed in Roosevelt's lower spinal cord and that this was the cause of his symptoms. Keen later changed his diagnosis and suggested that the paralysis was caused by a "lesion of the spinal cord."[7] He recommended massage of the leg muscles to improve circulation and maintain tonus.[8] Although it caused terrible pain, Eleanor and Howe vigorously massaged Roosevelt's legs. Despite misdiagnosing Roosevelt's condition twice in a few days, Keen did not hesitate to send a bill for the astounding amount of $600,[9] the equivalent of $9,300 in 2022.

Roosevelt's fever continued for almost a week, and his inability to urinate and move his bowels persisted for two weeks. Although the weakness in his arms started to improve, the paralysis of the legs from the hips down continued.

It was not until August 25 that a correct diagnosis was made. Dr. Robert Lovett, chair of the Harvard Infantile Paralysis Commission in Boston, traveled to Campobello and examined Roosevelt. Lovett declared that the "physical findings" provided "perfectly clear" evidence that Roosevelt suffered from poliomyelitis.[10] Lovett recommended that the massages of Roosevelt's legs that were utterly painful and did not seem to be helpful be stopped, and he advised that a trained nurse be hired to care for the patient.[11]

On September 14 Roosevelt was transported to New York City, where he was admitted to Presbyterian Hospital for rehabilitation under the care of Dr. George Draper, who, like Lovett, was a renowned expert on poliomyelitis and who knew Roosevelt from Groton School and Harvard. It would be another two weeks before Roosevelt could be transferred to his home at East 65th Street.

Draper tried to be optimistic about the prognosis, at least in front of the patient. At one point he stated, "you can say definitively that he will not be crippled. No one need have any fear of permanent injury from his attack."[12] Despite the rosy

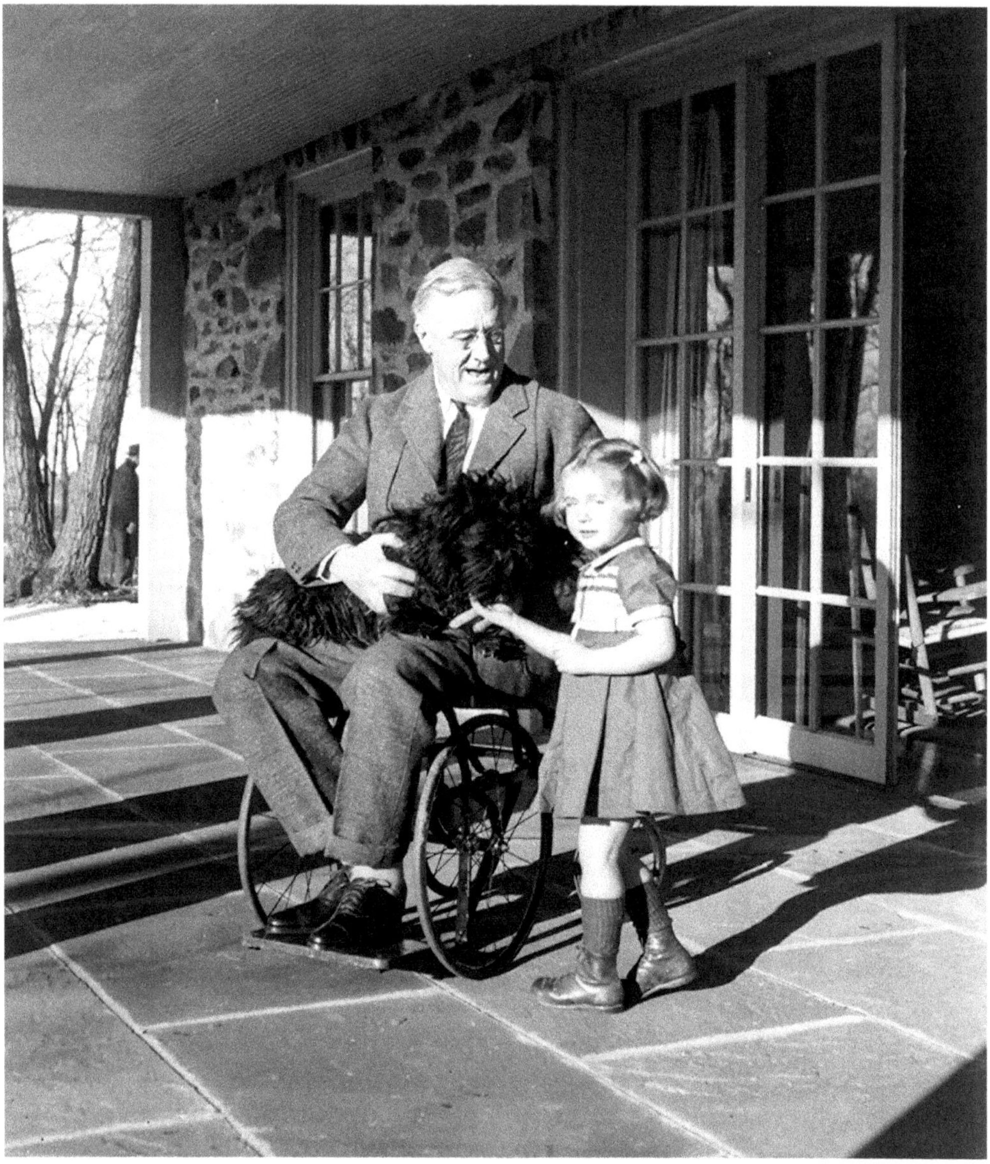

FDR at Hill Top Cottage in Hyde Park, New York, in 1941, together with his Scottish terrier Fala and Ruth Bie, the three-year-old granddaughter of the cottage caretakers. The photograph was taken by Franklin D. Roosevelt's friend and distant cousin Margaret "Daisy" Suckley in February 1941. Collection: FDR Photos, Franklin D. Roosevelt Library Photographs.

prediction, Roosevelt would remain paralyzed from his hips down for the rest of his life. Even though this was a devastating blow, he decided not to give up his ambitions for a political career. He worked hard on physical therapy but also spent much energy on efforts to hide his condition from the public. It was important to regain strength of his upper body muscles; they would be essential for his support when standing up, getting in and out of his wheelchair and cars, and when "walking." When giving speeches standing up, he gained support by holding on to a reinforced lectern.

Swimming became one of Roosevelt's favorite activities. He traveled for the first time to Warm Springs, Georgia, in the fall of 1924. Warm Springs became like a second home for Roosevelt, where he could retreat, enjoy hydrotherapy, undergo physical exercises, and, of course, swim. He encouraged other patients with polio to keep "swimming in warm water—lots of it."[13] Amazingly, he learned how to walk short distances while wearing long heavy steel braces extending from the heels to above the hips and locking at the knees and by swiveling the body in a "two-point walk." To make this propelling walk possible, he used the support of a strong person (often one of his sons) on his left side and a cane on his right side. Even if he was able to take these steps, he seldom displayed this ability publicly.

Although many were aware of Roosevelt's disability, most Americans were fooled by the illusion created by Roosevelt, his family, and his advisers. The press helped him with the scheme and seemed to adhere to a gentlemen's agreement not to show Roosevelt in what he would consider compromising pictures. His public appearances were arranged to prevent the press from seeing his arrivals and departures and to block the public from seeing him getting in or out of cars and trains. Privately, Roosevelt used a wheelchair, but only a few official pictures exist of Roosevelt in a wheelchair. Roosevelt's efforts to conceal his condition were also vigorously supported (and encouraged) by his longtime political counselor Howe and later, when in the White House, by Stephen Early, Roosevelt's assistant secretary in charge of press relations. Even the Secret Service pitched in and occasionally ripped the film out of the cameras of overzealous journalists showing Roosevelt in a wheelchair or being helped in or out of a vehicle.

So successful were the efforts to hide Roosevelt's disability from the public that many political figures in Europe remained unaware of his disability for years. John Gunther, a renowned author and journalist stationed in Europe during the ten years leading up to World War II, reported, "I repeatedly met men in important positions of state who had no idea that the President was disabled."[14]

Did a Tonsillectomy Play a Role in Roosevelt's Poliomyelitis?

Roosevelt underwent a tonsillectomy (surgical removal of the tonsils) in December 1919.[15] Two years prior, he had been hospitalized with a peritonsillar abscess.

In the 1940s and 1950s, several medical articles were published suggesting that a tonsillectomy increased the risk of an individual being afflicted by poliomyelitis. For example, in 1957 Dr. Noah D. Fabricant of Chicago, Illinois, highlighted the fact that Roosevelt's poliomyelitis was preceded twenty-one months earlier by a tonsillectomy. In his article, Fabricant concluded that "it is conceivable that his tonsillectomy could have been a contributing factor in Franklin D. Roosevelt's poliomyelitis attack."[16]

Partly explaining why a tonsillectomy may increase the risk for poliomyelitis is the fact that the virus can enter the body via the mouth, with the infection beginning in the intestines. Water or food contaminated by an infected person can spread the disease. With the disease eradicated from most parts of the world, the number of papers addressing tonsillectomy as a risk factor for poliomyelitis has dwindled over the last several decades.

Still, there has been more recent research into the role of tonsillectomy in poliomyelitis. As late as 1990, different potential mechanisms of tonsillectomy-associated poliomyelitis were discussed in medical literature.[17] Two main theories were reviewed, one being that virus present in the throat may enter nerve fibers exposed during the surgery and travel to the central nervous system via the nerves, and the other being that the nasopharyngeal immune response is decreased following tonsillectomy (as manifested by reduced pharyngeal IgA production). Although some observations may seem to support these theories, the whole concept of increased susceptibility to poliomyelitis following tonsillectomy remains controversial.[18]

Even if there were speculations in the 1940s and 1950s that Roosevelt's tonsillectomy in 1919 may have played a role in his paralytic illness, it seems unlikely or at least not possible to prove.

Did Roosevelt Have Poliomyelitis or Guillain-Barré Syndrome?

Despite the fact that Roosevelt's paralytic illness was finally diagnosed as poliomyelitis (after initially having been misdiagnosed as a "heavy cold" or a blood clot in the lower spinal cord), recent publications have challenged the diagnosis. Instead, it has been proposed that Roosevelt may have suffered from Guillain-Barré syndrome.

Guillain-Barré syndrome is named after two of the authors who provided a detailed description of the condition in 1916. In that year, the French neurologists Georges Guillain (1876–1961) and Jean Alexandre Barré (1880–1967), together with André Strohl (1887–1971), a future professor of physiological medicine, published a paper describing two French soldiers presenting with ascending paralytic illness.[19]

The fact that Roosevelt's paralysis was ascending, starting in the lower extremities and propagating upward to ultimately affect the chest, shoulders, and arms, was a significant (but not the only) observation that supported the argument that Roosevelt's paralytic illness was caused by Guillain-Barré syndrome. The condition characterized by an ascending paralysis was previously called Landry's ascending paralysis, so named after a report by Octave Landry (1826–1865) in 1859.[20] The two patients described by Guillain, Barré, and Strohl had indeed been diagnosed with Landry's ascending paralysis (although Guillain was unwilling to accept that Landry's ascending paralysis belonged to the same syndrome he described). It was the examination of the cerebrospinal fluid (obtained by a lumbar puncture, or spinal tap) from these patients that confirmed that Landry's ascending paralysis (later to become known as Guillain-Barré syndrome) was separate from poliomyelitis. The cerebrospinal fluid from the two French soldiers contained only a few white blood cells (leukocytes) but did contain high concentrations of protein, findings that were opposite to those in poliomyelitis.

André Strohl, the last name in the list of authors of the 1916 paper and whose name for some reason was dropped from the future eponym of the syndrome, performed novel myographic studies of tendon reflexes and documented important electrophysiological abnormalities in the two patients. Historians have provided several possible reasons why Strohl was dropped from the name of the syndrome. He was not a neurologist, was quite young at the time of the 1916 report and may not have been respected by established neurologists, and seems to have been dismissed by Guillain himself in public speeches and articles. There may also have been political reasons. Strohl not only had a German name but was also born in Alsace, a French province heavily influenced by German culture and traditions, and it is possible that he was subjected to anti-German sentiments after World War I.[21]

At the time of Franklin Roosevelt's paralytic illness, the awareness among American doctors of the report by Guillain, Barré, and Strohl was low. The few articles published early after the original report had come mainly from Europe, and the fact that the 1916 paper was in French probably did not stimulate wide readership in the United States. Also, the experts on poliomyelitis who cared for Roosevelt, Drs. Lovett and Draper, had published their treatises on the condition around the same time as the French report had appeared,[22] which may explain why they may not have paid full attention to other potential causes of Roosevelt's paralytic illness.

It would be more than eighty years before Roosevelt's diagnosis was challenged and the theory was put forward that he may have suffered from Guillain-Barré syndrome rather than poliomyelitis. In a paper from the University of Texas published in 2003, Dr. Armond Goldman and coauthors performed a detailed review of Roosevelt's symptoms during those fateful days in August and September 1921 and subjected the observations to a so-called Bayesian analysis.[23] (Bayesian analysis is a statistical method named after the English mathematician Thomas Bayes [1702–1761] that allows for the calculation of "posterior probabilities" or, in the case of Roosevelt, a retrospective estimate of the diagnostic probabilities of the cause of his paralytic illness). In their analysis, the authors assessed eight symptoms that Roosevelt experienced or lacked during his paralytic illness, including the presence of an ascending, nearly symmetric paralysis that progressed for ten to thirteen days, facial paralysis, prolonged bladder and bowel dysfunction, numbness and dysesthesia (abnormal sense of touch of the skin, often a painful feeling of "skin-on-fire"), "absence of meningismus" (head and neck pain and necks stiffness), fever, descending pattern of recovery from the paralysis, and permanent paralysis. In their research, the authors determined that six of the eight "posterior probabilities" supported the diagnosis of Guillain-Barré syndrome and concluded that the outcome of the analysis "strongly favored Guillain-Barré syndrome."[24] Expressed in another way, the same group of researchers later stated that the overall probability that Roosevelt had Guillain-Barré syndrome was around 99 percent.[25]

Notwithstanding that a spinal tap and determination of the white blood cell count and protein levels in the cerebrospinal fluid would have provided more definitive evidence of Roosevelt's diagnosis, most historians seem to agree that it is unlikely that he underwent the test. According to one source, however, a spinal tap was performed four days into Roosevelt's illness in hopes of decreasing cerebrospinal pressure.[26] Regardless, laboratory results from any spinal tap have not been made public. This is why researchers have had to rely on clinical signs and symptoms when analyzing the likelihood of Roosevelt's diagnosis, leading to the conclusion that "over 80 years after his illness, the cause of FDR's paralysis cannot be established with certainty."[27]

Even though the report in 2003 and subsequent publications by the same authors have generated a great amount of interest among historians and other nonmedical writers, others have been less impressed, and some have rebuked the idea that Roosevelt's paralytic illness was caused by Guillain-Barré syndrome and strongly argued for the correctness of the diagnosis of poliomyelitis.[28] The controversy has resulted in an academic feud with sometimes aggressive and bitter comments. For example, in a recent publication authored by a group of specialists in physical medicine and rehabilitation, the possibility that Roosevelt's paralytic illness was caused by Guillain-Barré syndrome was called a "newly contrived controversy" that should be "put ... to rest."[29] The authors dismissed the 2003 paper by calling it an example of "a common academic hobby."[30] They also alleged that the "analysis ... contains serious flaws"[31] and strongly argued for the validity of the diagnosis made by Lovett and Draper, the leading experts on poliomyelitis in America at the time of Roosevelt's paralytic illness, and concluded that "it is apparent in reviewing FDR's initial clinical presentation, subsequent medical management, and his partial recovery that the diagnosis of poliomyelitis was neither made casually nor by physicians and therapists unfamiliar with this then-common disease."[32]

It may of course be argued that the question of the underlying illness of Roosevelt's paralysis is merely of academic interest. After all, no effective well-proven treatments were available for either condition at the time of Roosevelt's disease. However, his poliomyelitis (if that is what he had) had enormous social and economic consequences. He became a symbol for the fight against polio at a time when the disease was still active and feared. His efforts at Warm Springs lay the foundation for a major new field of medicine: the specialty of physical medicine and rehabilitation. Because of Roosevelt's disability and despite his efforts to keep it out of sight, Americans' view of disabled people changed. His fundraising through the March of Dimes supported research that resulted in effective vaccines, preventing the death of millions all over the world.

Regardless of the cause of Roosevelt' paralytic illness, it is indeed remarkable that someone facing so many challenges would go on to become a two-term governor of the state of New York and a four-time president of the United States.

Dr. Ross T. McIntire, Personal Physician to the President

When Roosevelt first took office as president, he needed to appoint someone to the position of White House physician. Dr. Joel T. Boone, who had served as personal physician to presidents Warren Harding, Calvin Coolidge, and Herbert Hoover, was hoping to stay on. He was surprised to learn that the new president had other plans.

Roosevelt conferred with Dr. Gary Grayson, who had been the physician to President Woodrow Wilson and who was also a close friend to Roosevelt. Grayson recommended Dr. Ross McIntire for the job as the new White House physician. Grayson and McIntire knew each other from the time they had worked together at the U.S. Naval Dispensary in Washington in the 1920s and at the U.S. Naval Hospital in the 1930s.

When Dr. McIntire, a specialist in ophthalmology and otolaryngology, was appointed personal physician to President Roosevelt, he was struck by "a complete surprise."[33] Indeed, he questioned whether it was prudent that someone with his qualifications should serve as the president's physician. When Grayson heard about the doubts, he wrote McIntire a letter explaining that "the President is as strong as a horse with the exception of a chronic sinus condition that makes him susceptible to colds. That's where you come in."[34] In addition, it was argued, McIntire was an excellent choice because "he knew how to keep his mouth shut," a quality highly valued by Grayson. After all, Grayson had been successful in his cover-up of President Wilson's medical condition after a massive stroke in 1919 had made him incapable of fulfilling his duties as president.

McIntire understood the importance of doctor-patient confidentiality and would prove willing to apply that also when the patient was the president of the United States. He was of the opinion that the "health of the chief-executive ... is his own private business."[35] Being able to keep his mouth shut made McIntire a long-lasting White House physician. He remained in the position throughout Roosevelt's entire time as president. Seeing the chief executive once or twice every day for twelve years brought them close and gave McIntire influence over Roosevelt. It was said about the doctor that he was "the only man who gives orders to Franklin Roosevelt."[36]

Several historians and physicians have given varying assessments of McIntire and his job as President Roosevelt's personal physician. McIntire was described by some as "a forty-three-year-old career Navy medical officer of no particular distinction."[37] His management of Roosevelt's hypertension and heart failure was considered incompetent by the president's cardiologist.[38] McIntire's involvement in the mysterious (maybe even criminal) disappearance of Roosevelt's medical records from Bethesda Naval Hospital as well as other places has, at least indirectly, been implicated by some.

On several occasions, McIntire gave less than truthful statements about the president's health, for which he has been called a downright liar. "This was not the first time nor the last that the admiral [McIntire] lied to the press, to the Roosevelt family, and to all concerned."[39] When McIntire in his book *White House Physician* continued to claim that Roosevelt had always been "in excellent condition for a man of his age,"[40] some historians commented that "there is no other way to characterize McIntire's statement except as a bold-faced lie."[41] The same authors also raised the possibility that McIntire shortly after Roosevelt's death had destroyed the president's complete medical file because he "had the most to lose if the records ever were made public."[42]

Not surprisingly, when McIntire was assessed in an essay by a fellow otolaryngologist, the verdict was kinder. "The career of Dr Ross T. McIntire, otolaryngologist and personal physician to the 32nd president of the United States, engenders a sense of honor to our profession."[43]

An additional colleague who praised McIntire was the world-renowned Boston surgeon Dr. Frank Lahey. In January 1945 he wrote in a letter to an acquaintance that the president's personal physician was "the most satisfactory man to work with.... He has a breadth of vision that is refreshing.... I have never known a more completely unselfish individual in such a high and influential position."[44] Realizing that he may be too positive and exaggerating in his assessment of McIntire, Lahey added, "If you think there are unduly laudatory remarks, as you well may, you could easily find out that I am quite a hard-boiled person."

Minor Surgeries While in Office

Although Roosevelt was protective about his health situation and, as we have seen, worked hard on concealing his disability for the American people, he thought it was okay to disclose a few minor surgical procedures he underwent while in office.

In mid-November 1937, Roosevelt developed sever pain from an abscessed tooth. The misery was accompanied by high fever, with his temperature reaching 103°F.[45] It was obvious that the tooth needed to come out.

The day before the procedure, the president was called on in his bedroom by several individuals who needed to discuss pressing political issues. Postmaster General James A. Farley was among the visitors. He later recalled the encounter with the president. "I was shocked by his appearance," Farley said, and added, "His jaw was swollen.... During the entire interview he kept an ice bag to his jaw to relieve pain."[46]

The recovery from the tooth extraction took longer than expected. Some three weeks after the operation, the president was still having pain. "If anybody punched me there I would be sore," he told reporters at a press conference on December 5. "Putting it as a layman, I would say that it has not healed."[47] It did, of course, ultimately heal, and Roosevelt would not need another operation until almost seven years later.

Roosevelt had noticed a swelling on the back of his head for about twenty years. Doctors had diagnosed the swelling as a sebaceous cyst (a "wen" in laymen's language). It had progressively increased in size over the years and started to become a nuisance when his hat band rubbed against it. Now, he wanted it removed. A surgical procedure was scheduled for February 2, 1944, at Bethesda Naval Hospital.

Most surgeons would consider the excision of a sebaceous cyst a minor procedure, often performed in the office under local anesthesia. But this time it was different; after all, the patient was the president of the United States. No less than seven doctors were in attendance in the operating room on that day in February 1944.[48] Another source quoted six doctors (one of them an anesthesiologist for the local anesthesia) and two nurses.[49] The patient remained seated in his wheelchair, with his head resting against a support constructed especially for the event. The operation was performed under local anesthesia. The lesion was "about the size of a hen's egg and almost exactly in the midline."[50] Eight stitches were needed to close the incision.

The scalp is a blood-rich area of the body, and bleeding from the operation soiled the president's undershirt, which had to be replaced with a clean one. Despite that, "everything went off beautifully."[51]

Words about Roosevelt's surgery quickly leaked to the news media. White House press secretary Steve Early was awakened several times in the middle of the night by journalists asking if it was true that the president had been undergoing surgery. Early kept repeating that "the President wants to tell you about it himself."[52]

At a press conference two days after the surgery, reporters were excited and bombarded the president with questions. They of course wanted to know if he had been under the knife. Roosevelt tried to deflect the attention to his operation and move on to more important issues by joking about it. "Sure, I was under the knife. I am under the knife whenever I cut my fingernails."[53] The journalists caught on to the humor and asked, "Mr. President, did those Naval 'gims' permit you to smoke while they did their hacking?" Roosevelt replied, "No, but I yelled for a cigarette right afterword."[54]

The following day, the president's surgery was mentioned in the newspapers but did not create big headlines. The *New York Times* had a small headline, one column wide: "Went Under Surgery, Roosevelt Discloses; But It Was Only for an Old Wen on His Head, He Says."[55] The *Washington Post* used the headline "Roosevelt Recovers from Minor Surgery."[56] Other newspapers throughout the country also mentioned the operation with small articles.

No further questions regarding the president's operation were raised by the press, and the event was soon forgotten.

Uncontrolled Hypertension and Heavy Smoking: A Dangerous Combination

In January 1944, Roosevelt complained of frequent headaches. He was also fatigued and generally did not feel well. Roosevelt's secretary, Grace Tully, had noticed "the Boss occasionally nodding over his mail or dozing a moment during dictation." She added, "as it began to occur with increasing frequency I became seriously alarmed."[57] Eleanor and daughter Anna also became increasingly worried about Franklin's health and urged McIntire to consult other doctors. McIntire referred the president to Bethesda Naval Hospital for a complete medical checkup. He was scheduled for an appointment at 11 a.m. on March 27, 1944, with the cardiologist Dr. Howard G. Bruenn. When Bruenn examined Roosevelt, he found the president to be in poor condition. "He appeared to be very tired, and his face was very gray."[58] Even light movements resulted in "considerable breathlessness."

When Bruenn reviewed Roosevelt's previous medical records, he noticed that the president's blood pressure had been elevated since at least 1940. When Roosevelt was examined at Bethesda Naval Hospital on March 27, 1944, his blood pressure was 180/108 mm Hg. Physical examination as well as fluoroscopy and X-rays revealed "considerable increase" of the size of the president's heart. Bruenn also noted that the patient "coughed frequently during the examination but produced no sputum." Dr. Bruenn diagnosed Roosevelt with "hypertension, hypertensive cardiac disease, cardiac failure (left ventricular), and acute bronchitis."[59]

Lacking today's modern and effective medications for hypertension, Bruenn prescribed a mixture of lifestyle changes, a heart medicine, and medicine to reduce the coughing:

> The patient should be put to bed for 1 to 2 weeks with nursing care.
> Digitalization should be carried out: 0.4 g of digitalis every day for 5 days; subsequently, 0.1 g every day.
> A light, easily digestible diet. Portions were to be small, and salt intake was to be restricted. Potassium chloride in a salt shaker could be used as desired for seasoning.
> Codeine, ½ grain, should be given for control of cough.
> Sedation should be taken to ensure rest and a refreshing night's sleep.
> A program of gradual weight reduction.[60]

Although it may have been frustrating for doctors in those days to be unable to treat high blood pressure effectively, the dangers of hypertension were actually not well recognized at the time. In several contemporary textbooks on heart disease, it was pointed out that "hypertension may be an important compensatory mechanism which should not be tempered with, even were it certain we could control it," and that "people with mild benign hypertension with levels up to 210/110 need not be treated."[61] This is obviously quite different from today's recommendations of trying to keep the blood pressure not higher than 120/70 (and maybe even lower).

Remarkably, Bruenn did not initially comment on Roosevelt's smoking habits and did not include recommendations to stop or at least reduce the use of tobacco. Physicians and people in general had not started to fully understand the dangers of tobacco. Later during the care of Roosevelt, however, it was recommended that "cigarettes were to be curtailed"[62] and that consumption should be cut down to "six cigarettes a day."[63] At the time, Roosevelt smoked two packs a day of unfiltered Camels.[64]

For unclear reasons, McIntire initially resisted Bruenn's recommendation to start treating the president with digitalis. This put Bruenn in a difficult position. As one author commented, "FDR was in heart failure and was receiving inadequate treatment because a medically unsophisticated superior officer, who was basically an administrator, was in charge of the case."[65] After meetings with a team of additional doctors, McIntire finally agreed to start the president on the heart medicine. This resulted in a robust improvement of Roosevelt's condition, noticeable already after a week, although it did not normalize his blood pressure. The hypertension would continue to worsen during the remaining year of Roosevelt's life and cause his death. When Roosevelt arrived at Warm Springs at the end of March 1945, his blood pressure was 240/130 mm Hg. Although relaxing at the resort seemed to have an initial positive effect, shortly after 1 p.m. on April 12, Roosevelt had what most likely was a massive cerebral hemorrhage. Immediately after the event, he was examined by Bruenn. Roosevelt's blood pressure had skyrocketed. The systolic blood pressure was "well over 300 mm Hg; diastolic pressure was 190 mm Hg."[66] At 3:35, the president was dead.

Allegedly, no autopsy was performed. Several explanations for this have been offered. Dr. James Paullin of Atlanta, a former president of the American Medical Association, pointed out that "there were no facilities whatever to performing an autopsy."[67] It has been suggested that Eleanor opposed an autopsy, but there are no records that she prevented a postmortem examination. McIntire argued that "there was no useful purpose to be served by it."[68] Reports from an autopsy would obviously have been extremely important and would have prevented speculations about Roosevelt's illness and cause of death. Without that, historians have had to rely on circumstantial evidences when trying to determine what actually felled the president.

Did Roosevelt Die with (or from) a Metastasizing Cancer?

The narrative about Roosevelt's death from a stroke went unchallenged for almost thirty-five years. In 1979 Dr. Harry S. Goldsmith, an acclaimed surgeon and medical historian, published a sensational peer-reviewed article suggesting that other factors may have been in play.[69] Based on extensive research of both documents and photographs of Roosevelt, Goldsmith proposed that Roosevelt suffered from a metastasizing malignant tumor the last couple of years before his death and that a malignant melanoma may have been the primary source of the spreading cancer.

In his article Dr. Goldsmith recalled how he, as a surgical resident at the Memorial Sloan Kettering Cancer Center in New York City, had attended a talk given by Dr. George T. Pack in 1963. Pack, who died in 1969 at the age of seventy, had also had his training at Sloan Kettering and was now one of the most respected surgeons in New York and a world-renowned cancer surgeon who boasted many famous people among his patients. For example, he had performed surgery on Eva (Evita) Perón in Argentina in 1951. The subject of Pack's talk was illnesses in world leaders and the impact on world events. One of the subjects discussed during the talk was Franklin D. Roosevelt.

In his talk, Pack reported that a friend of his, Dr. Frank H. Lahey of Boston, another renowned surgeon and educator, had seen Roosevelt in consultation in 1944 and advised Roosevelt against running for a fourth term as president, since he had "a metastatic tumor" and would not survive a new term.[70] Goldsmith found this statement extremely interesting and went up to Pack after the talk and asked when this information would be published. Pack replied that he did not know but pointed out that the information was in his personal records, which would be released after his death.

Several months after Pack's death, Goldsmith contacted Pack's widow asking when the records would be published. "This would be done in the future" was the answer.[71] After another five years and without hearing from Pack's estate, Goldsmith again reached out to Mrs. Pack requesting information about her late husband's records. This time he was informed that "circumstances had prevented the publication of the journals."[72] He was also told that most of the journals had "either been lost or misplaced over the years." Goldsmith was offered the opportunity to review what was left of the records and needed only two and a half hours to go through the documents.[73] He found no information at all about Roosevelt.

At this point, Goldsmith started to question his own recollection of Pack's lecture in 1963. Had Pack really said that Roosevelt suffered from a metastasizing tumor? Goldsmith started contacting colleagues who he knew had been in the audience in 1963. Although some remembered the event and Pack's words, others could not recall the story about Roosevelt's malignant tumor. A colleague surgeon practicing in California, however, reassured Goldsmith that his recollection was correct. The California surgeon who had trained at Sloan Kettering at the same time as Goldsmith and had attended the same talk in 1963 confirmed that Pack had indeed mentioned that Roosevelt had a metastasizing tumor. The same surgeon added that in 1965, he had been invited by Pack to a dinner at the Strollers Club (a social club in New York City with many doctors among its members), where Pack gave a speech titled "Medicine in World History." In the speech, Pack repeated the story about Roosevelt's health that both had heard during the talk in 1963.

Now convinced that Pack had indeed reported that Lahey had been concerned about Roosevelt's metastasizing tumor and puzzled by the fact that he had not been able to find any original documents supporting the story, Goldsmith started to dig deeper. He contacted the U.S. Naval Hospital in Bethesda, where Roosevelt for sure had been a patient on many occasions. Curiously, Goldsmith was informed that "there were no records of Franklin D. Roosevelt available at that institution."[74] Not being ready to give up on his quest to find medical records of Roosevelt, Goldsmith contacted by phone and letter Walter Reed Medical Center, the Armed Forces Institute of Pathology, the National Archives, and the National Personnel Records Center in St. Louis (maintaining records of all former government workers), all with the same negative results: they had "no record of Franklin D. Roosevelt."[75]

Similar fruitless attempts to find written records of Roosevelt's medical care were reported already in 1970 by Roosevelt's cardiologist, Dr. Howard Bruenn. In an article published in the *Annals of Internal Medicine*, he reported that "the original hospital chart in which all clinical progress notes as well as the results of the various laboratory tests were incorporated was kept in the safe at the U.S. Naval Hospital, Bethesda, Md. After the President's death this chart could not be found,"[76] and it "has never been recovered."[77] In his 1979 report, Goldsmith pointed out that Dr. McIntire was one of the few who had access to the safe. This started to smell like a conspiracy. Had McIntire removed (and destroyed) the chart? Goldsmith and others seem to have implied that McIntire was behind the disappearance of Roosevelt's medical chart,[78] but if so, why?

In the absence of evidence as to how the medical records vanished and who may have removed them, it can only be speculated as to why it happened. If indeed McIntire was guilty of the removal (or even destruction) of Roosevelt's journals, it may be speculated that he did it on the request of Roosevelt's family, who wanted to preserve the image of Franklin Roosevelt to the afterworld as a healthy man (except for the paralytic illness, of course). This may also explain why Eleanor allegedly blocked an autopsy of her diseased husband.[79] Roosevelt's cardiologist made an interesting comment: "An autopsy was not performed at the expressed wish of Mrs. Roosevelt (despite the urgent request of the Russian authorities who thought that the President might have met foul play)."[80]

It has also been speculated that McIntire wanted to preserve his own reputation. It seems obvious that as a specialist in ophthalmology and otolaryngology, he did not manage the president's hypertension and heart failure in an optimal fashion. Also, McIntire on several occasions had made false statements about Roosevelt's condition and claimed that the president was in excellent health despite weight loss and other signs of failing health. McIntire was known as always wanting "to present the President of the United States as being completely healthy and disease-free," and he "never admitted, either before or after the death of Roosevelt, that the President ever had anything wrong with him outside of an occasional bout of flu or bronchitis."[81] It may of course be argued that McIntire's deceptions were justified, considering the political and military situation in the world, and may actually have been conducted on the direct order of the president; the enemies would have been delighted if Roosevelt was terminally ill during the endgame of World War II.

If indeed Roosevelt had metastasizing cancer and one of the metastases was in his brain, historians have pointed out that Roosevelt's ability to stand up against Joseph Stalin at Yalta may have been affected. There are many testimonies, in both writing and images, of the president's unhealthy appearance at the Yalta Conference. According to some historians, "photographs taken of Roosevelt at Yalta show a dying man."[82] This was obvious even though the media tried to hide it. "Because of careful screening of pictures before their release for publication, his physical condition was even worse in reality than what the public was shown."[83] A member of the American delegation commented that "we had the feeling that Roosevelt was not holding up our interest to the best" and then added that he "was giving way, giving into the Russians on almost everything."[84]

Questions and speculations about Roosevelt's health toward the end of his life will probably never be fully answered unless, of course, his medical charts would miraculously surface somewhere.

Roosevelt's physical status had started to deteriorate already the year before he was running for his last reelection. According to Judge Samuel Rosenman, presidential adviser and speechwriter credited with coining the term "New Deal," Roosevelt's physical decline began at the time of the Tehran Conference in November 1943.[85] Historians seem to agree that Tehran was a turning point for Roosevelt's health. Already in October, Roosevelt had experienced increasing "pain in his right side," interpreted by some as "the first evidence that [a] melanoma had metastasized to his abdomen."[86]

The Tehran meeting was the first summit between the three major Allied leaders, but things did not seem to go well for Roosevelt. During a steak dinner hosted by Roosevelt on November 28, he became acutely ill with abdominal pain, and "suddenly, in the flick of an eye, he turned green and great drops of sweat began to bead off his face."[87] The president was quickly wheeled to his room and examined by Dr. McIntire. To everyone's relief, the word came back that it was "nothing more than a mild attack of indigestion." The president, however, did not return to the dinner.

Even more worrisome was Roosevelt's apparent mental decline. When Winston

Churchill was asked whether Roosevelt had been engaged during the conversations with Stalin, the British prime minister commented that "the president was inept. He was asked a lot of questions and gave the wrong answers."[88]

People close to the president had started to realize that he was a sick man. Six years after Roosevelt's death, James A. Farley, a former member of Roosevelt's cabinet, wrote in a letter to the *New York Times* that "in 1944 it was widely known that FDR was a dying man."[89] The decline of Roosevelt's health continued during 1944 when, against the advice of Dr. Frank Lahey,[90] he was running for his fourth term as president. When Roosevelt's son James saw his father in December 1944, he "realized with awful irrevocable certainty that we were going to lose him."[91] Roosevelt had lost his appetite and complained "can't eat—cannot taste food."[92] He had dropped an alarming thirty pounds in weight and looked like "an extremely sick man."[93] Despite this, McIntire continued to claim that "the President's health is excellent, I can say that unqualifyingly."[94] The president had also started to complain of abdominal pain.

At Yalta in February 1945, "signs of physical decline of Roosevelt were clearly obvious, and there were many at this meeting who believed that his mental deterioration was also evident."[95] Many observers testified to Roosevelt's both physical and mental decline. Sir Alexander Cadogan of the British Foreign Office commented that he "got the impression that most of the time he [Roosevelt] hardly knew what it was all about."[96] The president was seen "looking straight ahead with his mouth open, as if he were not taking things in."[97] Lord Moran, Churchill's private physician, commented that "the President appears a sick man.... I give him only a few months to live."[98]

After Roosevelt's return to the United States, his health continued to worsen. When delivering a report to Congress on March 1 about his meeting with Churchill and Stalin, Roosevelt "looked gaunt and emaciated and dark shadows circled his eyes."[99] By now, he had lost at least forty pounds in weight. The president, "a man of magnificent intellect and rhetorical skills," had difficulties delivering his speech. "Time after time he stumbled over the text, making mistakes that sometimes were simple and at other times were substantial."[100] And remarkably, he gave his speech sitting down, a first for the president!

Despite deliberate efforts by the White House and newspaper editors to block unfavorable pictures of the president, multiple pictures appearing in the press showed a Roosevelt who certainly looked ill. The images portrayed evidence of severe weight loss and surely supported Dr. Lahey's alleged warning to the president that he should not run for reelection in 1944 because he had a "metastatic tumor."[101]

In an additional interesting twist to the hunt for documents describing Roosevelt's health during the last couple of years of his life and the advice he had received not to run for reelection in 1944, it took a legal battle to unveil a memorandum written by Dr. Lahey on July 10, 1944.[102] The Lahey memorandum was written for the records to protect the doctor's reputation if he was criticized in the future about his medical treatment of the president, in particular if he would be accused of not trying to advise Roosevelt against running for reelection. The memorandum was deposited in a law office by Lahey's trusted business manager, Linda Strand, with strict orders that it could not be published unless Lahey was accused of mismanaging the president's health.

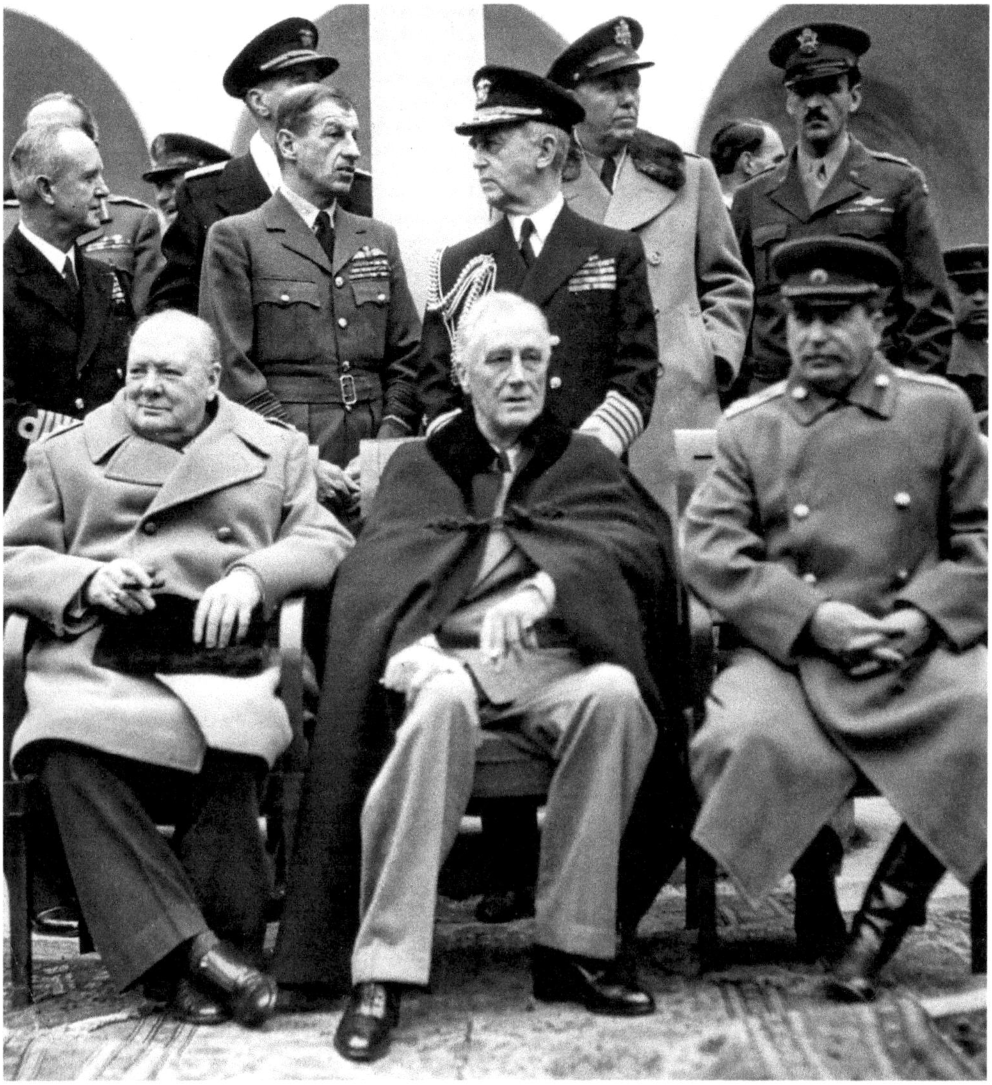

President Roosevelt at Yalta looking tired and frail and with clear signs of weight loss. Collection: FDR Photos, Franklin D. Roosevelt Library Photographs.

In the early 1980s Dr. Goldsmith learned about the document, and in 1983 he asked Strand to try to get the memorandum made public. She requested that the law firm where she had deposited the document release it, but the law firm refused. After a fierce legal battle going all the way up to the Massachusetts Supreme Court, the judges determined in 1986 that Lahey's conditions for disclosure had been fulfilled and that the document should be released. Strand handed over the document to Goldsmith,[103] but not until 2005 were parts of it made public.

In the memorandum, Lahey started by declaring that "I wish to record the following information regarding my opinions in relation to President Roosevelt's condition and to have them on record in the event there comes any criticism of me at a later date. I want to do this after having seen him in consultation as a private record."[104] Lahey then stated that on July 8, 1944, he had informed Dr. McIntire about his opinion that because the president was "if not in heart failure, at least on the verge of it," he thought that "over the four years of another term with its burdens, he [Roosevelt] would again have heart failure and be unable to complete it." Lahey also pointed out that he felt "it was not my duty to advise concerning whether or not such a term was undertaken" but that "it was Admiral McIntire's duty to inform him concerning his capacity."

Lahey's memorandum differed from the narrative provided by Dr. Goldsmith in 1979 in some aspects. As we have seen, Goldsmith remembered that Dr. Pack in his talk at the Memorial Sloan Kettering Cancer Center in 1963 had mentioned that Dr. Lahey "in 1944 … had informed the President that he had a metastatic tumor and advised him not to run for a fourth term, since he would not survive this term in office if elected."[105] The Lahey memorandum stated that he had not directly advised Roosevelt against running for reelection but that the recommendation had been given to McIntire.

In addition, nowhere in the memorandum does Lahey mention "metastatic tumor," but he does state that risk of heart failure was the reason he felt that Roosevelt may be "unable to complete" a fourth term.[106] This makes us wonder whether the rumors of cancer were just that, rumors only. Lomazow and Fettman strongly argue that Lahey's omission of the suspicion of cancer does not rule out that Roosevelt was indeed suffering from widespread cancer and quote several reasons for that opinion. First, multiple images from 1944 and 1945 showed a president who definitively looked ill and had lost weight. Second are "repeated credible firsthand reports from reputable physicians, several of them closely associated with Lahey, who all quote him as definitely reporting that the president had cancer."[107] And third, because the war was in what everybody was hoping its final stage, giving the enemy information suggesting that Roosevelt was terminally ill would be disastrous. Putting the information about Roosevelt's health in print or even thinking it was totally unacceptable. Cancer would remain "FDR's deadly secret, not even to be hinted at and certainly never be acknowledged in writing."[108]

It was about this time, late 1944, that Douglas MacArthur met with the president and later commented, "I had not seen him for a couple of years, and physically he was just a shell of the man I had known. It was clearly evident that his days were numbered."[109]

Historians have wondered why Roosevelt decided to run for a fourth term despite obvious signs of physical decline and against medical advice. In conversations with his son James, Roosevelt partly answered the question: "I don't dare shake the faith of the people, that's why I ran again, Jimmy." Roosevelt added, "The people elected me their leader and I can't quit in the middle of the war."[110]

Another and perhaps equally important reason that Roosevelt decided to run for reelection in 1944 was that he wanted to see his dream of the United Nations come true while still in the White House. He understood that it would be easier to get approval for the organization by the Senate as the president rather than as an ex-president.

Even if one accepts the theory that Roosevelt during the last few years of his life was afflicted by a metastasizing tumor, the question is what the primary tumor may have been. Several books and articles have argued that metastases from a malignant melanoma may have killed the president.

Did Roosevelt Have Surgery for Melanoma?

Although the evidence was circumstantial, Goldsmith in his 1979 article argued that a strong "hypothetic instance can be constructed that a pigmented lesion over the left eye of Roosevelt could have been a melanoma."[111] His publication was a sensation and was viewed by many as a new revelation. Of note, however, a pigmented suspicious-looking skin lesion above Roosevelt's left eyebrow had actually been reported almost a decade earlier. The historian Hugh L'Etang mentioned in his book *The Pathology of Leadership* (1969) that a pigmented skin lesion had been spotted above Roosevelt's left eyebrow.[112] L'Etang also reported that another historian had pointed out already in 1961 that the "pigmented naevus [above Roosevelt's left eyebrow] did not appear in photographs after 1943" and concluded that it had been "removed surgically."[113]

The appearance—and subsequent disappearance—of Roosevelt's "brown blob" have been documented by numerous photographs beginning in the early 1920s. In a photograph on the cover of *Time* magazine published on May 28, 1923, a small "dark spot" was seen above Roosevelt's left eyebrow.[114] Photographs over the next decade showed how the spot increased in size and became darker and ultimately started to grow into the eyebrow. It seemed to have reached its greatest size in 1939. Then surgical scars started to show up in the area, and the lesion became smaller over the next couple of years. "By September 1941 the patch was barely distinguishable, and by the middle of 1942, it had virtually disappeared completely."[115]

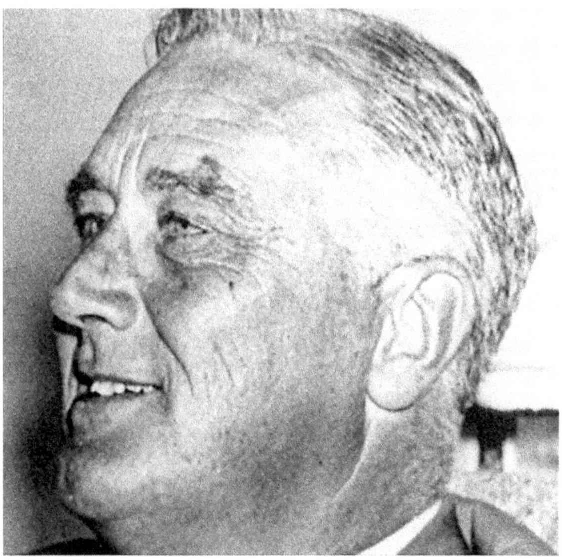

Roosevelt in August 1938 (age fifty-six years) with an asymmetric brown, slightly raised plaque above the left eyebrow. The pigmented skin lesion was larger than in a picture from 1933. A photograph in 1940 revealed changes consistent with partial surgical removal of the lesion. The photograph appeared as figure 3 in Ackerman and Lomazow, "An Inquiry into the Nature of the Pigmented Lesion Above Franklin Delano Roosevelt's Left Eyebrow," and is reprinted with the permission of the Journal of the American Medical Association Network.

Historians and medical experts have concluded that there is "solid evidence that the 'brown blob' had undergone changes that can only be attributed to surgical procedures."[116] Dr. McIntire (an ophthalmologist and ear, nose, and throat surgeon) never wanted to admit that the president had had any serious illnesses or had undergone any surgical procedures (other than extraction of an abscessed tooth) and has been implicated in the removal of Roosevelt's pigmented skin lesion. Some authors have bluntly stated that "it is undeniably certain that Ross McIntire continually was burning, carving, and scraping away at the malignant lesion above FDR's eye until it disappeared."[117] Other historians and medical experts are in agreement that the skin lesion had most likely been removed surgically and have stated that it would be "unusual" and "unlikely" for the "lesion above the left eyebrow to have undergone complete regression in the rather short space of 4 years (i.e., in the period from early 1940 to 1943)."[118]

At the time of Roosevelt, a malignant melanoma was often thought to be a death sentence, considered one of "the most malignant of all tumors," with prognosis worse "than that of any other type of malignant neoplasm."[119] Modern therapy, most notably different types of immunotherapy, has improved the prognosis, but the disease is still feared, in particular when metastases have developed.

Several observations are especially pertinent for the story about Roosevelt's suspected melanoma. Among patients who die from the disease, about 90 percent have developed metastases to the brain.[120] Indeed, the third most common cancer metastasizing to the brain is malignant melanoma.[121] Furthermore, brain metastases from melanomas are known to have a high incidence of spontaneous bleeding, accounting for the death of between a quarter and half of all deaths in patients with melanoma.[122] Taken together, these observations have led some authors to imply that Roosevelt's catastrophic cerebral hemorrhage on April 12, 1945, was a bleeding from a melanoma brain metastasis.[123]

Another intriguing observation is that malignant melanomas often metastasize to the gastrointestinal tract, in particular the small bowel.[124] This is why abdominal pain in a patient with malignant melanoma may raise the suspicion of spread to the abdomen. It is therefore not far-fetched that some of Roosevelt's symptoms have been used to support the suspicion of malignant melanoma, "like recurring bouts of excruciating pain caused by the cancer that had metastasized to his bowel."[125] When the president was examined by Dr. Lahey in March 1944, the surgeon was "particularly interested in the gastrointestinal tract."[126] At the time, Roosevelt had experienced severe abdominal pain on several occasions. At one point, his son James described how his father suddenly "began to groan, [and] his face took on an expression of suffering."[127] Roosevelt was exhausted by the pain and said to his son, "Jimmy, I don't know if I can make it. I have a horrible pain." From a surgeon's perspective, these symptoms would raise the possibility of crampy pain caused by a tumor obstructing the bowel.

As if vague hints in the medical and historical literature and many intriguing images of Roosevelt's "brown blob" above his left eyebrow are not enough to shroud his last years in a veil of mystery, there is also the story about the pathology conference at St Louis, Missouri, in 1949. At that meeting, a paper was presented by surgeons from Walter Reed General Hospital addressing the treatment of malignant melanoma. L'Etang described in his book how "all the slides and specimens shown had a serial number with one exception … which only bore a date: 14 April 1945."[128]

The specimen shown on that slide was a section of a brain with a metastatic melanoma that measured 4.5 × 5.25 centimeters.[129] Curiously, the date on the slide lacking a serial number was the date when Roosevelt's body arrived at Washington from Warm Springs, making "this observation rather more than a mere coincidence."[130]

Although this seemed to make a strong case for a presidential melanoma brain metastasis at the time of L'Etang's publication, it turns out that L'Etang based his conclusion on a report by an American surgeon, Francis Massie, who had interpreted a label on the slide, "A-14–45," as meaning April 14, 1945. Recent research, however, suggests that the label actually may not have meant April 14, 1945, but rather "the fourteenth autopsy performed at Walter Reed in 1945."[131]

More Mysteries

The last couple of years of Roosevelt's life were associated with several more mysteries than covered in this chapter. The secrecy and deceptions would continue for decades after his death (and have still not been completely resolved). Many hidden facts about Roosevelt are related to his medical conditions, whereas other secrets are part of his relationships with women other than Eleanor.

In this book, we have discussed in some detail controversies related to Roosevelt's paralytic illness (was it polio or Guillain-Barré syndrome?); the "brown blob" above his left eye (was it melanoma?); his loss of appetite, weight, and energy; recurrent bouts of severe abdominal pain (did he have metastasizing cancer spreading to his abdomen, causing blockage of his bowels?); and the way he died (was it a "garden-variety" of cerebrovascular catastrophe caused by hypertension, or was it bleeding into a metastasis from a malignant melanoma?).

Although this list of medical mysteries is long, Roosevelt's medical riddles are not limited to the catalog of potential diagnoses provided here. Additional rumors include those suggesting that Roosevelt's metastasizing tumor may have been prostate cancer and that radiation of the primary tumor may have caused rectal bleeding and severe anemia, even necessitating blood transfusions.[132]

Roosevelt's frequent "seizures" toward the end of his life have also been surrounded by controversy. Despite having been observed by many close to the president, the short-lasting episodes of unconsciousness were not even mentioned in the "definitive" account of Roosevelt's clinical course.[133] Other writers, however, have reported on a series of "little strokes" during Roosevelt's final years.[134]

Of course, the question must be asked as to why there was so much secrecy and deception? While it is easy to understand that disclosure of the president's health problems toward the end of World War II would have risked the outcome of the conflict, it may be more difficult to comprehend the rationale for why the secrecy has continued even after Roosevelt's death.

Historians have given several explanations. One reason for concealing Roosevelt's health status provided by several writers has been that physicians, in particular Dr. McIntire, wanted to protect their own reputations and ward off accusations that their management of the president's health may have been inept.

Several researchers have also pointed out that full disclosure of Roosevelt's physical and mental decline toward the end of his life would propagate the narrative about the "sick man at Yalta" and his inadequate (according to some) representation of the interests of the United States during the final meeting between the three Allied leaders. Indeed, the hesitancy by the president's daughter Anna and her husband Dr. James Halsted when Dr. Bruenn wanted to publish an article about his involvement in the medical care of the president may support that notion. In negotiations conducted before Bruenn finally published his paper in 1970, Anna and her husband argued that "whatever documents he [Bruenn] had should remain closed to outsiders 'for a considerable period yet to come'—suggesting twenty-five years as an appropriate time span."[135] Of course, even if a long time span would have lifted the restrictions to release certain documents, due to the mysterious disappearance of Roosevelt's medical records, we probably would have learned nothing meaningful.

Dr. Goldsmith's Research and Writings

Dr. Harry S. Goldsmith is arguably one of the most insightful medical historians dealing with the health of Franklin D. Roosevelt. A renowned surgeon with a long and illustrious clinical and academic career and a deep interest in medical history, Goldsmith has spent decades researching and writing about Roosevelt. As Goldsmith explained in his 1979 article on the subject, his interest of Roosevelt's health was initiated by a talk he listened to as a surgical resident at the Memorial Sloan Kettering Cancer Center in 1963 during which the speaker claimed that Roosevelt was suffering from a metastasizing tumor during 1944 when running for his fourth term in the White House. The curiosity sparked by that talk has had a great impact on Goldsmith for more than five decades. His continued research has generated one book and several peer-reviewed articles in medical literature.

Goldsmith's initial paper, published in December 1979, was a sensation. It was reported on the evening news of all major TV networks and created headlines in newspapers across the country. *Time* magazine wrote about the publication that "now a doctor has raised anew the suggestion that Roosevelt had terminal cancer, knew it, but chose to run for re-election in 1944 anyway."[136]

During many years, Goldsmith has spent long hours searching for the truth about Roosevelt's health. Goldsmith has followed leads and tracked down numerous individuals all over the country who had knowledge about President Roosevelt. The efforts have resulted in exciting reading, sometimes akin to page-turning detective novels. It is amazing that during the same time, Goldsmith has been able to develop a successful academic surgical career and publish close to three hundred articles and book chapters in the surgical field. Remarkably, he continues to produce unique academic articles proposing novel, "out-of-the-box," treatments for malignant brain tumors, including the use of abdominal tissue (the momentum) to increase the blood flow and delivery of chemotherapeutic drugs to the area of the brain where a tumor has been removed.[137]

Considering the secrecy surrounding Roosevelt's medical care, it is not surprising that Goldsmith has come across many controversies and discovered new facts that have made him modify statements and conclusions made during the early years of his investigations. Some of those stories will be highlighted here to illustrate the complexity involved in the research of a field rich in secrecy, deceptions, and controversies.

In his pivotal article 1979, Goldsmith suggested that based on his research, "a hypothetical instance can be constructed that a pigmented lesion over the left eye of Roosevelt could have been a melanoma."[138] More recently, however, Goldsmith has modified his opinion of Roosevelt's pigmented lesion. For example, in 2009 Goldsmith stated that "based on these observations [renewed inspection of images of Roosevelt and the scar caused by the surgical removal of the pigmented lesion], there appears to be insufficient evidence to believe that FDR had a primary melanoma involving his left eyebrow."[139]

An additional interesting discrepancy between Goldsmith's 1979 paper and some of his later writings is related to Dr. Lahey's alleged statement that he had advised the president not to run for reelection because "he had a metastatic tumor."[140] In the same article, Goldsmith reported that his colleague, surgical resident Dr. Kiley, who had attended the same talk as Goldsmith in 1963, had "confirmed that we had both heard Doctor Pack make statements that Franklin D. Roosevelt had a terminal malignant condition" and that in a subsequent talk Dr. Pack had again given "the same information to his audience on the health of Franklin D. Roosevelt that we both previously had heard."[141] Later in the 1979 article, Goldsmith implied that a melanoma above Roosevelt's left eye may have been the primary location for his metastatic tumor.[142]

In a book published almost thirty years after the 1979 article,[143] Goldsmith again tells the story about Dr. Pack's 1963 talk at the Memorial Sloan Kettering Cancer Center. This time, however, there is a difference: in the 2007 book, the reason for Lahey's advice to the president against running for reelection (that Roosevelt had a metastatic tumor) was omitted.

In his work published in 2007, Goldsmith quotes a letter from Dr. Kiley written in 1977 (two years before the 1979 article) in which Kiley claims that Lahey had told Roosevelt that he had "a metastatic carcinoma primary in the prostate, advising him not to run for re-election as he would never complete his term in office."[144] The possibility that Roosevelt had metastasizing prostate cancer was not mentioned in the 1979 paper.

The apparent discrepancies exemplified here illustrate the difficulties that arise when original documents (Roosevelt's medical records) have gone missing. Such lack of secure information and primary sources adds to the mysteries surrounding Roosevelt's health issues. Indeed, Dr. Goldsmith pointed out in his original article that "throughout the course of my study on the health of Franklin D, Roosevelt, I have noted numerous discrepancies concerning his health written by individuals who had direct knowledge of his condition. All of these discrepancies, however, would have become meaningless if President Roosevelt had had an autopsy performed. Tragically, this was not done."[145]

Conclusion

Although extraction of an abscessed tooth and removal of a sebaceous cyst are the only documented surgical procedures that Roosevelt underwent during his presidency, numerous pieces of circumstantial evidence indicate that he may have had surgery for malignant melanoma and may even have died with (or perhaps of) metastases from this malignant lesion. Whether true or not, the speculations and stories about Roosevelt's "brown blob" have kept historians and medical experts busy and generated numerous articles and books throughout the years.

In a recent commentary, Dr. Goldsmith pointed out that "most individuals are totally unaware that all of FDR's medical records disappeared within several days of his death and have never been recovered" and that "without any histological confirmation it will be impossible to gather precise knowledge of FDR's final health condition."[146] Dr. James E. Wiedeman, another surgeon and medical historian, described recently how, in the hunt for knowledge about Roosevelt's final diagnosis, he had contacted Eleanor Roosevelt II (niece of First Lady Eleanor), ninety years old at the time of Wiedeman's interview. She informed him that "her family never mentioned the possibility of cancer, but knowing her 'Uncle Franklin' he would never have allowed this to be disclosed and affect his goal to end World War II and rebuild Europe."[147]

Chapter Seven

Dwight D. Eisenhower

Did Eisenhower Have Crohn's Disease?

The Thirty-Fourth President

January 20, 1953–January 20, 1961

Dwight David Eisenhower had several encounters with surgeons throughout his life. As a young man, he underwent an appendectomy and would later undergo three additional abdominal surgeries. A heart attack after his last operation felled Eisenhower in March 1969.

Early Life

Eisenhower was born on October 14, 1890, in Denison, Texas, and moved with his family to Abilene, Kansas, at one and a half years old. He would consider Abilene his hometown for the rest of his life. He grew up under poor circumstances in a family that "had to struggle to survive."[1] He was the third of seven sons. One of his brothers died in early childhood from diphtheria, but the other boys lived into adulthood. It is almost impossible to imagine that one of the Eisenhower sons, "Little Ike," growing up in poverty, would one day be instrumental in saving the world from Hitler's tyranny and ultimately go on to become a two-term president of the United States.

Eisenhower grew up in a religious

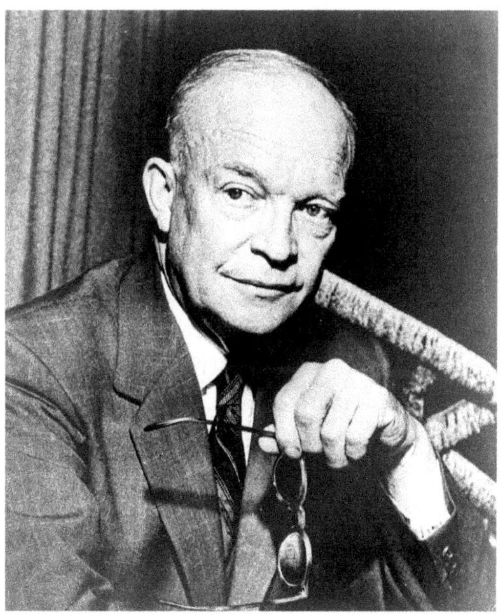

Dwight D. Eisenhower. Library of Congress, Prints and Photographs Division, Washington, D.C.

family, with time devoted every day at breakfast and dinner for Bible reading. His father, David, of Dutch immigrant descent, was strict and reinforced his discipline whenever needed.[2] David was described as "a figure more to be feared than loved by his sons."[3] Dwight's mother, Ida, was a softer soul and the person in his early life who stood for love and embracement. Although the Bible was Ida's favorite reading material, she also had an interest in history. Her collection of history books was popular reading material for young Dwight and became the source for his early and lifelong interest in military history. Little did Ida know that her son would make a career in the army. Being strongly against war and other violence, she might have kept the books away from her son had she been able to look into the future. Eisenhower's decision to enter West Point "left his mother, a pacifist, in tears."[4]

Biographers have described how Dwight showed bravery and stubbornness during his early years. As a telling story, they have described how at the age of sixteen he refused to follow his doctor's order to have his leg amputated. He had scratched his left leg when running home from school one day, and although the wound was superficial, after a couple of days it became infected.[5] The youngster developed high fevers and signs of life-threatening gangrene and sepsis. When blackness and swelling of the leg were creeping up to the knee, the family doctor explained that the leg needed to be amputated to save Dwight's life. Dwight refused, explaining to the doctor that "I'd rather die."[6] When the doctor had departed, Dwight took his brother's hand and pleaded, "You've got to promise you won't let them do it. You've got to promise. I won't be a cripple. I'd rather die."[7] Miraculously, after a couple of days' additional suffering, things turned around, and the fever, swelling, and blackness of the leg subsided. Three weeks later, Dwight was up walking around, with the leg still in place.

Despite the seriousness of the leg infection in his youth, Eisenhower seemed to have been able to forget the incident later in life. During a press conference forty years later he declared, "Rarely have I known any time in my life when I had to be concerned about my own physical feeling outside of flu or cold or something like that."[8]

Historians have also told stories showing that Dwight angered easily, even to the point of violence, when growing up. In a fight with one of his brothers, Little Ike hurled a brick toward his brother's head. Luckily enough, the sibling ducked just in time to avoid being hit. It was obvious, however, that in the heat of the brawl, Dwight "had fully intended ... to do damage with that brick."[9]

Eisenhower's temperament and tendency to get easily angered would stay with him into adulthood with detrimental consequences, both socially and medically. This would result in disciplinary actions by his superior officers while at West Point and explain the large "numbers of demerits he received."[10] One time when Eisenhower was pulled away from the golf course to take a call from Secretary of State John Foster Dulles and it turned out that the call was a mistake, Eisenhower's "anger became so real that the veins stood out on his forehead like whipcords."[11]

After Eisenhower's heart attack in 1955, his doctors warned against losing his temper.[12] The president finally understood that his bad temper could be dangerous, and he became "both dutiful and successful in following his doctors' orders to control his emotions."[13] After a short time it was reported that "not once in these months did there explode one of those outbursts of raging impatience so familiar in the past."[14]

Personal Life

Eisenhower married Mamie Doud in 1916. They had two sons. Tragically, their first son, "Ikky," died of scarlet fever at three years old. Their second son, John, was born in 1922. One of John's children, David (who, together with his great-grandfather, was the namesake of Camp David), would marry Richard Nixon's daughter, Julie, in 1968.

Some of Eisenhower's hobbies included golf, card games (particularly bridge), and oil painting (mainly landscapes but also portraits, including studies of Mamie, their grandchildren, British field marshal Bernard Law Montgomery, George Washington, and Abraham Lincoln). Even if most people probably think of golf when remembering Eisenhower's free-time activities, some were of the opinion that "the President plays better bridge than golf."[15] Golf, however, was number one for Eisenhower. He spent so much time on the golf course that "a great number of Americans ... [felt] that he should have spent more time as president and less as a golfer."[16]

It would be difficult to talk about Eisenhower's personal life without telling the story about Kay Summersby.

Kay Summersby

When Eisenhower arrived in London in May 1942, there was a beautiful woman waiting for him. Eisenhower did not know anything about the arrangement, and Kay Summersby did not know who Eisenhower was.

The pretty thirty-three-year-old fashion model had been waiting for almost three days for a group of high-ranking U.S. military officers to arrive. She was there together with other members of the Mechanised Transport Corps who had been assigned as private chauffeurs for the Americans. The officers were delayed because of bad weather. When they finally arrived, Kay was disappointed that she would be the driver for "an obscure major general named Eisenhower."[17] She was actually quite annoyed when she realized that her assignment had given her someone who was "a mere two-star ... just another flunky general of no importance." The assignment of the drivers was competitive, and to be designated the chauffeur for a high-ranking officer "was considered a mark of prestige (and snobbery) among the drivers."[18] Little did Summersby know how famous her passenger would end up being and how closely their names would be linked when history was written.

During the numerous hours Eisenhower and Summersby spent together in the car driving around in war-torn North Africa and Europe, they developed a close relationship. Eisenhower became dependent on Summersby's skills as an efficient private chauffeur and later as his personal secretary. Summersby had already proven herself to be an excellent driver, finding her way around the London streets during blackouts and fog. Eisenhower's biographer Carlo D'Este pointed out that "Eisenhower was extremely fond of Kay Summersby and valued—even treasured—her company."[19]

Summersby admired Eisenhower and, in particular, was amazed by his work ethics and his ability to put in endless hours on his tasks. As time went on, she became increasingly smitten with the general. They spent time together not only in the automobile but privately as well. Photos started to appear in the press showing them together, and rumors began to fly on both sides of the Atlantic. Later in life, Summersby would allege that they had indeed developed an intimate relationship. She claimed that they began a romance during the summer of 1943 that "included everything but sex."[20]

When Mamie Eisenhower started to see pictures in the press of her husband together with Summersby and also heard gossips about an affair, she became worried. Although she kept most of her concerns to herself, Eisenhower had an inkling about her fears and tried to reassure her about his love and faithfulness. In a letter to his wife penned in June 1943, Eisenhower wrote, "Your letters often give me some hint of your loneliness, your bewilderment and your worries in carrying on your own part in this emergency.... Just please remember that no matter how short my notes I love you—I could never be in love with anyone else—and that you fill my thoughts and hopes for the future always. You never seem to comprehend how deeply I depend upon you and need you."[21]

It is a matter of controversy how deep the relationship between Eisenhower and Summersby was. Although Summersby herself in her book *Past Forgetting: My Love Affair with Dwight D. Eisenhower* asserted that their affections had indeed been serious, others have been less convinced and have pointed out the fact that the book was written by a ghost writer at the time when Summersby was terminally ill with cancer and that most of the sensational claims likely were fabrications.[22] The rumors about the romance between Eisenhower and Summersby were dismissed as "fanciful allegations" by D'Este.[23]

There is no evidence that Eisenhower and Summersby saw each other again after the war despite the fact that Summersby, now a naturalized U.S. citizen, had moved to America. Although Mamie had had some angst about her husband and Summersby, she stayed with him, and the marriage remained intact.

Even though we may never learn all the facts about the relationship between Eisenhower and Summersby, there is no doubt that their time together during World War II became an important part of Eisenhower's personal life.

Military and Political Careers

Despite eagerly wanting to, Eisenhower was never deployed out of the country during World War I, a fact that disappointed him greatly.[24] Instead, he was stuck in the United States serving in the infantry at different camps in Texas and Georgia. His first command was with a unit training tank crews at Camp Colt in Gettysburg, Pennsylvania.

World War II would offer quite different engagements, with Eisenhower gaining ever-increasing importance. As supreme commander and a five-star general, he led the Allies in Operation Overlord and secured the defeat of Germany by successfully directing the D-Day Normandy landings on June 6, 1944. Eisenhower became an iconic hero for the defeat of the Nazi regime.

After landslide victories over Democratic candidate Adlai Stevenson, Eisenhower led two successful administrations, 1953–1961. Some of the events and achievements that stand out in people's memory from those years include the Cold War and tensions with the Soviet Union, the Korean War (1950–1953), the Suez Crisis of 1956, the launching of Sputnik in 1957 (starting a fierce competition in space with the Soviets), and the 1960 U-2 incident involving the capture and imprisonment of spy plane pilot Gary Powers. We are still reminded on a daily basis when driving on one of the highways about the Interstate Highway System authorized by President Eisenhower in 1956. The idea for this connective road system was born when Eisenhower, as a young officer in the 1920s, led a team of motorized troops coast to coast to show the need for highways across the continent.

Historians and scholars like to remind us of a warning that Eisenhower gave during his farewell address to the American people from the Oval Office on January 17, 1961, at the end of his second term: "we must guard against the acquisition of unwarranted influence, whether sought or unsought, by the military-industrial complex."[25] This statement is as well founded today as it was then.

Heavy Smoking and Heart Problems

When entering West Point in 1911, Eisenhower began chain-smoking. His cigarette addiction would continue for decades and was at its worst during the stressful days of World War II. Summersby had to put up with a lot of cigarette smoke filling the car when chauffeuring the general during the war. In her book *Eisenhower Was My Boss,* she commented that "two packs a day were quite normal."[26] One of Eisenhower's biographers made the following assessment of the general's smoking: "For years, he smoked like a furnace—60 cigarettes a day or more."[27]

The heavy smoking would finally catch up with Eisenhower. In 1948, he started to experience irregular heartbeats. In March 1949 his friend and personal physician, Howard Snyder, strongly advised Eisenhower to cut down on his smoking from four packs of cigarettes to one.[28] After a couple of days Eisenhower found that counting his cigarettes was worse than smoking, so he decided to quit "cold turkey." To prove to himself what a strong character he had, he played a funny game: "I decided to make a game of the whole business and try to achieve a feeling of some superiority.... So I stuffed cigarettes in every pocket, put them around my office on the desk ... [and] made it a practice to offer a cigarette to anyone who came in ... while mentally reminding myself as I sat down, 'I do not have to do what that poor fellow is doing.'"[29] Even though he quit smoking, damage had already been done, as would become evident from multiple cardiovascular events later in life.

In September 1955, two years into his first term as president and while on vacation at his in-laws' house in Denver, Colorado, Eisenhower suffered a serious myocardial infarction (the first of what would be about seven such events). The anger outburst after being interrupted during a golf game may have precipitated the heart attack.

It soon became clear to Dr. Snyder and his colleagues that the president had suffered a myocardial infarction. Despite that, Eisenhower's press secretary was initially instructed to announce that the president had had an episode of indigestion. Soon, however, the truth would be told. When the press was informed that the president had suffered a "moderate" heart attack, "a 3 on a 5-point scale,"[30] the news generated both political and economic consequences.

When the information hit the newsstands, it generated a precipitous sell-off on Wall Street. The Dow Jones index saw a dramatic fall, reducing the value of stocks by some $12 billion in the most serious collapse since the crash of 1929.[31]

The heart attack in September 1955 complicated Eisenhower's deliberations regarding whether to run for a second term. He had stated the year prior that "I don't want a second term. Four years in the White House is enough for one man."[32] But he was under constant pressure to try to keep the White House for one more term. Mamie tried to convince her husband to run again; she was concerned that he would become bored and depressed as a retired man. Some of his doctors were also supportive and thought that Eisenhower had healed his heart well enough to be able to sustain a grueling campaign in 1956 followed by an additional four years in the White House.

Eisenhower announced his plan to run for reelection on February 29, 1956. Despite obstacles, including the need for major surgery in the midst of the campaign, he went on to defeat Adlai Stevenson for a second time in a victory that was an even greater landslide than in 1952.

As a result of the heart attack in 1955, Eisenhower developed a ventricular aneurysm (an out-bulging of the heart wall as a result of the weakened heart muscle at the site of the infarction). Although there was disagreement between Eisenhower's doctors about whether an aneurysm had developed, after Eisenhower's death his autopsy confirmed "a large, thick and calcified walled aneurysm, ... the highly calcified wall indicating it had been present for years."[33] Indeed, "the pathologist agreed that it had probably existed since 1955."

The aneurysm became the site of a blood clot formation, and when a piece of the clot traveled to the brain, the president suffered a mild stroke on November 25, 1957. Eisenhower lost his ability to complete sentences and speak clearly and had difficulties moving his right hand. He was already on a blood thinner. After being kept in seclusion for three days, he regained most of his abilities although not completely. During a press conference he showed some remaining difficulties with his speech, and then as now the press was merciless, and some journalists made fun of the president and counted the number of goofs.[34]

More cardiovascular events were to happen. Eisenhower suffered several additional heart attacks after leaving office. A particularly severe attack afflicted the ex-president in August 1965. Four years later after his final surgery, Eisenhower suffered a postoperative myocardial infarction that resulted in his demise on March 28, 1969.

In addition to cigarette smoking, Eisenhower's health was probably also impaired by heavy alcohol consumption. Some of his drinking habits were illustrated by a story told by British prime minister Harold Macmillan's biographer, Charles Williams. During a visit to England in 1959, Eisenhower was invited for dinner to the prime minister's residence at Chequers. Before dinner, Dr. Snyder kept an eye on the president and saw him consume "several gin and tonics, and one or two gins on the rocks" as well as "three or four wines with the dinner."[35]

Even though Kay Summersby had also taken note of Eisenhower's drinking, she seemed to be less concerned than some of the doctors. In one of her biographies, she commented that "with General Ike liquor was only a social custom, necessary, but pleasantly enjoyable after one becomes hardened to it; he treated it lightly but with respect." She reassured the reader that "there is no likelihood that anyone will ever see General Eisenhower drunk. He handles liquor as respectfully and carefully as an old soldier handles a gun—a loaded gun."[36]

Most likely, Eisenhower's smoking and drinking habits weighed heavily on the surgeons' shoulders when they assessed risks involved in the surgeries the ex-president needed during his later years.

Appendectomy

In 1923, Eisenhower had his appendix taken out. During several years prior, he had experienced episodes of right lower abdominal pain. Because the pain typically resolved by itself, no further actions had been taken. Occasionally, however, the suspicion of appendicitis had been raised. Some medical historians have also raised the possibility that the recurring bouts of abdominal pain may have been early manifestations of Crohn's disease.

While on leave from his military duty in Denver in the late summer of 1923 with Mamie and son John, Eisenhower again was bothered by abdominal discomfort. He went to nearby Fitzsimmons Army Hospital, where he underwent an appendectomy. The actual circumstances around the appendectomy, including the indication for surgery, are somewhat unclear. One of Eisenhower's biographers reported that "a common myth is that Eisenhower, with single-minded determination to ensure that nothing would prevent him from playing a role in a future war, deliberately had his appendix removed."[37] The fact that Eisenhower had seen one of his friends die from acute appendicitis is a more likely reason why he was pushing for his appendix to be removed.[38] Although it is not known whether Eisenhower urged the surgeons to remove his appendix "prophylactically" or whether his abdominal examination prompted the procedure, his appendix was removed.

Notwithstanding that the microscopic examination of the appendix was reported as showing "chronic catarrhal appendicitis,"[39] an inflammation affecting the superficial layer of the appendiceal mucosa, one of Eisenhower's biographers mentioned that "the organ turned out not to be diseased."[40] Mamie remembered that the diagnosis was "not definite."[41]

Another and perhaps even more peculiar detail about Eisenhower's appendectomy is that he did not inform his wife when he sought treatment at the Fitzsimmons Army Hospital; she was notified only after the procedure.[42] After spending fifteen days in the hospital following the appendectomy, Eisenhower returned to military duty. Two weeks of hospital stay after an appendectomy may seem unusually long, but those were the days before same-day surgeries and short hospital stays after most surgical procedures.

In addition to his appendix, Eisenhower also lost his tonsils early in life. After having been hospitalized for a severe throat infection in 1919, he returned to the hospital for a tonsillectomy (the surgical removal of the tonsils). Seventeen years later he had another episode of throat infection and underwent a second tonsillectomy, with "removal of remnants of his tonsils."[43]

General Eisenhower's "Melanoma"

An anecdote about the removal of a skin lesion was provided by a dermatologist who was a witness to the event in 1944. Dr. Donald M. Pillsbury was a consultant in dermatology to the Committee of Medicine of the National Research Council and was responsible for dermatologic morbidity in the U.S. Army. In the fall of 1944 after the liberation of the French capital, Pillsbury was stationed at the Office of Chief Surgeon in Paris. One morning when he noticed some unusual tension and excitement in the office, he asked one of the surgeons what was going on. He was informed that the supreme commander had a melanoma on his trunk and that the surgeon was going to the headquarters at Rheims to "cut it out."[44] Pillsbury wished the surgeon success and saw him depart "speedily in a staff car."

When the surgeon returned late in the afternoon, he proudly showed Pillsbury a bottle containing a good-sized specimen of fat and skin. When Pillsbury, with his dermatologic expertise, saw a blackish nodule on the skin side of the specimen, he told the surgeon that "this is an absolutely typical seborrhoic keratosis, and I'll wager you 100 to 1 on it."[45] Instead of being celebrated for the successful removal of a malignant skin lesion on the supreme commander, the surgeon was criticized for performing unnecessary surgery! The microscopic examination confirmed Pillsbury's diagnosis, and "those with knowledge of the original diagnoses heaved sighs of relief."[46]

But the story didn't end here.

Years later when Pillsbury was presiding over the Annual Meeting of the Society of Medical Consultants to the Armed Forces at Walter Reed Hospital, President Eisenhower happened to be at the hospital for his annual physical checkup. Pillsbury described how "through the good office of my friend, Dr. I.S. Ravdin, the President agreed to appear at our meeting."[47] During his short remarks from the podium, Eisenhower said that he "owed a debt to some consultants because they had probably saved his life by getting rid of a malignant growth on his skin." Clearly, Eisenhower still believed that the dark spot had been a melanoma. Pillsbury thanked the president for his presence but did not make any further comments. In his mind, however, he contemplated "never underestimate the persuasive powers of a general surgeon who regards all darkly pigmented lesions as melanoma,"[48] probably remembering a favorite saying of many surgeons: "When in doubt, cut it out."

President Eisenhower's Operation for Bowel Obstruction Caused by "Regional Enteritis"

June 8, 1956, got off to a bad start for the president. The new day had just begun when at 12:30 a.m. Eisenhower began experiencing abdominal pain. The evening before he had attended the annual banquet of the White House Press Photographers Association, where Bob Hope had provided entertainment and drinks and food had been had. When Eisenhower woke up from the belly pain he initially suspected that he was suffering from indigestion, but when the pain became excruciating, Mamie asked Dr. Snyder to come and see his patient. When the doctor arrived at 2 a.m., both he and the president were hoping the pain would go away by itself, as it had on so many previous occasions. But this time would be different. The pain did not show any signs of abating; if anything, it grew worse. The abdomen started to become distended, and the president started to feel nauseated and ultimately vomited. What happened over the next twenty-four hours has been well documented in the medical literature. Here, we will rely on detailed descriptions provided by surgeons who were directly involved in the care of the president during the hours leading up to the surgery, performed the procedure, and took care of the patient after the operation.

Eisenhower had been diagnosed multiple times previously with partial small bowel obstruction, and the cause of the problems had been suspected to be intra-abdominal adhesions (scar tissue) that had formed after his appendectomy in 1923. At least on one previous occasion, Eisenhower was close to having surgery for his intestinal problems. While stationed in the Philippines in the 1930s, working under Douglas MacArthur, Eisenhower had a new encounter with abdominal pain. He checked into a hospital in Manila on January 28, 1938, with severe abdominal pain caused by an intestinal obstruction so severe that his abdomen was distended like that of a "dying frog."[49] The surgeons explained to Eisenhower that he had a dangerous "stoppage of the bowel" and made preparations to operate. Eisenhower reportedly fainted from the pain and woke up on the operating table just when he was about to be put to sleep. He stopped the procedure, explaining that "I think I would like to go to the toilet." The visit to the bathroom relieved Eisenhower from some of his pain and distention, and the surgery was called off. Later when back in his sickroom, Eisenhower was able to "expel the rest of the gas." This was done in the presence of a nurse stationed at his bedside, an event that made the private Eisenhower terribly embarrassed. When remembering the ordeal, he looked back at the tribulation as "the tortures of the damned."[50]

Although Eisenhower was able to avoid surgery in 1938, eighteen years later when having another small bowel obstruction, he was less lucky and could not escape the knife.

Further investigations of the recurrent bouts of bowel obstruction had been performed in May 1956, and the results suggested that there may be an additional reason, other than adhesions, for the problem. A "small bowel series" (abdominal X-rays with contrast in the small intestine) revealed a narrowed area in the most distal part of the small bowel, interpreted as being consistent with regional enteritis, or Crohn's disease, a pathological entity described in the literature only about twenty-five years earlier, and this was considered the likely cause of the president's more recent episodes of abdominal discomfort.[51]

When Dr. Snyder arrived at the White House in the wee hours of June 8, he found the president to be in significant discomfort. On examination, the abdomen was distended and tympanitic but without localized tenderness. The president was able to get some sleep during the early morning hours but woke up again with worsening pain that had now become colicky. A tap water enema at 6 a.m. did not relieve the pain, and later in the morning the president vomited 1.5 liters of bile-stained fluid.

The patient's condition deteriorated, and he became "listless, apathetic, perspiring freely, with his skin somewhat cool and clammy and with his normal ruddy color absent."[52] His pulse rate was 120 per minute, and his blood pressure had fallen to 100/76 mm Hg. The signs of threatening shock were alarming, and after he was stabilized with intravenous fluids, he was transferred by ambulance to Walter Reed General Hospital at 1:30 p.m.

On the president's arrival at the hospital, his abdomen remained distended. When listening to the abdomen, the doctors noticed that the bowel sounds were "hypoactive, with occasional high-pitched sounds,"[53] findings that indicated that the bowel was working against a blockage.

A surgical team consisting of Drs. Leonard Heaton (commander at Walter Reed), Isidor Ravdin (chairman of surgery, University of Pennsylvania, Philadelphia), Brian Blades (chairman of surgery, George Washington University, Washington, D.C.), and John Lyons (considered the premier private practice surgeon in Washington at the time) was assembled at the hospital by 6 p.m. It was now obvious that the president had another bout of bowel obstruction, which was also confirmed by an X-ray of the abdomen at 1 a.m. on June 9, revealing significantly dilated loops of small bowel.[54] Something had to be done, but the decision to operate was not an easy one. The surgeons were dealing with a patient who was sixty-five years old, had suffered a serious heart attack only nine months earlier, and was on anticoagulant therapy. And on top of all that, he was the president of the United States in the midst of a campaign running for reelection. Although Dr. Lyons initially felt that observation rather than immediate operation would be the best approach, when Eisenhower's condition did not show any signs of improvement, Lyons agreed with his colleagues, and the team of surgeons unanimously felt that they had no choice but to recommend surgery.[55] The angst felt by the surgeons was reflected by a note in the patient's chart written by Dr. Ravdin:

> There can be no doubt that the President has intestinal obstruction of an acute nature. The films made of his large and small bowel on May 11, 1956, disclose areas of the terminal ileum which are identical with those seen in an area of regional enteritis with "skip areas."
>
> He has drained moderately from his gastric tube, but in spite of this the number of loops which are distended has increased as recorded in the last x-ray over that taken at 1830 hours.
>
> The abdomen is softer. Peristalsis is present at times. The pulse has shown a tendency to become more rapid.
>
> He has passed no gas by rectum. Urinary output of 490 cc. shows that his kidneys are functioning.
>
> The dilemma facing us is whether to delay operation further or to go ahead and side-track

> the area of obstruction. Because the distended gut area has increased, because the condition has existed for 24 hours, because operation with the patient in good condition is safer than waiting until the necessity of operation is forced upon us, I favor intervention.
>
> The only alternative to this would be long tube (Miller-Abbott) intubation, which, if it gives evidence of emptying the small gut is defensible. If it does not give such evidence promptly, I would again favor laparotomy.[56]

The president was brought to the operating room and put to sleep at 2:20 a.m. on June 9, 1956. The incision was made at 2:57 a.m., and the surgery took about two hours. When Eisenhower's abdomen was opened, the surgeons confirmed the cause of the obstruction. The terminal thirty to forty centimeters of the ileum "presented the typical appearance of chronic so-called dry enteritis. That is, the involved area was grayish-red, thickened, indurated, and contracted." That this part of the bowel was the cause of obstruction was evident from the finding that "the small bowel immediately proximal to the involved area was greatly dilated." Luckily, the bowel had not been injured by the obstruction, because "the color (of the distended bowel) was pink."[57]

Although resection (removal) of the diseased area of the bowel could have been an option, the surgeons decided to perform an ileotransverse colostomy (connecting and creating an opening between the ileum above the area of obstruction and the transverse portion of the colon), thus bypassing the narrow area and allowing intestinal content to flow freely from the small bowel to the colon.

Overall, the president did well after the surgery. He was out of bed on the first postoperative day. He was able to pass gas after five days and was allowed to resume regular food intake a week after surgery. The president started to transact official business on the fifth postoperative day. He received official visitors in his hospital room, including Secretary of State Dulles and Chancellor Konrad Adenauer of West Germany. Except for a minor wound infection on the eleventh postoperative day, Eisenhower did not have any complications from the surgery. He was discharged from the hospital 21 days after the operation.

Although from his surgeons' perspective Eisenhower had a basically uneventful postoperative course, the pain he experienced from his abdominal incision was significant. His vice president commented that the president "suffered more pain over a lager period of time" and "looked far worse than he had in 1955 [after the heart attack]."[58] When Eisenhower's son visited the hospital, he found his father in a lot of pain and stated that "Dad was suffering severely."[59]

Unsurprisingly, word about Eisenhower's illness and his transfer to Walter Reed spread rapidly and made headlines the same day. Front-page banners were screaming "IKE ILL, TO UNDERGO MAJOR SURGERY," followed by "Friend and Foe Hope for Quick Recovery."[60] Other headlines described that Eisenhower needed the surgery to ease bowel obstruction.

In addition to the concerns for the president's health and wishes for a speedy recovery, the press also became flooded with analyses of the political and economic aspects of Eisenhower's illness. The news of Eisenhower's surgery resulted in a "nervous fall" on Wall Street, although many of the losses were recovered before the end of the day. Similar fluctuations on the stock market had been seen about half a year

THE AMERICAN PAPER FOR AMERICANS

Chicago Daily Tribune

THE WORLD'S GREATEST NEWSPAPER

Founded June 10, 1847

★★★SPORTS FINAL

VOLUME CXV—NO. 138 | [REG. U.S. PAT. OFFICE: © 1956 BY THE CHICAGO TRIBUNE] | SATURDAY JUNE 9, 1956 | THIS PAPER CONSISTS OF FOUR SECTIONS—SECTION ONE | F | FIVE CENTS—PAY NO MORE

OPERATE ON IKE!

Quit Germany, Bulganin Urges

U. S. Consigned 'to Grave' by Khrushchev

BY WILLARD EDWARDS
(Chicago Tribune Press Service)

Washington, June 8—Nikita Khrushchev, Communist party boss in Russia, told Red leaders in Warsaw shortly before the Geneva conference last year that peaceful co-existence between east and west was impossible and that the United States must be "pushed into the grave."

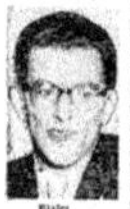

Bialer

This sharp contradiction between Khrushchev's public and private utterances was revealed to the senate internal security subcommittee by Seweryn Bialer, an escaped Polish Communist party official, whose defection was announced yesterday. He crossed the border into West Germany last Jan. 31 and arrived in the United States May 4.

Names Spies in United States

The 29 year old witness not only disclosed the Kremlin's secret policies but aired new details of the liquidation of the Russian police chief, Beria, and the removals of Molotov and Malenkov from office.

"Stalin and Beria are gone but the same terroristic methods remain," he testified, thru an interpreter. His defection is regarded by American intelligence as the most important in many months and his testimony was recorded for broadcasting by Radio Free Europe to Russia and its satellites.

Others Eager to Defeat

Bialer also revealed the identities of two Russians who served in the United States as soviet spies. One, he said, was Col. Melchior of the Kremlin's military intelligence who assumed the "cover" of vice consul at the Polish consulate in New York City from 1949 to 1955.

The other espionage agent, Bialer said, was Capt. Samuel Ehrlich of Russian military intelligence, who was sent to the United States in 1951 with an assignment to obtain a post at an American university and spend two years here.

Bialer had told the subcommittee in executive session

[Continued on page 4, col. 5]

Tribune Features

News summaries on page 4

Asks 4 Nations to Join in Calling Home Troops

O. K. SLASHED AID BILL
House votes tentative O.K. for 3.8 billion dollar foreign aid program, cut more than 1 billion below what President Eisenhower asked. Story on page 3.

BY ROBERT YOUNG
(Chicago Tribune Press Service)

Washington, June 8—Russian Premier Bulganin proposed to President Eisenhower in a letter which the White House made public tonight that the United States, Britain, and France join the soviet union in withdrawing part of their military forces from Germany as a concrete move toward possible general disarmament.

The Bulganin letter dealt generally with world disarmament, asserting the soviet premier thought Mr. Eisenhower would agree "that at the present time, the problem of disarmament continues to be one of the most important and urgent international problems."

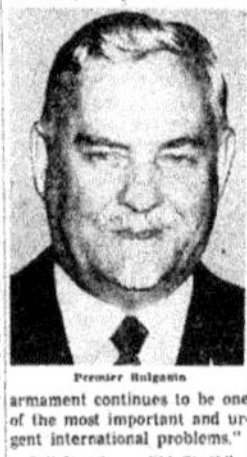

Premier Bulganin

Call It "Same Old Stuff"

Bulganin spoke of the vast sacrifices and losses of World War II and the threat of "mass destruction" by nuclear weapons in the future. The letter, Bulganin said, "makes the necessity of solving the problems of disarmament particularly urgent."

Despite Bulganin's assertion that the soviet union has decided to "make a new approach to the solution of the disarmament problem" in view of the Kremlin's conviction that international tension is easing and the "cold war" is "becoming a thing of the past, top Eisenhower administration sources dismissed the latest letter as "the same old stuff."

Skips Over Ike's Proposals

These sources said the latest letter from Moscow to President Eisenhower on the subject of disarmament was, in their opinion, nothing more than another attempt to "exploit" the maximum propaganda gain from Russia's announcement May 14 that it would reduce its military strength 1,200,000 troops by May, 1957, and would make further cuts if this country, Britain, and France also would reduce their armed strength.

The soviet union, the sources continued, gave no assurance in the Bulganin letter that anything would be done to lessen the threat of nuclear weapons and nothing to implement

[Continued on page 4, col. 1]

'SHOOT TO KILL' HUNT IS ON FOR TRIPLE KILLER

16 States Alerted for Fugitive

A 16 state police alarm was sent out yesterday for an ex-convict with a shotgun who killed two men and a woman in a burst of gunfire in a north side cabaret.

Police were ordered to "shoot on sight" Lawrence Neumann, 29, of 6150 Rockwell st. He was believed heading for Mexico in his cream and brown 1953 model car.

Twenty teams of detectives searched the area around the Screwball club, 3320 Broadway, where he was reported seen as late as 9:30 a. m. yesterday, more than seven hours after the shootings. A bartender there reported a man matching Neumann's description made a telephone call from the tavern and left in the car of a stranger who arrived five minutes later.

Description Is Given

Police broadcast this description of Neumann: 6 feet 1 inch tall, weighing 190 pounds, brown hair and brown eyes, and ruddy complexion. He was wearing a light blue shirt, blue slacks, and a blue striped cap such as worn by railroad engineers and firemen.

Victims of the shooting in Mickey and Maxie's Miracle cabaret, 1114 Argyle st., were Max Epstein, 50, of 5009 Sheridan rd., bartender and part owner of the tavern; Mrs. Lois Gates, 27, of 925 Carmen av., a divorcee and dice girl; and John Keller, 49, of 4746 Kenmore av., a news dealer.

Grudge Is Nursed

Mrs. Gates and Keller were innocent victims of Neumann's wrath against Max Epstein and his brother, Mickey, 36, also of 5009 Sheridan rd. and part owner of the cabaret, police said.

The Epsteins had Neumann arrested on a disorderly conduct charge May 9 as the result of an altercation. He in turn had them arrested on a charge of assault with intent to kill. Altho all charges were dismissed May 16 in Town Hall court, police said Neumann

[Continued on page 7, col. 1]

THE WEATHER

SATURDAY, JUNE 9, 1956

CHICAGO AND VICINITY: Fair and warm today; high, in 80s, except lower near lake; low tonight, 62; variable winds, becoming light northeasterly. Partly cloudy tomorrow; high, in 80s, lower near lake.

ILLINOIS: Fair and warmer today; partly cloudy tomorrow and continued warm; chance of scattered thundershowers in northwest tomorrow afternoon or tomorrow night.

TEMPERATURES IN CHICAGO

7 a. m....60	3 p. m....80	11 p. m....70
8 a. m....66	4 p. m....†81	Midnight....67
9 a. m....69	5 p. m....80	1 a. m....67
10 a. m....74	6 p. m....81	2 a. m....66
11 a. m....75	7 p. m....78	3 a. m....*65
Noon....77	8 p. m....77	4 a. m....*64
1 p. m....77	9 p. m....74	5 a. m....*63
2 p. m....79	10 p. m....72	6 a. m....*61

†High. ‡Low. *Unofficial.

THE MOON

New June 8 · Waxing June 9-14 · First Qu. June 15 · Full June 23 · Last Qu. July 1 · Waning July 24

Sunrise, 5:16. Sunset, 8:24. Moonrise, 7:18 a. m. tomorrow. Morning stars: Mars and Mercury. Evening stars: Jupiter, Saturn, and Venus.

For 24 hours ended 7:30 p. m., June 8: Mean temperature, 74 degrees; normal, 68; month's deficiency, 20; year's excess, 136. Precipitation, none; month's deficiency, 1.06 inches; year's deficiency, 2.25 inches. Highest wind velocity, 13 m. p. h. Relative humidity: 7:30 a. m., 80 per cent; 1:30 p. m., 43; 7:30 p. m., 35. Barometer, 7:30 a.m., 29.99; 7:30 p. m., 30.02.

[Map and other reports on page 12]

Concern for President, in Hospital Again

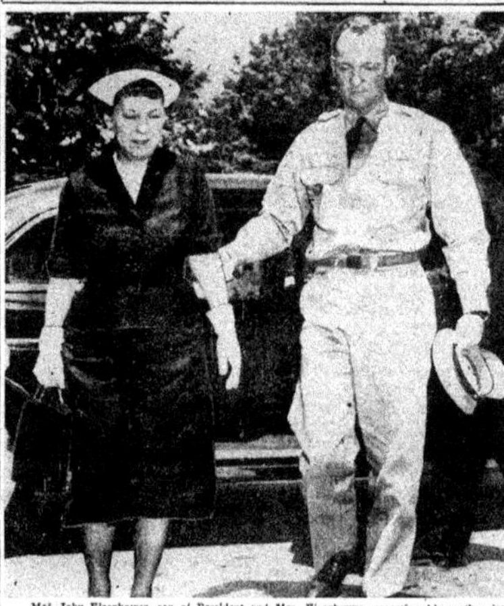

Maj. John Eisenhower, son of President and Mrs. Eisenhower, escorting his mother into Walter Reed hospital in Washington yesterday after President was stricken with intestinal ailment and was taken to hospital. [United Press Telephoto]

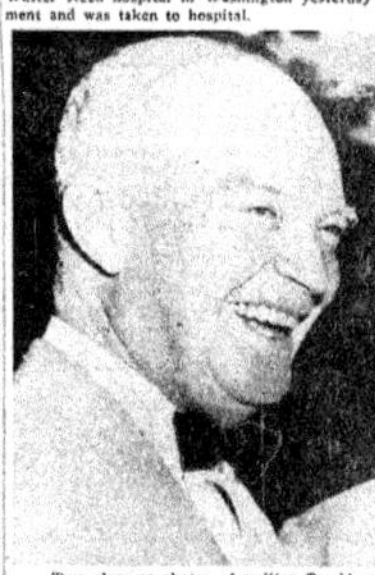

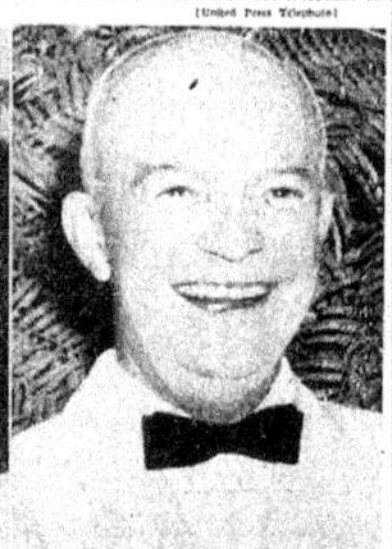

Two close-up photos of smiling President taken Thursday night at Washington Press Photographers dinner before he became ill. [Associated Press Wirephoto]

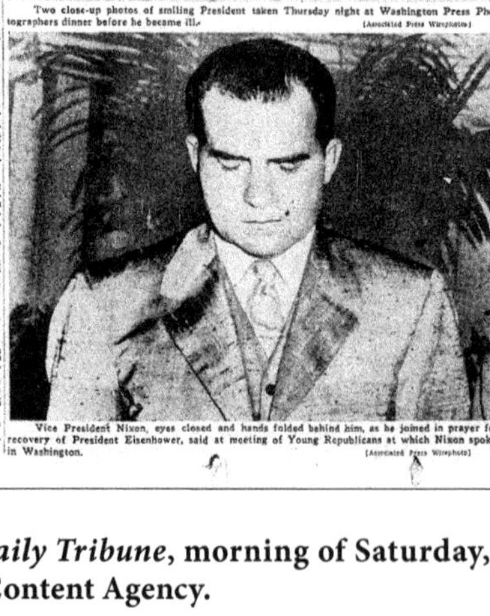

Vice President Nixon, eyes closed and hands folded behind him, as he joined in prayer for recovery of President Eisenhower, said at meeting of Young Republicans at which Nixon spoke, in Washington. [Associated Press Wirephoto]

EXPLORATORY SURGERY TO EASE OBSTRUCTION

President Stricken During Night; Rushed in Ambulance to Army Hospital

MAMIE FOLLOWS IKE TO HOSPITAL
Turn to back page for picture of Mrs. Eisenhower as she accompanied ambulance taking stricken President to hospital. Other pictures pertaining to President's illness are on pages 2, 3, and back page.

BY WALTER TROHAN
(Chicago Tribune Press Service)

Washington, June 9 [Saturday]—President Eisenhower this morning was under operation for an obstruction of the lower intestine. The operation was decided upon by a team of consulting doctors.

A team of four doctors performed the operation in operating room No. 6 on the third floor. The President underwent general anesthesia.

The operation began at 1:59 a. m. Chicago time.

The operation was described as exploratory to discover and relieve the cause of the obstruction.

The decision to operate was announced by Hagerty in a statement to reporters keeping vigil at the hospital. He said:

"It is the considered opinion of the physicians in attendance that since the previously mentioned partial obstruction in the terminal portion of the small intestine has persisted, an exploratory operation is necessary."

List Four Surgeons

Those engaged in the operation were Maj. Gen. Leonard D. Heaton, commanding general of the hospital; Isadore Ravdin, professor of surgery at the University of Pennsylvania medical school; Col. Robert T. Gant, chief of surgery at Walter Reed, and Lt. Col. Max Smith, assistant chief of surgery at Walter Reed.

The doctors present as observers were Dr. Brian Blades, professor of surgery at George Washington university, and Dr. John H. Lyons, Washington surgeon.

The operating doctors were attended by a medical staff of assistants.

The operation was decided upon after a midnight consultation at which the 13 participating doctors ordered a third X-ray. The X-ray was called for in order to determine whether surgery should be undertaken.

Earlier at 8:35 p. m. yesterday, it had been announced that there was "no indication for immediate surgery" when Mr. Eisenhower was reported to be progressing satisfactorily.

Mamie, John Present

Mrs. Eisenhower was standing by in the hospital with her son, Maj. John Eisenhower, who is stationed at nearby Fort Belvoir, Va. Dr. Milton Eisenhower, President of Pennsylvania state college, was also standing by.

Hagerty repeatedly refused to go beyond the statement he read to reporters:

"I think you can understand my position," he said.

The operation was reported to have begun a short time after Hagerty made his announcement to newsmen, who settled down for their vigil.

Hagerty was asked if there was any consideration of malignancy involved. He replied that has not been considered at any time.

The only evidence of the drama of a President who had

NATURE OF IKE'S AILMENT TOLD BY VAN DELLEN

BY DR. THEODORE R. VAN DELLEN
(Health Editor of The Tribune)
(Drawing on page 2)

The ilium is the last third of the intestine and its inflammation [ileitis] leads to a swelling of the wall with narrowing of the passageway. A moderate swelling of the wall produces a partial obstruction, whereas a marked swelling blocks the opening of the intestine completely.

The early stage of ileitis mimics appendicitis with pain in the lower abdomen, nausea, and vomiting. With the onset of obstruction, the pain becomes more colicky and the abdomen is distended. X-rays are needed to locate the obstruction.

Cause Is Unknown

The most common type of ileitis is regional ileitis. It is more prevalent in young persons and the cause is not known.

Patients with this type of ileitis usually require surgery in time and recurrences are likely. Other causes for inflammation include tuberculosis and typhoid fever. Cancer of this part of the intestine seldom occurs. Mechanical obstructions caused by hernia, adhesions, kinking, and constipation are more common.

The treatment of an obstruction of this nature depends upon the nature and extent of the inflammation.

May Subside Spontaneously

President Eisenhower's physicians will be as conservative as possible because of his recent heart attack. There is a good possibility that the inflammation in his case will subside spontaneously or respond to intestinal antiseptics.

A simple emergency lifesaving operation is done occasionally to allow the intestinal contents to escape thru an artificial opening in the abdominal wall.

In this way, the obstruction is bypassed and the inflamed loop of intestine is put out of commission temporarily and given a rest.

The front page of the *Chicago Daily Tribune*, morning of Saturday, June 9, 1956. Published with permission of the Tribune Content Agency.

EDITORIALS — THE DAILY PRESS

NEWPORT NEWS • HAMPTON • WARWICK, VA., SATURDAY MORNING, JUNE 9, 1956

Political Aspects Of The President's Illness

Although we are sure nobody wanted it that way, Democratic chances for capturing the presidency in the November elections have been given a big boost by Mr. Eisenhower's unfortunate illness.

The health issue is bound to be a strong factor if Ike is the candidate. Even the optimistic Republican National Chairman Leonard Hall conceded that it would be an issue in spite of the remarkable recovery the President made from his heart attack last September. But it is bound to be a much more persuasive issue now; even if it turns out as we all hope and pray it will, that there is no cardiac connection to this illness. But it will raise doubts in the minds of many voters that Mr. Eisenhower enjoys the robust health that he once did. It will be suspected that he is "brittle."

Many of us have had the uneasy feeling lately that Mr. Eisenhower was doing too much. Those 27 holes of golf he played no more than ten days ago was convincing evidence of that; the Richmond News Leader's scolding editorial convinced us that it was a foolhardy thing for him to do. And you have only to look at that double-page spread in the U. S. News and World Report of June 1, labelled: "In One Week Ike Did These Things, Saw These People" to convince you that the President was over-doing it.

Was he trying to contradict those political adversaries who had been charging that he was a "part-time President?" We don't think so. We are told that even under doctors' orders Mr. Eisenhower does not always find it easy to go slow. He is a naturally active man.

He finds he cannot suppress all his old habits without seeking release of energy in other trivial habits. He still toys with his glasses, nibbling at the bows, when in a reflective mood. In the privacy of his White House home, Mr. Eisenhower had a habit of occasionally mounting stairs two steps at a time. That was a practice doctors ordered him to stop. But sometimes lately he forgets these orders. He was seen striding up stairs two steps at a time.

We are sure the President will not permit the Republicans to renominate him if he is convinced in his own mind that his health would not permit him to be a "full time President" for another four years if he was reelected in November. But his chances of reelection undoubtedly have been set back considerably by this illness. Under the circumstances we are reluctantly forced to the conclusion that it would be better if he changed his mind about running again. There is no point in his staying on such a trying job if it is going to kill him.

Editorial, the *Daily Press*, Saturday, June 9, 1956, page 4. Published with permission of the Tribune Content Agency.

earlier when the losses in conjunction with the president's heart attack were followed by a surge in stock values after his doctors declared Eisenhower fit.[61] The main political question in June 1956 was whether Eisenhower's illness would influence the upcoming presidential election in November. Some journalists speculated that "the Democratic chances for capturing the presidency in the November elections have been given a big boost by Mr. Eisenhower's unfortunate illness."[62]

Eisenhower's Surgeons Criticized by Colleagues

Disappointingly, it did not take long before Eisenhower's surgeons were criticized for their performance both privately and publicly by colleagues, "many of them surgeons but many of them from decidedly remote specialties."[63] For example, the president's surgeons described how a professor of preventative medicine voiced the opinion that that he "did not think that the bypass we had created could possibly prove competent." The president's surgeons were outraged by the criticism from many colleagues. They felt that that "only surgeons with a close-up view of the Eisenhower peritoneal cavity had any right to comment on what had been done within it."[64] Some people, however, were supportive of the surgeons. For example, "one reporter stated it quite well when he wrote that criticism multiplied in direct ratio to the distance of the critics from the operating room and from the patient."[65]

There were mainly two issues surrounding the surgery that were subjected to disapproval. First, some of the critics questioned whether it was necessary to subject the president to an emergency operation instead of giving more time for the condition to resolve spontaneously (as had happened on previous occasions). The other issue was the choice of the bypass procedure instead of resection (removal) of the diseased part of the bowel, potentially risking renewed abdominal problems in the future from the retained segment of the intestine. The first issue was preemptively addressed by the note in the patient's chart written by Ravdin before taking the president to the operating room. The other point of disagreement was addressed vigorously by the surgeons by explaining that the main goal of the operation was to relieve the bowel obstruction and that it needed to be done expeditiously, with the patient on the operating table for as short time as possible (a resection would undoubtedly have taken longer time than the bypass). The surgeons felt vindicated by the fact that the president had a smooth postoperative course and that there had been no evidence of persisting or recurrent problems from the terminal ileitis, at least not up to seven and a half years when the article was written in which they defended their procedure.[66]

Was It Crohn's Disease?

Although most previous reports in medical literature reported that the cause of Eisenhower's bowel obstruction in 1956 was "regional enteritis" (a term strongly indicating Crohn's disease), at least one medical historian, Adrian Marston, has questioned the diagnosis.[67] In doing so, several factors were listed as to why the obstruction in the president's intestine may not have been Crohn's disease. Among those factors were the patient's age at the time of his operation (it is less common that a patient experiences the first symptoms and manifestations of Crohn's disease at the age of sixty-six); the findings on the small bowel X-ray on May 11, 1956, which in retrospect may not have been typical for Crohn's disease; and the fact that no additional lesions developed after Eisenhower's surgery in 1956 and that the narrow area in the terminal ileum remained unchanged on multiple X-rays over the following decade.

If the obstruction resulting in Eisenhower's operation in 1956 was not caused by Crohn's disease, what else could it have been? Marston, in his writing, proposed that it may have been scar tissue resulting from ischemia (reduced blood flow) secondary to a drop in blood pressure when the president had his myocardial infarction in 1955. In support of his theory, the author quoted examples from medical literature where such a mechanism had resulted in ischemic strictures of the intestine. A detailed documentation of Eisenhower's blood pressure on September 24, 1955, revealed that his systolic blood pressure fell precipitously from 180 to 90 mm Hg immediately after the heart attack.[68]

Because Eisenhower's surgery was performed primarily to relieve his bowel obstruction, rather than to remove the diseased part of the intestine, it may be argued that the discussion about the underlying cause of the obstruction is merely an academic exercise. However, the distinction between an inflammatory and ischemic lesion causing the obstruction and necessitating an emergency operation in a patient as prominent as an American president adds an important footnote to history and may be worth contemplating.

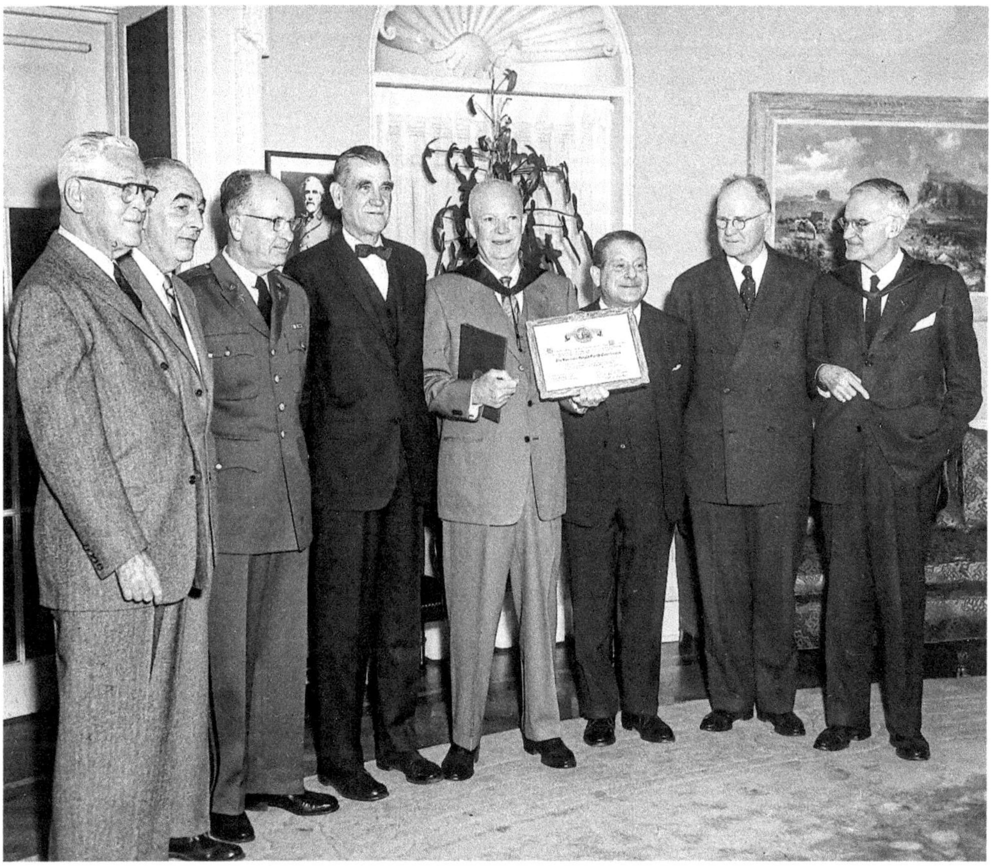

President Eisenhower receiving an Honorary ACS Fellowship in the White House with his medical team, February 6, 1958. From left: Dr. Howard Snyder, Dr. Brian Blades, Dr. Leonard Heaton, Dr. John Lyons, President Eisenhower, Dr. Isidor Ravdin, Dr. Frank Barry, and National Security Advisor Robert Cutler. University Archives, University of Pennsylvania, Ravdin Papers, box 14, folder 4. Published with the permission of University Archives and Records Center, University of Pennsylvania.

The American College of Surgeons and the President's Operation in 1956

The American College of Surgeons (ACS) is a prestigious and influential organization of surgeons in North America founded in 1913 to promote the quality and safety of surgical care. All surgeons on the team taking care of Eisenhower in 1956 were fellows (members) of the ACS. One of the surgeons, Dr. Isidor Ravdin, had a leadership role in the ACS and was actually presiding over an ACS Board of Regents meeting in Chicago on June 9, 1956, when he was summoned to Washington by his wartime friend Dr. Leonard Heaton to attend to the president.[69] Although Ravdin was formally reprimanded in a letter from the Board of Regents for practicing "itinerant surgery," in the same letter he was praised for bringing honor to the ACS.[70]

After the surgery, Eisenhower in a telegram dated October 5, 1956, gratefully acknowledged the ACS for the assistance its surgeons provided during his illness.[71] The ACS reciprocated the president's kind words by appointing him an honorary fellow of the organization at a White House ceremony in February 1958.

Removal of Eisenhower's Gallbladder

Eisenhower started to have symptoms of gallstones in August 1966. He was bothered by indigestion, belching, abdominal pain, and discomfort, sometimes radiating up behind his breastbone. An X-ray of the gallbladder showed multiple gallstones.

Because of continued symptoms and because they could be difficult to differentiate from cardiac disease (particularly important in Eisenhower's case, considering his medical history of multiple heart attacks), a cholecystectomy (removal of the gallbladder) was recommended.

After consultations with Eisenhower's cardiologists, the surgeons took him to the operating room on December 12, 1966, and removed the gallbladder through a right "subcostal incision," an incision placed below and parallel to the right costal margin. These incisions typically measured between three and five inches in length (laparoscopic, minimally invasive, cholecystectomies, so-called "key hole surgeries," using small incisions measuring about half an inch, were still twenty years in the future). A diseased gallbladder containing sixteen gallstones was removed "without difficulty."[72] Knowing about Eisenhower's previous bowel surgery, the doctors were curious about what the area of that procedure would look like. In particular, they wanted to check the connection between the ileum and the colon created by the ileotransverse colostomy created in 1956, but adhesions prevented access to the right upper abdomen and examination of the bowel; "these adhesions were not disturbed."[73]

Eisenhower had an uneventful recovery after the cholecystectomy. He was out of bed the day after surgery. The stitches could be removed on the fifth postoperative day. "The patient elected to remain in the hospital until the 15th day after operation to regain his strength and for further cardiac evaluation."[74]

The Final Surgery

When Eisenhower underwent his final operation in 1969, he was an extremely high-risk patient. The year prior, he had suffered multiple heart attacks during a prolonged hospitalization. He suffered his fourth myocardial infarction in April 1968, and during the remainder of the year he had three additional myocardial infarctions. In August his heart went into ventricular fibrillation (an especially dangerous heart arrhythmia), requiring defibrillation on fourteen separate occasions from August 16 through August 24. In a medical report, it was dramatically declared that "it is scarcely an exaggeration to state that he 'died' 14 times."[75]

Such was Eisenhower's medical history when he again arrived at the hospital with evidence of small bowel obstruction. Early on the morning of February 21, 1969, Eisenhower woke up with "severe sharp non-colicky pain just to the right of the umbilicus."[76] Even though the surgeons were probably praying and hoping they would not have to operate on this high-risk patient and that the obstruction would resolve spontaneously as it had on several previous occasions, it became evident after a couple of days' observation that the obstruction was not going to settle. After consultations between the surgeons and the cardiologists, it was determined that surgery was needed, despite Eisenhower's extreme cardiac risks.

The ex-president's final operation commenced at 9:20 p.m. on February 23, 1969.[77] The surgeons found that the small bowel was blocked by adhesions that had formed between the intestine and the inside of the abdominal wall. The blockage was released by dividing the adhesions. The anastomosis (connection) between the ileum and the colon created thirteen years earlier was found to be open. The diseased segment of intestine left behind in the patient's abdomen when the bypass procedure was performed did not show any evidence of progressive disease, vindicating the surgeons' decision to perform a bypass procedure rather than resection in 1956.

After the operation, Eisenhower was monitored extremely carefully—and nervously—by the surgeons and cardiologists. The first couple of weeks, the patient seemed to be doing relatively well. The nasogastric tube (a tube inserted into the stomach through the nose to evacuate fluids from the stomach) could be removed four days after surgery. The patient was able to sit up in bed after two additional days. But then the heart started to act up again. Eisenhower's cardiac status began to deteriorate in mid–March, and despite the efforts of the cardiologists, President Eisenhower expired at 12:25 p.m. on March 28, 1969.

The Autopsy and the Surprising Pheochromocytoma

At the postmortem examination, the opening (stoma) between the small and large bowels created when the ileotransverse colostomy was performed in 1956 was wide open, measuring four centimeters. The narrowed area of the terminal ileum that had been bypassed by the surgeons thirteen years earlier seemed to be "essentially unchanged." When it was opened, it was thick-walled and fibrotic and showed microscopic changes consistent with a "burned-out, dry type of chronic ileitis."[78]

Microscopic examination of the intestine just above the terminal ileum showed "changes characteristic of relatively quiescent Crohn's disease."

Unexpectedly, a 1.5-centimeter tumor was found in the left adrenal gland. Microscopic examination of the tumor revealed that it was a pheochromocytoma.[79] A pheochromocytoma is a tumor that in most cases is located in one of the adrenal glands and produces catecholamines. Pheochromocytomas are most often benign but can also be malignant. High levels of catecholamines can result in rapid heartbeats and high blood pressure, with these manifestations often being intermittent. A nonphysician historian made a comment about the adrenal gland tumor almost three decades after Eisenhower's death: "For many years, he suffered from transient hypertension, a condition that may well have been caused by the small tumor discovered in one of his adrenal glands during his post-mortem in 1969."[80] This remark piqued interest among a group of physicians who, with the permission of Eisenhower's son John, retrieved the microscopy slides from 1969. One of the doctors, a Harvard pathologist, reexamined the slides and confirmed that the adrenal tumor was indeed a pheochromocytoma.[81] This prompted further research, mainly investigating whether Eisenhower's elevated blood pressure and heart attacks may have been related to the pheochromocytoma.

Findings from the research indicated that Eisenhower had suffered from episodes of hypertension for decades. Seemingly compelling evidence for an association between Eisenhower's heart attack in September 1955 and fluctuating hypertension was found; shortly before the myocardial infarction, Eisenhower's systolic blood pressure had been critically increased into the range of 160–180 mmHg.[82] The authors added a cautionary note, pointing out that although "a preexisting (ischemic) cardiomyopathy can be worsened by a catecholamine excess[,] ... in the case of President Eisenhower, the exact sequence of events cannot be determined by a retrospective chart analysis."[83]

When John Eisenhower was informed about the results of the research, he wrote a "gracious" letter to Dr. Kevin Loughlin, one of the doctors in the research group, and commented that he found the information of "considerable interest."[84] He went on to make the following comments regarding his father's health: "Dad seemed to give every [medical] department a crack at him. I always attributed his high blood pressure—and his heart attacks—to his very heavy smoking, but you may have discovered another complication. Fortunately, he seemed to be quite philosophical on medical matters. He declared that his health was the responsibility of the Army medics. I hope he was as serene as he appeared." Eisenhower's son then finished the letter to Loughlin with the following lines: "I hope that your discoveries regarding pheochromocytoma will lead to significant results in our medical knowledge."[85]

It is noteworthy that even if *Presidents Under the Knife* tells stories about several deceptions surrounding presidential surgeries, Eisenhower's hypertension also generated misleading statements from his doctors. On one occasion, his physician told him that his "diastolic BP was 80 to reassure him. I did not want him to go down to dinner with a concern for his BP."[86] His doctor obviously was hoping that Eisenhower did not understand the difference between systolic and diastolic blood pressure or would not notice the ambiguity in his statement.

The deceptions surrounding Eisenhower's cardiovascular health worked both ways. Ann Whiteman, the president's personal secretary, at one time commented, "The doctors think that he has been fooling with the anti-poly saturated diet[;] … meanwhile I noticed that DDE, who really seems to be feeling fine, had two sausages this morning for breakfast."[87]

Chapter Eight

Lyndon B. Johnson

Workaholic and Chain-Smoker

The Thirty-Sixth President

November 22, 1963–January 20, 1969

The Early Years

Lyndon Baines Johnson was born in Stonewall, Texas, on August 27, 1908, into a family that had its share of conflicts and struggles. He was the first of five children who saw the family harmony frequently ruined by their father's drinking habits. Their mother, Rebekah Baines, was "strong-willed," and although the father, Sam Ealy Johnson, could be "caring," he was also "heavy-drinking."[1]

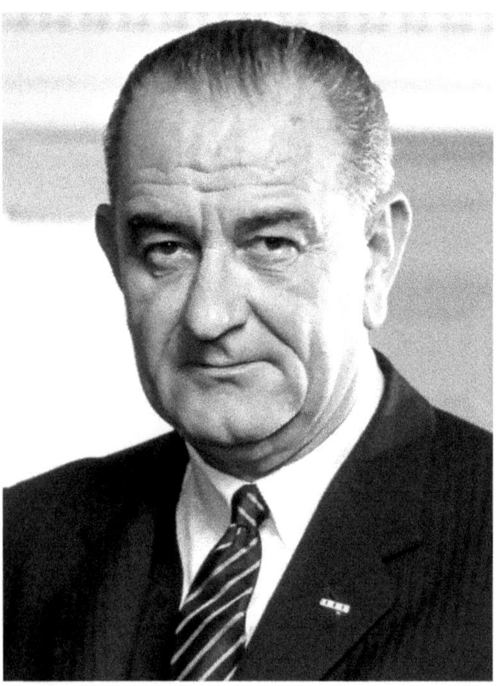

Lyndon B. Johnson. Alamy Stock Photo. Credit: Pictorial Press Ltd.

The home was not always a happy one. When Sam Ealy was out drinking and unable to provide for the family, Rebekah "cried a lot."[2] At one point, Lyndon recalled that "there was nothing Mother hated more than seeing my Daddy drink. When he had too much to drink, he'd lose control of himself. He used bad language. He squandered the little money we had on the cotton and real estate markets. Sometimes he'd be lucky and make a lot of money. But more often he lost out.... When [my mother] got upset, she blamed our money problems on my father's drinking ... especially when he stayed out all night."[3]

Lyndon revered his mother and thought of her as a "saintly woman to whom I owe everything."[4] Both parents were strict disciplinarians, and the father did not hesitate to spank the children when he felt there was a need for it. Lyndon remembered how his father would "take a razor strip and just whip the hell out of us."[5] Despite his father's many shortcomings, Lyndon could not help admiring him and wanted to follow in his footsteps when he was sober and showed some of his good sides. He acknowledged that "I wanted to copy my father always, emulate him. Do what he did.... He loved political life [serving several terms in the Texas legislature] and I followed him."[6]

Health Problems

Johnson had several factors working against him when it came to health. Ever since college he was a heavy smoker, initially smoking the pipe (which was the cool thing to do in those days), later cigarettes, up to the point that he was a chain-smoker. His biographer Robert Caro commented, "he seemed ... always to be holding a cigarette and his fingers were stained yellow with nicotine."[7] Johnson was known for being a workaholic, never allowing a break and always "pushing himself and everyone else mercilessly."[8] Johnson's brother, Sam Houston, at one point commented that Lyndon continued "to drive himself at a furious pace."[9]

Lyndon's eating habits were also not healthy. He always rushed through his meals even when growing up. One biographer commented that Lyndon's "table manners when he was a child were so atrocious that at times his mother was in tears."[10] When in college and having a meal in the cafeteria, "he would rush ahead of everyone else, grab a tray, rush to select his food, rush to his table, and gulp down his food."[11]

Later in life, Lady Bird was particularly unhappy with her husband's eating habits. On the campaign trail in 1937, she complained that "he ate very irregularly and had very unbalanced meals, which made me very angry.... He would just stop at some country store and buy a can of sardines and some crackers, or some cheese."[12] Johnson kept the poor eating habits throughout life and became "overweight and flabby."[13]

It would be another five years before Johnson's dietary habits would improve. In 1942, Lady Bird hired Zephyr Wright as a maid and—importantly—as a cook. Zephyr's husband, Sammy, was employed as a driver. The Wrights would stay loyal to the Johnsons for more than a quarter of a century and would become like family members. They were with the Johnson family at both the ranch in Texas and in Washington during Johnson's congressional years, vice presidency, and ultimately in the White House.

Zephyr's most popular cooking was southern. She soon became a favorite in the family—not surprising considering what she put on the table: "homemade spoon bread, fried chicken, steak, shrimp curry, hash, brownies, and homemade ice cream with cooked custard and fruit."[14] To make Lyndon happy, she would whip up a chocolate soufflé. Her Sunday breakfasts included delicatessen fare such as "deer sausage, cured bacon, popovers, grits, scrambled eggs, homemade peach preserves, and coffee."

Although these lists of temptations would seem to be impossible to surpass, a dish that made her even more beloved was her chili, "the second most famous Texas food after ribs."[15] What made her chili so celebrated (other than the taste, of course) was its dependability. Whenever it was served, it was a humongous success. Zephyr's recipe was "a straight forward, no-frills mix of coarsely ground meat, onion, tomatoes, salt, cumin seed, oregano, chili powder, garlic cloves, and hot water."[16]

Johnson soon got hooked on southern cooking, including the barbecued ribs. He started to understand the political value of food and frequently hosted dinners for foreign dignitaries and national politicians. Many of these events took place at the Stonewall ranch, but he often offered southern cuisine in the White House as well. And so it was that Johnson, once known for sloppy and unhealthy eating habits, became known for his "Barbecue Diplomacy."[17] He lived up to the saying that "Nothing is more political than food. Nothing."[18]

The concern for Lady Bird was no longer that her husband ate too little and too hastily; it became the opposite. With Zephyr in the kitchen, Lyndon "steadily" gained weight. He became concerned himself and tried to go on a diet. Zephyr wished to help him by serving smaller potions and low-calorie foods. Even though Johnson tried to follow the new rules, he soon began complaining about the small helpings. To show who was the boss at the stow, Zephyr at one point put a note under Johnson's plate: "You have been my boss.... Now I'm going to be your boss.... Eat what I have put in front of you and don't ask for any more and don't complain."[19] Johnson got the message, and to a group of senators he commented, "When I feel the arrogance of power, Zephyr will take it out of me."[20]

During his time in Congress, the Wrights accompanied Johnson and his family several times back and forth between the nation's capital and Stonewall. On one occasion in 1948 Johnson, now being a newly elected senator, asked Zephyr and Sammy to drive from Washington to Austin in Texas to join him for an event. Zephyr refused and described her previous experiences: "When Sammy and I drive to Texas and I have to go to the bathroom, like Lady Bird or the girls, I am not allowed to go to the bathroom. I have to find a bush and squat." She continued, "When it comes time to eat, we can't go to the restaurants. We have to eat out of a brown bag. And at night Sammy sleeps in the front of the car with the steering wheel around his neck while I sleep in the back." She put her foot down: "We are not going to do it again."[21]

Johnson was stunned and never forgot the event. He invited Zephyr to the ceremony on July 2, 1964, when he signed into law the Civil Rights Act. After signing the bill, the president handed the pen to her and said, "You deserve this more than anybody else."[22]

Given Johnson's challenges of heavy smoking, poor dietary habits, and managing his weight as well as the fact that he never exercised regularly and had a strong family history of heart disease, it is easy to understand that he had the cards stacked against him, something that would become clear throughout his political career; as Caro explained: "Almost every great crisis of his career had been accompanied by a crisis in his health."[23] It was not surprising that Johnson would die from his failing heart. He was ultimately felled by a heart attack in Johnson City, only fifteen miles from Stonewall, where he had been born sixty-four years earlier.

In addition to his heart problems, Johnson had several encounters with surgical procedures during his lifetime. Most of those were one way or another related to his political career.

Running for Congress and Having an Appendix "on the Point of Rupture"

In 1937, Johnson was in "his first desperate campaign as an unknown candidate for Congress."[24] Several days before the election he began to suffer increasing abdominal pain, nausea, and vomiting but refused to cancel or postpone his campaign. On April 8, two days before the election, the pain was reaching a climax, but he decided to keep going and gave a speech at a rally in the Travis County Courthouse in Austin, Texas. At this time the candidate was really feeling sick. His pain was nearly unbearable. He was sweating and had to hold on to the railing of the lectern while giving his address. In the midst of the discourse, Johnson doubled over from pain and had to sit down. After a short while, he got back up again and finished his speech.[25] At the end of the rally, Johnson shook hands with the listeners but then finally gave up and allowed himself to be taken to the hospital. He underwent emergency surgery and had his appendix removed. His surgeon explained that Johnson's appendix had been "on the point of rupturing."[26]

Johnson won the election with a comfortable margin. Some of his political enemies accused him of having faked the illness for political gains, but the finding at the surgery of course proved the accusation wrong. Ironically, the illness, which was real, may have helped Johnson to his victory; one of his aides pointed out that "it got us an unexpected top-page headline … [and a] … last-minute burst of publicity."[27]

Johnson's eleven years in the House of Representatives were not happy years. The new congressman had higher ambitions and felt trapped in his career. It was not a surprise that he decided to run for the Senate in 1948 despite having lost a try for the same position seven years earlier.

Multiple Kidney Stones

Johnson had several bouts of renal colic during his career. In most of those instances, he had stones that traveled down the ureters from the kidneys. When they got stuck they caused tremendous pain, which resulted in multiple hospital admissions. Whereas most of the stones passed spontaneously, on some occasions surgeons were needed to remove them.

While campaigning for a Senate seat in 1948, Johnson developed severe pain in his left flank. He was concerned that yet another kidney stone had formed (he had had kidney stones in March and October 1946) and was traveling down the ureter and that it would derail his bid for the Senate seat. When the stone remained stubbornly caught in the ureter and continued to cause severe pain and when fever developed, even Johnson understood that he needed help. He was admitted to one of the hospitals in Dallas, where the doctors explained that the stone was too big to pass spontaneously. Because the fever signaled infection of the kidney with risk for damage to the organ, he was advised to have the stone removed surgically. As expected, Johnson wanted none of that and did not even want to discuss the possibility of an operation. Because previous stones had passed, he was adamant in his conviction that this one would as well. He kept repeating, "I'll pass it, I'll pass it,"[28] and he got upset when the need for surgery was brought up: "I have had this before. Just leave me alone."[29]

Not until Lady Bird arrived did things start to quiet down. Johnson was advised to be flown to the Mayo Clinic to be seen by the chief urologist, Dr. Gershom Thompson, world-renowned for being able to remove kidney stones through a cystoscope rather than an open operation. With this technique, a cystoscope is inserted into the bladder through the urethra, and a nylon loop or basket is inserted into the ureter and used to pull out the stone. The only problem in Johnson's case was that the stone seemed to be too big and located too high up in the ureter to be treated with this method. Because there was evidence of a complete blockage of the ureter complicated by infection of the kidney, the doctors strongly advised Johnson to undergo surgery. He again refused and asked for a couple of additional days to allow the stone to pass.

Johnson used those days to do everything imaginable to help get the stone to move. He was driven around on bumpy Minnesota roads, hoping to shake loose the stone. He ran up and down in stairs and even jumped up and down as forcefully as the pain allowed. He also kept begging the urologist to try to remove the stone via the cystoscope despite having been informed that the stone was too big for that approach. He desperately needed to avoid an open operation with an extended time in the hospital and a protracted period of postoperative convalescence. It was vital to get back on the campaign trail as soon as possible to win that Senate seat; otherwise, he feared, his political career would be over.

Finally, on May 30 the surgeon gave in and agreed to try to remove the stone via the cystoscope. When the doctor came out after forty-five minutes and triumphantly announced that the procedure had been successful, everyone sighed a deep breath of relief. Not only would the doctors and nurses get rid of a high-profile and unusually demanding patient after a week in the hospital that to the staff "seemed more like a year,"[30] but, more importantly, Johnson would be able to resume his campaign and would win the Senate seat.

Whereas in 1948 Johnson was lucky and could have his kidney stone removed without a big operation, he was less fortunate seven years later when an even bigger stone had formed in the left kidney. This stone was too big to even make its way into the ureter and remained in the kidney, causing pain and discomfort. At this time

Johnson was the newly appointed majority leader in the Senate, and the new kidney stone was to be even more disruptive on his political life than the previous stones. In January 1955, Johnson underwent removal of the stone (a left nephrolithotomy) at the Mayo Clinic through a fairly big incision in the left flank. The surgery required a longer stay in the hospital and an extended time of convalescence. He was not able to return to the Senate until March. It was a frustrating experience for the workhorse from Texas to be forced to stay away from his busy political life in Congress for two months. The defeat of his first significant effort as majority leader—a tax reduction bill— during his absence from the Senate of course made life even more frustrating.[31]

Actually, the entire year of 1955 would continue to plague Johnson with forced times away from work. Already two months after his kidney operation Johnson was back in the hospital, this time for a heart attack.

Johnson's Heart Attack in 1955

Johnson had several heart attacks during his lifetime. The first heart attack struck him at the age of forty-seven in 1955, and the last one killed him eighteen years later.

We have already seen that Johnson had a number of risk factors that made him predestined to suffer heart problems. According to one biographer, "all of the men in the Johnson family had died early of heart disease."[32] Johnson's genetic background and heavy smoking were probably the most important factors, but excessive alcohol consumption, unhealthy food served in big helpings (such as Mrs. Wright's fried southern food, creamy sweet desserts, and homemade ice cream), and overweight certainly contributed to Johnson's cardiac problems. Constant stress, lack of rest and exercise, and an "aggressive Type A personality" were additional factors putting Johnson at high risk for heart disease.[33]

During most of his life, Johnson never allowed himself to slow down and rest or take time for any type of exercise. He was a true workaholic. Throughout his time in Congress and the White House, he had a "method of compressing two work days into one" by working "from dawn until 4, then nap until 5:50 and start all over again."[34] He had difficulties accepting that people were not always willing or able to work as hard as he did, resulting in frequent confrontations and angry exchanges. Johnson became known for being a man difficult to work with; one of his aides described his boss as "a bully, sadist, lout and egotist."[35] During his presidency, Johnson was often seen being in the face of congressional leaders giving them the "Johnson treatment," consisting of a mixture of "cajolery, flattery, indifference, coldness, insult, and even intimidation."[36]

The stress created by Johnson putting pressure on himself and his frequent frictions with people around him certainly did not improve the health of his heart.

At the time of Johnson's initial myocardial infarction on July 2, 1955, he was chain-smoking about sixty cigarettes per day. He initially blamed the chest pain on indigestion, but when the pain persisted and got worse, he said that he felt "like somebody's sitting on my chest."[37] He later commented that the pain from the heart attack was "the worst ... a man could have and still live."[38]

After initially refusing to have a doctor called (again, he would have nothing done that could impact his political career), Johnson finally gave in and was rushed to Bethesda Naval Hospital, "mad as hell" that he was going to be hospitalized.[39] A couple of hours after admission to the hospital, Johnson went into shock and came close to death.[40] It would be more than a month before he was released from the hospital and three additional months in convalescence at his ranch in Texas until he could go back to work in Washington. True to his character, Johnson was more concerned that the heart attack would put an end to his political career than to his life. Frustrated, he commented, "I'll never get a chance to be President now."[41]

Johnson was shaken by the experience and wanted to do anything possible to avoid it from happening again, so he quit smoking and managed to stay away from cigarettes until he retired.

Johnson's Gallbladder Surgery

In early September 1965 when on a visit to his ranch in Texas, Johnson developed pain in the right upper portion of his abdomen. Now president following the assassination of John F. Kennedy on November 22, 1963, Johnson did not want to make a big deal of his symptoms and dismissed them as being "related to something that he had eaten."[42] At first he did not tell his physician, Dr. George G. Burkley, about the belly pain. Johnson did, however, tell his wife, and when Lady Bird reminded him that he had experienced similar symptoms just before his heart attack in 1955, he took his symptoms more seriously and let Dr. Burkley know.

When the doctor was informed about the symptoms and examined the president, he initially agreed with Johnson that the problems may be related to indigestion. Burkley actually suspected that the symptoms were caused by "catfish poisoning, since the President had consumed large quantities of deep-fried catfish the previous evening."[43] Burkley soon changed his diagnosis to acute cholecystitis (acute inflammation of the gallbladder) but was also concerned that the symptoms may be caused by new kidney stones. And of course, like Lady Bird, Burkley understood that the symptoms may originate from Johnson's heart.

The president's symptoms subsided, and he was able to fly back to Washington. Burkley arranged for Johnson to have an X-ray performed in Washington. The test, an oral cholecystography, revealed that the gallbladder was not functioning properly, a finding that supported the diagnosis of cholecystitis. As an incidental finding, the X-ray also showed that the president had a kidney stone that was stuck in the middle portion of the right ureter.

Burkley realized that the president would probably need an operation for removal of the inflamed gallbladder but wanted that recommendation anchored with a specialist. Burkley therefore consulted Dr. James C. Cain, a renowned gastroenterologist at the Mayo Clinic. Cain agreed with the diagnosis and the recommendation for surgery. He suggested that Johnson undergo a cholecystectomy four to six weeks later. The interval would allow for the inflammation to "cool off" and would allow for an easier and safer procedure. (At the time, this was a common practice believed to result in fewer complications. Subsequent studies have shown that removal of the gallbladder can be safely performed during the first twenty-four to forty-eight hours of acute cholecystitis resulting in shorter overall hospitalization time and avoiding the need to come back later for the surgery. This has now become the most common way to manage patients with acute cholecystitis.)[44]

Once the recommendation for cholecystectomy had been made and the president had consented, it was a matter of identifying the appropriate surgeon. Dr. Cain recommended that one of his colleagues at the Mayo Clinic, Dr. George A. Hallenbeck, should be given the honor. Hallenbeck accepted the challenge and decided to have one of his younger colleagues, Dr. Donald McIlrath, assist him. The surgical team would also include Dr. Ormand Culp, a well-known urologist from the Mayo Clinic who would help out with removal of the kidney stone in the right ureter if needed. Dr. Cain initially wanted Johnson to have his surgery at the Mayo Clinic, but the president preferred to have it done at Bethesda Naval Hospital. It was closer to the White House and, importantly, was the hospital where Johnson had been treated for his myocardial infarction in 1955 and had been admitted on several additional occasions to have his heart and general health checked.

The surgery was scheduled for October 8. The president informed the press about his diagnosis and scheduled surgery on October 5.[45] The timing of the press release was decided in order not to detract from the visit to the United States of Pope Paul VI, which ended on October 4.

When Dr. McIlrath later recounted the circumstance around Johnson's gallbladder surgery, he provided some interesting details, reported in a recent article.[46] Johnson wanted to keep his upcoming surgery secret as long as possible, mainly not to rattle the stock market. The two doctors from the Mayo Clinic were to fly to Washington, D.C., two days before the operation to see the president and discuss the procedure. They had booked seats on a commercial flight, but when the Secret Service heard about the plans, the arrangements were changed. There was concern that if the Mayo surgeons were seen flying to the capital, rumors would spread quickly. The surgeons were instead informed that they would travel in an unmarked government plane flown up from Washington to pick them up. The plan was to have the plane land at Rochester precisely at the time of the surgeons' arrival at the airport, which would minimize the risk of the doctors being spotted. Unbelievably, however, the Secret Service had forgotten that Rochester is in the central time zone, which was why the plane arrived one hour early. In order to avoid having a government plane sitting in full view on the tarmac for an hour, it was ordered to take off and circle the airport until the surgeons arrived and could board the plane in secret.

After arriving in Washington, the surgeons were taken to the White House. When they met with the president, he seemed less interested in the surgical details than in other aspects of his upcoming operation. He wanted to know how long he would be under general anesthesia, an important question, since the 25th Amendment had not yet been signed into law. Johnson had asked his vice president, Hubert Humphrey, to be available "in case the President was not able to resume his official functions immediately after the operation."[47] In addition, Johnson wanted to know how long he would be bedridden and how long it would be before he could be seen in public. The president had decided to have his surgery on a Friday to be able to recover over the weekend before being seen by the press. In addition, Johnson was convinced that a Friday operation would have less impact on the stock market.

Although the president seemed to be more concerned about the political and financial fallouts of the operation rather than any surgical aspects and risks for complications, the surgeons, of course, had more of those worries on their minds. Johnson was lucky to be blessed with surgeons who were extremely experienced and had great confidence in themselves. Even so, they realized that as with any surgery there were risks involved, but they wanted the president to feel assured that they would be careful and do anything they could to avoid mishaps. When leaving the meeting with the patient, Hallenbeck turned around and reassured Johnson: "Mr. President, I can assure you that your operation is one that we do not want to flub."[48]

The president was brought to the operating room for removal of his gallbladder on the morning of Friday, October 8. The operating room was crowded. In addition to the principal surgical team, the room was filled with seven additional doctors, nurses, and three Secret Service men. After general anesthesia had been induced, a "generous, right subcostal incision was made."[49] When the abdomen had been opened, the surgeons found that the gallbladder had a "substantial amount of associated acute inflammation."[50] After the gallbladder had been removed, the kidney stone in the right ureter was taken out by Dr. Ormond Culp using the same abdominal incision that was made for the cholecystectomy. The operation went well and lasted about two hours.

Although the president's history of heart disease had been of great concern before the operation, there were no cardiac complications or "other untoward intra-operative events of records," despite some reports that circulated that the patient may have experienced cardiac arrhythmia during the operation.[51]

The president bounced back quickly after the surgery. He was described as "a good patient who complained very little."[52] He was able to take up governmental duties one day after the procedure and could meet with the press on Monday, reassuring the country that he was doing well after his operation. The stock market did not tank, and everyone was happy.

Johnson was released from the hospital on postoperative day seventeen. Before that he had managed to create additional headlines, one of which made a splash in America and quickly spread throughout the world; in today's parlance, one would say that it went viral. On the twelfth day after the operation, the president wanted to go outside the hospital walls to enjoy a beautiful and sunny day in Bethesda. It would also be a good day for a photo op. For that purpose, he was positioned at one of the putting greens of the golf course located on the grounds of Bethesda Naval Hospital. As usual, journalists were shouting questions. When one of the reporters asked how his scar was healing, Johnson pulled up his shirt, pointed at the scar, and explained that was where the surgeons did their job. Cameras were clicking, and a photo shot by Charles Tasnadi of the Associated Press became famous and traveled around the world.

Johnson's behavior was probably not as spontaneous as previously thought but instead was rather calculated.[53] Rumors were spreading after the operation that the

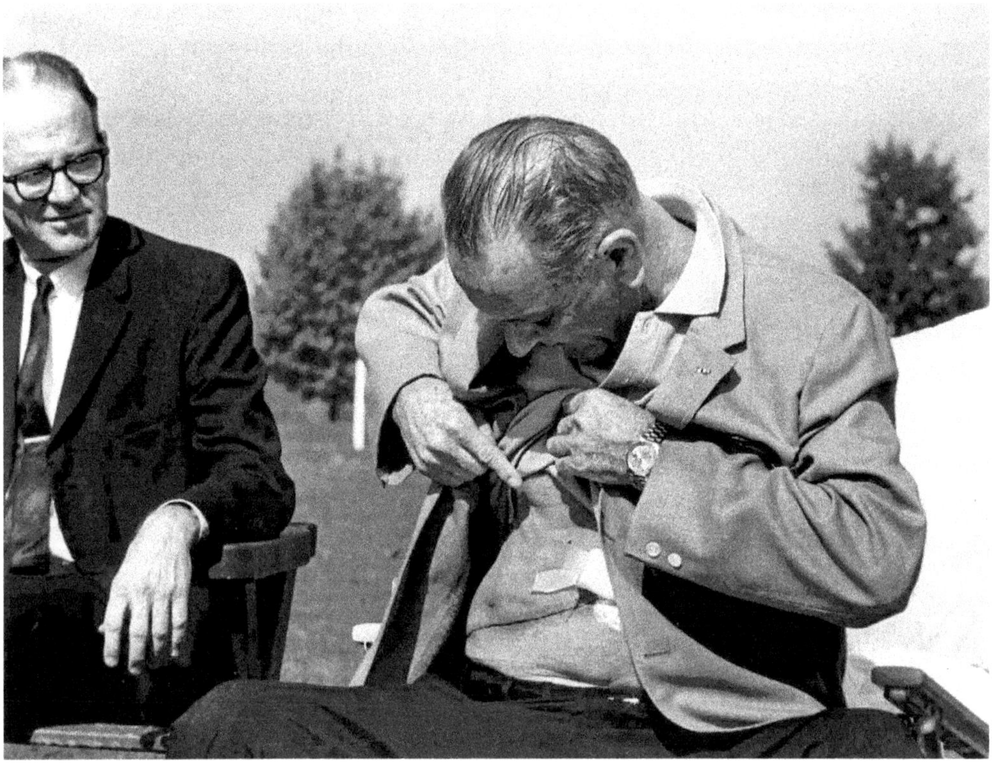

President Johnson pulling up his shirt and showing the scar after his gallbladder surgery performed twelve days earlier on October 8, 1965. Photo: Charles Tasnadi, Associated Press.

president had undergone cancer surgery rather than gallbladder surgery. When Johnson heard about the gossip, he immediately called Dr. Hallenbeck and asked if the incision he had used was typical for removal of the gallbladder. When the surgeon explained that surgery for cancer would have been performed through a midline abdominal incision, Johnson decided to show his scar to the

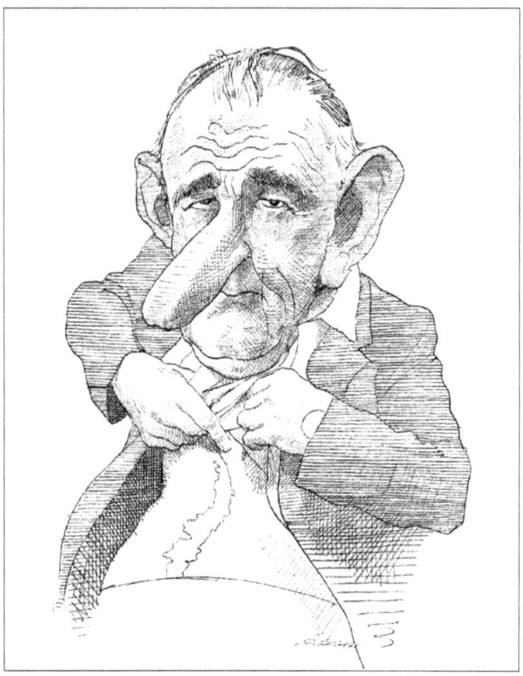

Cartoon of President Johnson showing the scar after his gallbladder surgery. Created by David Levine, published in the *New York Review of Books*, 1966, and held in the collections of the Billy Ireland Library & Museum at Ohio State University. Reprinted with permission of © Matthew and Eve Levine and the David Levine Archives.

reporters to quell any suspicion that anything other than a cholecystectomy had been performed. After the event the president happily commented, "That's one rumor taken care of."[54]

Regardless of Johnson's motive to show off his scar, the image of the president of the United States exposing his belly was mocked by many. Some complained that the behavior was not "presidential"[55] and made Johnson look like "a hayseed with a lack of social graces."[56] His political enemies relished seeing cartoons depicting Johnson with a Pinocchio nose and the scar looking like a map of Vietnam. This was, after all, during the time of the Vietnam War, with strong and sometimes violent protests against the conflict in Asia.

The Doctors Taking Care of the President's Gallbladder

It was indeed a seasoned and experienced group of physicians participating in the care of Johnson's inflamed gallbladder. His White House physician, Vice Admiral Dr. George Burkley, was somewhat of a veteran when it came to caring for presidents. He had been the physician in charge at Camp David under President Eisenhower. Burkley continued his service during the following administration and served President Kennedy, initially as the assistant and subsequently as the chief White House physician and Kennedy's personal physician.

Burkley had been in Kennedy's motorcade, riding behind the president's limousine, on that dramatic day in November 1963 and had the terrible duty of pronouncing President Kennedy dead at Parkland Memorial Hospital and then informing Mrs. Kennedy about her husband's fate.

Dr. Burkley had graduated from the University of Pittsburgh Medical School and had trained as an internist. He was sixty-three years old when Johnson (reluctantly) told him about his symptoms from the gallbladder. Burkley retired from his White House position at the end of Johnson's administration.

When Burkley suspected that Johnson's abdominal pain in September 1965 was caused by cholecystitis, he consulted Dr. Cain at the Mayo Clinic. Cain, who was not only a famous gastroenterologist but also happened to be a personal friend of Johnson, had graduated from the University of Texas School of Medicine in 1937. Cain had trained in internal medicine at the Mayo Clinic where he now practiced, specializing in diseases of the gastrointestinal tract. He had served as Johnson's personal physician since 1946.

In an interview on February 22, 1970, for the Lyndon Baines Johnson Library, Cain talked about his interactions with Johnson.[57] Cain and Johnson had first met in the 1930s when Cain's future wife, a good friend of Lady Bird, had introduced Cain to Johnson. Their meeting led to a lifelong friendship through Johnson's years as congressman, vice president, and ultimately president. Cain made a point of staying out of politics and was one of Johnson's most trusted medical advisers. Even when Johnson was president, Cain remained on a first-name basis with Johnson and kept calling him "Lyndon" rather than "Mr. President."

Cain kept a close eye on Johnson's eating habits throughout the years. During the interview, Cain talked about an informal meeting he had with Dr. Burkley and Bill Moyers, the president's press secretary. Johnson happened to pass by the room where the meeting took place and decided to sit in and join the conversation. To save time, the group ordered sandwiches for lunch rather than opting for a more formal meal. Cain recalled how "the President actually—by actual count—ate seven of these little half sandwiches."[58] Later on that day Cain confronted Johnson: "Now Lyndon, you've just got to cut down on your weight; you've just got to watch how much you're eating." Cain then commented, "He was up ten pounds or so above what he ordinarily weighed." Johnson did not seem or want to understand but said, "Jim, I really don't eat much," and then continued: "For example, I didn't have any lunch today." Cain reflected, "And he had just eaten seven sandwiches that I counted while he was doing it. But he didn't remember it at all. I mean, it's this type of problem."

The interviewer continued by asking Cain what type of exercises he prescribed for the president. Cain's answer was revealing in terms of both Johnson's lack of physical activities and his personality: "Walking, if he could; swimming, if he would. We tried all kinds of exercises. He's a man that nearly has to do two things at once and exercises—just doing exercise and doing nothing else is so boring that it is just very difficult for him to do this kind of thing."

During the interview, Cain also confirmed that the president was a hardworking man. For example, Johnson typically did "night reading."[59] Johnson would have "on his bed at night 50 or 100 items that if he didn't do them then they just stacked up," and he would have to do them the next day; "he's been one that liked to get his work done immediately. Tomorrow doesn't exist with him."

Although some found Johnson too demanding and difficult to work with, Cain commented that "the President is a very kind person and a very thoughtful person," always considerate to his staff.[60]

It turned out to be an easy task for Cain to identify Dr. George A. Hallenbeck as the surgeon to perform Johnson's cholecystectomy. Hallenbeck had graduated from Northwestern University in Chicago and then done his surgical residency at the Mayo Clinic. In addition to being a clinician and a famous surgeon, he was also an active and proliferative researcher and had obtained a PhD in physiology at the University of Minnesota.

Hallenbeck was fifty years old when he was consulted to perform the president's gallbladder surgery. At the time, he was chief of surgery at the Mayo Clinic and was admired both nationally and internationally for his surgical skills and scientific achievements. In addition, he had an attribute that certainly did not hurt him at the prestigious medical center: he had an impressive pedigree, with several members of his family having contributed in significant ways to the history of the Mayo Clinic. Hallenbeck was the grandnephew of one of the doctors who had participated in the founding of the Mayo Clinic, Dr. Christopher Graham. The business manager of the initial practice group at Mayo was Hallenbeck's grandfather. And Hallenbeck's father, Dr. Doer Hallenbeck, was a renowned internist who had spent his entire career at the institution. With a family tree like this and with his own accomplishments, the choice was easy. Dr. George A. Hallenbeck would be Johnson's surgeon.

Hallenbeck asked Dr. Donald C. McIlrath to come with him to Washington and be his assistant surgeon. McIlrath at the time was thirty-six years old. He was a product of the University of Kansas Medical School and had obtained his surgical training at the Mayo Clinic. He and Hallenbeck knew each other well from the clinical arena and from the time McIlrath had spent in Hallenbeck's research laboratory during his training. When they were flown from Rochester to Washington to meet with their patient, they were probably chuckling when they realized that the Secret Service had messed up and not remembered the time difference between the East Coast and Minnesota.

Johnson's Double Operation

On November 3, 1966, President Johnson held a news conference informing the media that he had been advised to undergo surgery for a "small bulge" that had developed close to the scar after the gallbladder operation the previous year. A small hernia had been noticed in April at the site where a Penrose drain had been placed at the conclusion of the cholecystectomy. A Penrose drain is a soft flexible rubber drain that is placed close to the operative site to prevent fluid accumulations after surgery. Placement of a drain after removal of the gallbladder was routine at the time of Johnson's gallbladder surgery but is seldom considered necessary nowadays. Where the drain is brought out from the abdomen, the abdominal wall can be weakened and a hernia may develop, and this is what had happened to the president about six months after the cholecystectomy.

At the press conference, Johnson explained that he had "experienced a continuing soreness and a drawing, pulling sensation" and that "the protrusion has enlarged recently and the soreness has recurred, and the doctors have therefore recommended surgery."[61] The president had just returned from a trip to Asia, and one of his physicians who participated in the press conference explained that during the trip "he was quite active in doing a lot of standing and walking and so forth, and this [the hernia] seemed to be enlarging very slightly." The surgeons therefore felt that they "ought to go ahead and repair" the hernia.

When one of the journalists asked whether anyone would "fill in for the period when the President is under anesthesia," Press Secretary Bill D. Moyers replied, "I don't believe so."[62] Obviously, this is quite different from what happens now even when only sedation is used during a routine colonoscopy.

The operation was performed on November 16 by the same surgeon who had removed Johnson's gallbladder about a year prior. Dr. Hallenbeck repaired the defect in the abdominal wall without any problems "with steel sutures in 19 minutes."[63]

During the press conference on November 3, Johnson additionally announced that "the doctors also intend at that time to remove a small polyp from my throat." Johnson had been bothered by hoarseness for some time and had been diagnosed with a benign-looking polyp on his right vocal cord in August 1966. When asked by the reporters what would cause it, a throat specialist present at the news conference explained, "In this instance, excess voice usage."

Johnson was known for being a constant talker. He was described as "a restless, incessant communicator" and "the most loquacious President of this century and maybe of all time."[64] After removal of the vocal cord polyp, Johnson was ordered to rest his voice for a couple of days. When his wife was asked if she could remember a time when her husband had been speechless, she answered, "No, and we are going to make the most of it."[65] She would not be able to enjoy a quiet husband for long, however, because within twenty-four hours, despite the doctors' orders, he was talking again with his near-normal voice.

Secret Surgery for Skin Cancer

On October 18, 1967, President Johnson had a skin lesion removed at his left ankle. A biopsy two days earlier had revealed that the skin tumor was a basal cell carcinoma (the most common type of skin cancer and the easiest to cure). The diagnosis and the operation were kept a secret and were denied by misinformation and lies for ten years "because of deep concern that public reaction to the word cancer would far exceed the seriousness of the medical situation."[66] The truth was finally told in an article in the *New York Times* on June 29, 1977.[67]

According to the *New York Times* article, the fact that Johnson had undergone surgery for skin cancer had been denied by Lady Bird as well as by the physicians involved in the president's care. This was yet another example of lack of transparency regarding a president's health, with information blocked for political reasons. Interestingly, it turned out that between thirty and forty tumors had been removed from Johnson's skin between 1965 and 1969, but all had been benign except the basal cell carcinoma at his left ankle.

Some of the political implications of Johnson's secrecy around his skin cancer were commented on in 1977. "The medical matters of Presidents and other political leaders are regarded as public information, and the charge of secrecy has raised questions about the openness of the Johnson Administration."[68]

Retirement in Texas

When Johnson decided not to run for reelection in 1968, he was a tired and aging man. He had come to realize that winning a reelection campaign was not a given and was even unlikely considering the situation in Vietnam. During his retirement years at his Texas ranch, he suffered occasional bouts of depression. He was also plagued by frequent chest pains and shortness of breath. People around him noted that he was "perceptively aged and worn."[69]

A historian pointed out that Johnson had begun "to stray from his diet and gained a considerable amount of weight" when he moved back to Texas.[70] Most concerning for his health, he had taken up smoking again after having stopped the habit following his heart attack in 1955; he was now back to smoking "excessively."[71] This, of course, did not help his heart, and in 1971, Johnson now sixty-three years old, had another episode of severe chest pain that put him in the hospital at the Brooke Army

Medical Center in San Antonio. The public was told that the former president had "only an attack of angina," but the suspicion has been raised that this was probably a new heart attack. At the time, Johnson was overweight (weighing 235 pounds) and was again chain-smoking. When friends encouraged him to quit smoking, he complained, "I am an old man, so what's the difference? I always loved cigarettes and missed them every day since I quit."[72]

While visiting his daughter Lynda in Charlottesville, Virginia, in April 1972, Johnson had another episode of severe chest pain. This time there was no question that the former president had suffered a massive heart attack. He was hospitalized and put in the intensive care unit. To the doctors' great concern (and against their advice), after only three days Johnson demanded to be flown to the Brooke Army Medical Center. Although he survived both the short stay in the intensive care unit and the flight back to Texas, he continued to suffer incapacitating chest pains and was in frequent need of oxygen, but he would not stop chain-smoking and eating "an abundance of unhealthful food."[73]

During the remaining months of his life, Johnson continued to suffer from severe chest pain on a daily basis. He consumed increasing amounts of nitroglycerin pills and frequently needed oxygen. In desperation, he saw the famous heart surgeon Dr. Michael DeBakey and asked if anything could be done. DeBakey, however, understood that the risks would be too high and declined to operate on Johnson.[74]

Friends understood that the end was approaching, and the former president understood it as well. At one time he uttered, "I've got an instinct."[75] President Richard Nixon also realized that Johnson was not doing well. Nixon had called Johnson on January 2, 1973, to let him know peace was finally coming in Vietnam. Johnson, however, was not able to voice any joy about Nixon's news and instead informed his successor that he had been suffering severe chest pain throughout the night and had just called his doctor for help. Nixon replied, "I called you at the wrong time."[76]

Johnson died on January 22, 1973. Not surprisingly, the autopsy the next morning found that the death was caused by severe coronary occlusions.[77] Johnson's risk factors for heart disease had conspired to kill the former president.

Two days prior to Johnson's death, Nixon's second inauguration had taken place.

Chapter Nine

Ronald Reagan

Reagan to the Surgeon, "Please tell me you are a Republican"

The Fortieth President

January 20, 1981–January 20, 1989

Ronald Reagan was indeed a lucky man. On March 30, 1981, a bullet fired by an assassin-to-be missed the president's heart by less than an inch, and Reagan became the only president who survived after being shot in an attempted assassination during his presidency. He also did well after removal of part of his large bowel for cancer in 1985, surviving for almost twenty years until the age of ninety-three without the cancer returning.

Although President Reagan had several additional procedures, the surgery following his assassination attempt and the operation for colon cancer are arguably the surgeries that stand out the most in the public's memory. They certainly attracted more attention in the news media and medical literature than his other operations combined and will occupy the major part of this chapter. First, however, let us recall some of the facts from his early life.

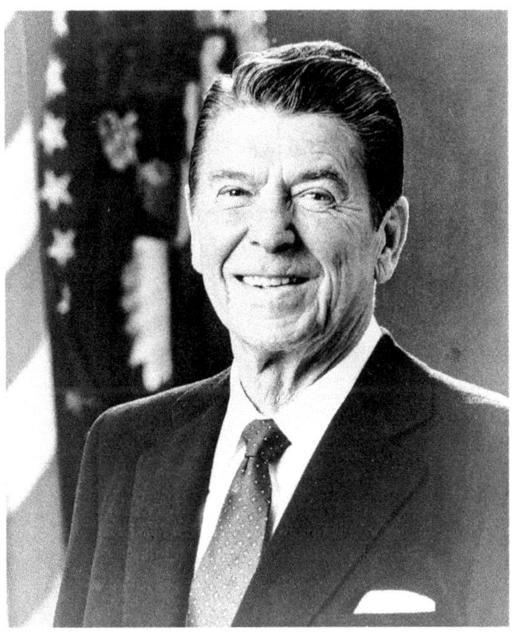

Ronald Reagan, 1981. Library of Congress, Prints and Photographs Division, Washington, D.C.

The Fat Little Dutchman

When Ronald Reagan was born in Tampico, Illinois, on February 6, 1911, he was a big baby, weighing ten pounds.[1] Reagan, in his autobiography, writes about the family legend that when his father first saw his newborn son, he exclaimed, "He looks like a fat little Dutchman." His father then, almost prophetically, added, "But who knows, he might grow up to be president some day."[2] Reagan did not think his name Ronald was good enough for a full-blooded American boy, so "as soon as I could, I asked people to call me Dutch."[3] His father continued to refer to his son as "the Dutchman."

Later in life, the nickname most commonly used for Ronald Reagan was "the Gipper." This was based on his acting as the football player George Gipp in the movie *Knute Rockne, All American*. In the movie, Gipp urged his teammates to give all they had and "win just one for the Gipper."

Reagan grew up in a family with few means. When reflecting on his childhood, he commented that "we were damn poor."[4] As a young man, he suffered profound nearsightedness and in adult life was handicapped by hearing loss, with nearly total deafness on one side.

Despite obstacles, Reagan would one day fulfill his father's prophesy to reach the highest position in the country. Before getting there, Reagan had been in Hollywood as an actor and as the president of the Screen Actors Guild. He had served as a two-term governor of California (1967–1975). In 1980, Reagan defeated Jimmy Carter to become the fortieth president of the United States.

The Attempted Assassination of President Reagan and His Dramatic Surgery in 1981

It was less than three months after his first inauguration as president of the United States when Reagan was invited to address the Construction Trades Council at the Washington Hilton Hotel, about 1.5 miles from the White House, on March 30, 1981. When Reagan reflected on the events that took place on that critical day in 1981, he commented, "On several previous occasions when I'd been out in public as president, the Secret Service had made me wear a bulletproof vest under my suit. That day, even though I was going to speak to some die-hard Democrats who didn't think much of my economic recovery program, no one had thought my iron underwear would be necessary because my only exposure was to be a thirty-foot walk to the car."[5]

After the president had finished his remarks at the Washington Hilton, he exited the building at around 2:30 p.m. He was walking toward the waiting limousine when someone in the crowd shouted, "Mr. President. Mr. President."[6] Reagan stopped for a moment, turned around, and waved to the people. That's when the shots were heard. The drama that followed in real life would surpass anything attempted by Hollywood to depict similar events.

When the shots were fired, Reagan did not understand what had just happened and did not realize he had been shot. He thought he had heard "two or three firecrackers ... just a small fluttering sound, *pop, pop, pop*."[7] He turned to the Secret Service agents and asked, "What the hell's that?"[8] His bodyguards, however, immediately understood what they had heard. The head of the Secret Service unit, Jerry

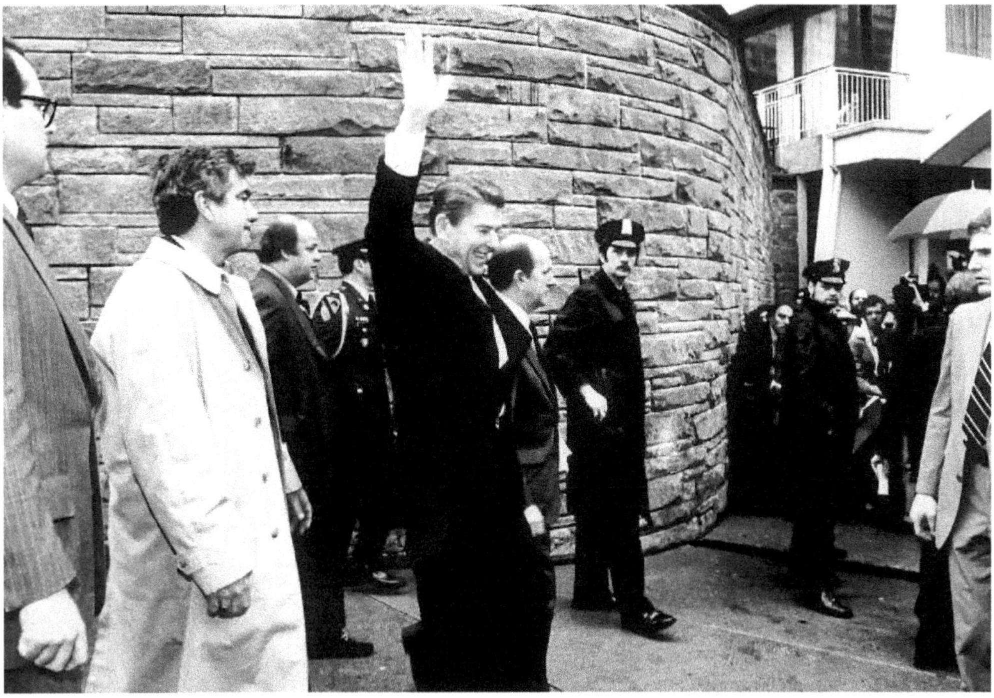

President Reagan exiting from the Hilton Hotel, Washington, D.C., on March 30, 1981. He was waving at the crowds just before being shot. Alamy Stock Photo, Credit: Maidun Collection.

Parr, pushed the president into the back of the limousine, threw himself on top of Reagan for protection, and ordered the driver to rush them to the White House.[9] Someone was shouting, "Haul ass! Let's get out of here!"[10]

In the car, Reagan complained of pain in his upper back that was "unbelievable. It was the most excruciating pain I had ever felt."[11] He blamed the pain on the less than gentle handling by Parr and told him, "get off, I think you've have broken one of my ribs." En route to the White House, the president had difficulties breathing and noticed blood in his mouth and on his hand when trying to cough. Reagan became increasingly agitated and told Parr, "You not only broke a rib, I think the rib punctured my lung."[12] When Parr realized that Reagan was coughing up blood, he made a decision that became one of the most important factors in saving the president's life. He shouted to the driver to take them to the nearby George Washington University Hospital instead of the White House.

When arriving at the hospital at 2:35 p.m., Reagan walked through the doors to the emergency department unsupported. To a nurse coming to meet him, the president complained that he was "having trouble breathing." He then fell down on one of his knees; "all of a sudden my knees turned rubbery."[13] Reagan was immediately lifted onto a stretcher and rushed into the emergency room. His pain continued, and in his autobiography he commented, "I guess I passed out for a few minutes."[14]

When examined by Dr. Joseph Giordano in the trauma room, the president was in distress, had a blood pressure of 80, was experiencing difficulties breathing, and had "ashen color and pallor."[15] What happened next has been described in the medical literature in an article based on extensive records made by the president's physician[16] and in a paper authored by the thoracic surgeon and radiologist who played prominent roles in the direct care of the president.[17]

In the emergency room, the president was noted to have blood in his mouth and on his teeth. When his chest was examined, a wound of one centimeter was noticed between the fourth and fifth ribs below the armpit on the left side, and it became obvious that the president had been shot. Because no exit wound was found, it was also realized that the bullet must be lodged in the chest. A chest X-ray confirmed the suspicions; in addition to evidence of blood in the left chest, a "metallic fragment" was noticed close to Reagan's heart. This, of course, was the bullet that had nearly killed the president. It was later described in Reagan's own words: "After they took it out of me, I saw the bullet. It looked like a nickel that was black on one side; it had been flattened into a small disc and darkened by the paint on the limousine. First the bullet had struck the limousine, then it had ricocheted through the small gap between the body of the car and the door hinges. It hit me under my left arm, where it made a small slit like a knife wound."[18] Later, it was determined that the projectile was a "devastator" bullet, designed to explode on impact, which luckily it did not do.

The president was immediately resuscitated with large volumes of intravenous fluids and blood transfusions that were aggressively pushed into him through multiple intravenous lines. A chest tube was inserted on the left side, rapidly emptying almost 1.2 liters of blood from the president's chest and continuing to pour out 200–300 milliliters of blood every fifteen minutes, totaling about 2.3 liters in the emergency room.

After the resuscitation the patient's condition stabilized somewhat, with the blood pressure restored to 160. The president felt a little better and was able to carry on a conversation with the doctors and nurses, even showing some of his typical humorous side. To one nurse who was holding his hand for comfort he quipped, "Does Nancy know about us?" This act of care was later remembered by Reagan. In his autobiography he regretted that he had never been able to personally thank the nurse, "Although I tried afterward to learn who the nurse was, I was never able to find her. I had wanted to tell her how much the touch of her hand meant to me, but I never was able to do that."[19]

First Lady Nancy Reagan arrived after about fifteen minutes. When Reagan saw his wife, he pulled up the oxygen mask and whispered, "Honey, I forgot to duck."[20] He was referring to Jack Dempsey, who had said the same thing to his wife after having lost against Gene Tunney in a heavyweight championship match.

Even though Reagan felt a little better at this point, his doctors did not. The president was continuing to bleed through the chest tube at a rapid rate, and Dr. Benjamin Aaron, chief of thoracic surgery at George Washington University Hospital, decided that surgery would be urgently needed to stop the bleeding. When realizing that he was being taken to the operating room, Reagan wisecracked to one of the surgeons, "I hope you are a Republican."[21] The surgeon, allegedly a devoted Democrat, replied, "Today, Mr. President, we are all Republicans."[22]

Reagan was taken to the operating room at 3:25 p.m., about an hour after the shooting had taken place. In the operating room Dr. Aaron, assisted by Drs.

Kathleen Cheney and David Adelberg, performed a "left anterolateral thoracotomy" (opening of the left chest from the front and side) by an incision through the space between the fifth and sixth ribs. After removing approximately 500 milliliters of blood from the pleural space, the source of the bleeding could be identified, and the hemorrhage could be stopped: "blood pulsated from a small artery.... The bleeding vessel was controlled by ligature."[23]

Because of the small size of the bullet, the projectile was initially difficult to localize. After identifying the entrance wound and probing the bullet track with a thin catheter, the ball was finally felt at the tip of the catheter and could be removed. With the help of the catheter, the path of the bullet could be reconstructed by the surgeons. It had ricocheted on the top of the left seventh rib, perforated the lung, and finally lodged close to the heart.

The actual thoracic part of the operation took one hour and twenty minutes, with the remainder of the two hours and forty minutes under general anesthesia being used for positioning of the patient, skin preparation, and "peritoneal lavage" to rule out bleeding in the abdomen.[24] Reagan was taken to the recovery room in stable condition at 6:45 p.m.

The patient gradually woke up from the anesthesia, and by 7:30 p.m. he was awake enough to start writing messages (he still had a breathing tube and so was unable to talk). The first note was written in desperation: "I can't breathe!"[25] Once the nurses had been able to explain to Reagan that the inability to breathe was caused by "the tube

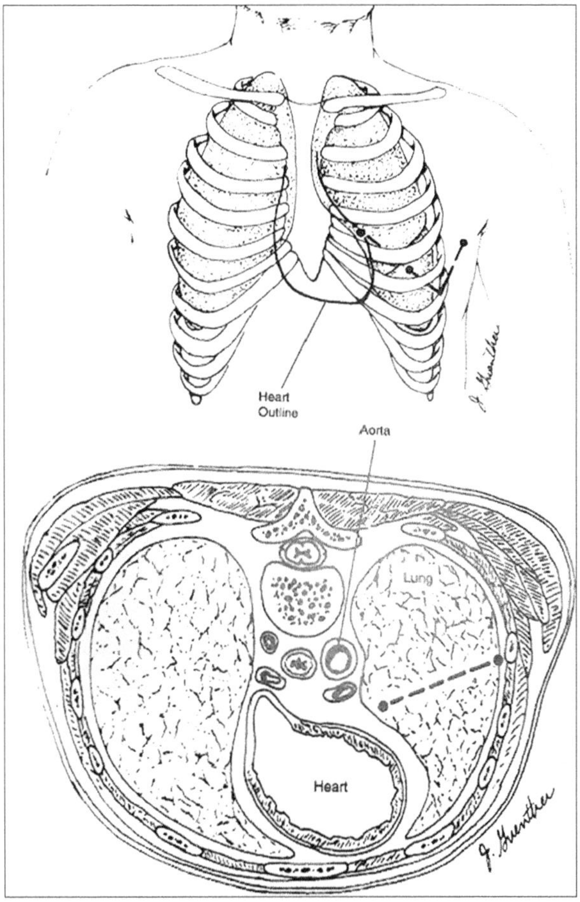

Diagram of Reagan's chest showing the path and location of the bullet as reported by his surgeon. The top image shows the bullet ricocheting off the top of the seventh left rib and lodging in the lung close to the heart. The bottom image shows a cross section of the chest and the path of the bullet, going through the lung and finally stopping close to the heart. Of note, the lower panel of the figure is just a diagram illustrating the path of the bullet through the left lung and does not illustrate the position of the president on the operating table. In fact, on the operating table, the patient was in the supine position (lying on his back). Reprinted from Aaron and Rockoff with permission of the *Journal of the American Medical Association* Network.

down your throat" and that the respirator was breathing for him, his anxiety was eased. He kept drifting in and out of sleep. Then he wrote another note: "I am still alive, aren't I?" As his wife later explained, "He cracked a number of jokes in the hospital, but this wasn't one of them. The writing on that note was so faint and wobbly I could barely read it."[26] Her husband later told her, "When I started to wake up and open my eyes, all I could see was white. The sheets, the walls, the coats on the doctors and nurses—everything was white. For a minute I wondered if I was in heaven and these were all angels."[27]

After emerging more from the anesthesia, the president did indeed start to crack real jokes. In one of them he wondered, "Can we rewrite this scene beginning at the time I left the hotel?"[28] After all, Reagan had been an actor with many years in Hollywood. He was now awake enough to remember what Winston Churchill had said at one point: "There is no more exhilarating feeling than being shot at without result." The breathing tube was removed at 2:50 a.m., and the patient was moved out of the recovery room to the intensive care unit at 6:15 a.m. At around 9 p.m., Reagan was moved to a "presidential suite" created by combining several adjacent hospital rooms on one of the hospital floors.

Except high fevers five to six days after the surgery, giving rise to concerns that the president had developed pneumonia, the postoperative course was smooth. Reagan quickly regained energy and his desire to work. Already after a day, Reagan sat in his hospital bed and penned a personal letter, eight pages long, to Soviet leader Leonid Brezhnev.[29] Reagan also continued to make jokes. For example, he told nurses who helped him brush his hair, "Now you can tell the world that I don't dye my hair."[30]

The president was discharged on April 11, twelve days after the attempted assassination. He was wearing a bulletproof vest when he left the hospital because "the threats on his life were continuing."[31] In his autobiography, Reagan reported that he had made the following entry in his diary on April 12: "The first day at home. I am not jumping any fences and the routine is still one of blood tests, X-rays, bottles dripping into my arms but I'm home."[32] In addition to all continued medical support and help with recovery, Reagan received home calls by his thoracic surgeon on two occasions.[33] The president's wounds were reported to be "healing well," and he was having "little pain and a good appetite." On his last follow-up visit in the White House six weeks after the emergency thoracotomy, Dr. Aaron found the president to be "fully recovered ... [and] participating actively in the affairs of state."[34]

Even though Reagan's recovery was impressive, some of the assessments may have been overly rosy. Four months after the assassination attempt, Reagan faced his first international meeting as president. When the annual G7 conference was held in Ottawa, hosted by Prime Minister Pierre Elliott Trudeau of Canada, in July 1981, Reagan also encountered French president François Mitterrand, British prime minister Margaret Thatcher, the prime minister of Italy and Japan, Giovanni Spadolini and Zenko Suzuki, and West German chancellor Helmuth Schmidt. All attendees were less than impressed by Reagan. In particular, Mitterrand and Trudeau were disappointed with what they considered Reagan's superficiality and "intellectual emptiness." Even if Reagan may have felt some of the other G7 participants' disdain, he did not appear to be bothered. But on the way back to Washington, he "seemed to collapse on Air Force One."[35] He was "exhausted nearly to the point of incoherence." One of his biographers commented that "sixteen weeks after his near-death experience, Ronald Reagan was not yet the man he had been" and wondered "if he indeed ever would be."[36]

Considering the dramatic events in the afternoon of March 30, 1981, it looked like a miracle that Reagan's life had been saved. Add to the president's arrival in the emergency room of George Washington University Hospital the admission of two additional victims of the shooting: the president's press secretary, James Brady, who had sustained a life-threatening head injury (but survived after emergency surgery), and Secret Service agent Timothy McCarthy, who had been shot in the chest (and also survived after surgery). A fourth victim of the shooting, Washington, D.C., police officer Thomas Delahanty, had been brought to the Washington Hospital Center and also underwent lifesaving surgery after sustaining a shot to his neck.

There were many heroes involved in the saving of President Reagan's life on that momentous day in March 1981. One of the most important actions of the day was Jerry Parr's redirection of the limousine from the White House to George Washington University Hospital. Although streets leading back to the White House were cordoned off in anticipation of the president's return after his speech at the Washington Hilton, when the limousine was redirected to the hospital, it "plunged through uncontrolled traffic, miraculously reaching the clinic in just three and a half minutes."[37] One of Reagan's biographers commented, "By general medical consent, Parr's decision to divert saved the life of the President of the United States."[38]

Other crucial actions included the immediate and aggressive resuscitation of the dying president performed by Dr. Joseph Giordano and his trauma team and Dr. Aaron's decision to take Reagan to the operating room urgently to stop the bleeding. Even though some identified individuals stand out as particularly important, there is no doubt that many unnamed doctors and nurses (including the hand-holding nurse who comforted Reagan in the emergency room) were essential for saving the president's life and those of the three additional victims brought to the emergency rooms of George Washington University Hospital and the Washington Hospital Center on March 30, 1981.

Ten years after the event, the emergency room of George Washington University Hospital was named for and dedicated to Ronald Reagan. During the ceremony, it was repeatedly made clear that the president's survival in 1981 was thanks to "his personal staff, his own fortitude, and the skill and attention of the staff of the GWUMC [George Washington University Medical Center]."[39]

"What happened to the guy with the gun?"

In one of the notes that Reagan scribbled when he started to wake up in the recovery room, he asked the questions "What happened to the guy with the gun?" and "What was his beef?"[40] The president would soon learn about the perpetrator, John Hinckley, Jr. Hinckley had an earlier career as a singer and songwriter. He was twenty-five years old when he shot the president. In the 1970s Hinckley had become obsessed with Jodie Foster, the young actress who had been featured in the 1976 film *Taxi Driver* in which the plot was the planning of an assassination of a presidential candidate. Hinckley started to seek opportunities to impress Foster and decided that killing a president would get her attention. In 1981, he started to plot the assassination of the newly elected President Reagan. Before the attempt Hinckley had written to Foster: "The reason I'm going ahead with this attempt now is because I cannot wait any longer to impress you."[41]

Outside the Washington Hilton Hinckley fired six shots at the president, hitting Reagan and three additional persons. At the trial in June 1982, Hinckley was found not guilty by reason of insanity, a verdict that resulted in an uproar of controversy and criticism. He spent the following thirty-four years in confinement at the mental institution of St. Elizabeth's Hospital in Washington, D.C. In 2016 Hinckley was conditionally released, one of the conditions being the requirement to live full-time at his mother's home. That and other conditions were reduced in 2018 when Hinckley was allowed to move out of his mother's house and live independently. He was fully released from court restrictions in June 2022.

Nancy Reagan commented in her memoirs that although she felt compassion for Hinckley's parents (who had sent a "moving apology" to the president's wife), she "could not find it in my heart to feel compassion for their son."[42] She then added, "Ronnie is different."

When contemplating his assassin-to-be, Reagan in his autobiography made several remarkable comments, showing an unbelievable ability for grace and forgiveness. When the president was fighting for his life in the emergency room and being readied to be brought to the operating room, he saw his press secretary James (Jim) Brady being wheeled by him, unconscious and on his way to the operating room. Someone told the president that Brady "was hit so badly he probably wouldn't make it." Reagan "quickly said a prayer" for Brady and added, "I didn't feel I could ask God's help to heal him, the others and myself, and at the same time feel hatred for the man who had shot us, so I silently asked God to help him deal with whatever demons had led him to shoot us."[43] A couple of paragraphs later Reagan added, "He was a mixed-up young man from a fine family. That day I asked the Lord to heal him, and to this day, I still do."

Who Was in Charge?

On the day Reagan was shot, not surprisingly, panic and confusion erupted at the White House. Vice President George H.W. Bush was on a visit to Texas, and it was unclear who was in charge in Washington. When government officials crammed into the Situation Room, Secretary of State Alexander Haig was the highest-ranking cabinet member and as such took on the role of spokesman for the government and became the focal point for most questions. He also incorrectly believed that he was next in line to the president after the vice president.

Haig was often looked upon as rough, self-important, and hard to get along with. He certainly seemed to enjoy his high-ranking position, and if not treated with full respect, he was known to let people know he was displeased. Nancy Reagan, for sure, did not like Haig and described him as "too power-hungry" and added, "He saw himself as the only person in the administration who should be making decisions on foreign policy."[44] There was also concern that he was dangerously trigger-happy. As Nancy Reagan commented, "If Ronnie had given him the green light, Haig would have bombed everybody and everything."[45]

Even the president, who usually put up with people who did not serve him well, lost his patience with Haig and at some point commented that "he didn't even want me as the president to be involved in setting foreign policy—he regarded it as his turf. He didn't want to carry out the president's foreign policy; he wanted to formulate it and carry it out himself,"[46] Reagan was only one year into his presidency when he accepted Haig's letter of resignation. Before leaving the White House, however, Haig had already made himself best remembered for his actions the day of the attempt on Reagan's life.

With the cabinet members assembled in the Situation Room, the confusion was obvious and growing. The reports from the hospital about the president's condition were fragmentary. Some of the news was obtained from the TV reporters who were constantly providing updates, sometimes contradicting each other and sometimes even themselves about the situation. One point of great confusion and concern was the condition of Press Secretary Brady, who was initially believed to have been killed. Donald Regan, the treasury secretary, for one thought that Brady had died and announced, "I've just received some sad news. Jim Brady is dead."[47] National Security Advisor Richard (Dick) Allen, a close friend of the Bradys, said, "Let's have a moment of silent prayer." Not until additional information was relayed back from the hospital did it become clear that Brady was still alive although with a serious brain injury.

When the White House spokesperson Larry Speakes was seen on television in front of the reporters being uncertain when trying to answer questions from the media about who was in charge, Haig became infuriated and stormed out of the Situation Room. A few moments later he showed up on television screens in front of the journalists claiming that he was "in control." Although later the rumor spread that he had said that he was "in charge," he never used those words.[48] His entire statement (as quoted by Larry Speakes) was "constitutionally, gentlemen, you have the President, the Vice President, and the Secretary of State, in that order, and should the President decide that he wants to transfer the helm, he will do so. He has not done that. As of now, *I am in control here* in the White House, pending return of the Vice President and in close contact with him. If something came up, I would check with him, of course."[49]

Although "in charge" and "in control" may seem basically synonymous, the phrase "in charge" stuck in people's memory thanks to the media's frequent use of it and the controversy that erupted. Interestingly, when Reagan nine years later recalled what he thought he had heard about Haig's behavior, he wrote that Haig had "claimed he was in charge of the country."[50] Mrs. Reagan got it right in her memoirs when she wrote that "Haig alarmed Ronnie's aides and much of the country with his famous statement 'As of now I am in control here.'"[51]

When the participants in the Situation Room meeting heard Haig's comments on television, they were angry and upset. Donald Regan asked Secretary of Defense Caspar Weinberger, "What's this all about? Is he mad?" Weinberger answered, "I can't believe this. He's wrong. He doesn't have any such authority."[52] No one seemed to know who had authority. When Haig returned to the Situation Room, his interpretation of the Constitution was challenged by Weinberger, to which Haig responded, "You'd better read your Constitution, buddy."[53] (Weinberger, of course, was correct. The Constitution made the vice president next in line to the president, followed by the Speaker of the House, the president pro tempore, and then the secretary of state.) As Regan pointed out, "We Cabinet members had never been instructed on the chain of Command under various circumstances."[54]

Even though Haig later tried to explain that he had never intended to give the impression that he believed he was in charge of the government, the damage was already done. The "in charge" incident would linger in many people's memory and negatively reflect on Haig's reputation for years. As Speakes, who took over as presidential spokesperson after Brady was shot, commented on Haig's statement about being in control, "Haig didn't realize it, but from a political standpoint he had just become history."[55]

Surgery for Colon Cancer

After Reagan's brush with death and dramatic surgery in March 1981, the president remained well for more than four years. Reagan had always lived a healthy life. He was an outdoor person, liked exercising, and was an ardent (and skillful) horseback rider. Sunny California had blessed him with a nice tan, certainly helping his good looks (important not only for an actor in Hollywood but also for a politician wanting to portray a healthy image to the public). He was proud of being able to chop wood at Rancho del Cielo. He was also keen on following the advice of his father-in-law, Dr. Loyal Davis, an acclaimed surgeon who "had always drummed into me the importance of having a yearly physical exam."[56]

As part of his annual checkups, the president was found to have occult (hidden) blood in his stool in March 1985. This prompted a flexible sigmoidoscopy (an examination of the inside of the lower parts of the large bowel using a flexible instrument, a sigmoidoscope). Although a sigmoidoscopy only examines a limited part of the colon as opposed to a colonoscopy, which examines the entire large bowel, it can still cause discomfort. When the flexible sigmoidoscope was "snaking and coiling" up the colon, Reagan, seldom missing an opportunity to crack a joke, asked if they were "looking for his larynx."[57] The examination revealed a small benign polyp. When repeat tests of the stool were performed, one sample showed a trace of blood, but on five additional tests the results were negative. Although that was somewhat reassuring, the president was advised to undergo a complete examination of his large bowel with a colonoscopy. Reagan was not too interested in that recommendation, but after some arm-twisting by his wife and Dr. John Hutton, former chief of surgery at Walter Reed Army Medical Center and appointed one of President Reagan's personal physicians in December 1984, a colonoscopy was finally scheduled for July 12, 1985.

Even if the president did not like the preparations needed for the colonoscopy, he had to do what any other patient must do: clean out his bowel. In his autobiography, Reagan described the ordeal: "After a Friday morning spent sipping eighty ounces of a medicinal concoction called Go Lightly, which is designed to clean out your system prior to certain procedures (and which it does with a vengeance), I went to Bethesda on Friday afternoon expecting to leave the following day."[58] The plan was for an overnight stay at Bethesda Naval Hospital and then go up to Camp David on Saturday. The plans, however, would have to be changed.

During the colonoscopy, an approximately five-centimeter villous tumor with an ulcerating center was identified in the cecum (the first part of the colon). It looked highly suspicious for cancer and would need surgical removal. Hutton commented to Speakes, "It's cancer, it's big, it's black, it's ugly."[59] During the colonoscopy the president's wife was in the waiting room, thinking about the upcoming weekend at Camp David. After the procedure the president was upbeat and joking, making people laugh. But when the doctors came out to report their findings, they were not laughing. Mrs. Reagan wrote in her memoirs how she felt that the doctors "were looking at me a little funny—especially John Hutton, who seemed to be avoiding my eyes."[60] One of the physicians said, "We have bad news for you." Nancy felt "as if I had been hit by a ten-ton truck."[61]

When the shocking news started to sink in, "Nancy and I and Dr. John Hutton ... held a strategy session" and discussed the options.[62] Three choices were considered: the president and his wife could continue to Camp David as they had initially planned, they could remain in the hospital and have the problem taken care of the next morning, or they could wait ten days and schedule the surgery after the state visit by President Li of China. Mrs. Reagan wanted the operation done as soon as possible (and had the support of Dr. Hutton): "All I cared about was getting the operation over with as quickly as possible. Now that we knew about the polyp, I couldn't stand the prospect of letting it stay inside Ronnie any longer than we had to."[63] But she was nervous that her husband would not like the idea of having major surgery the next morning. Because surgery the next morning was the only option when another round of Go Lightly, "which he absolutely hates,"[64] would not be needed, she decided to play that card and succeeded to convince her husband to have the procedure the following day. As the president explained, "I hated Go Lightly, so my decision was easy: Let's get it over with."[65]

The Colectomy and the Hospital Stay

The president was wheeled to the operating room the morning of Saturday, July 13, 1985. His wife accompanied him all the way into the operating room and gave him a kiss before he was put under.[66] Before being taken to the operating room, the president signed a letter addressed to the Speaker of the House of Representatives and the president pro tempore of the Senate invoking the Twenty-Fifth Amendment, temporarily transferring his powers to Vice President Bush, who became the acting president for the next eight hours and fifty minutes:

> I am about to undergo surgery during which time I will be briefly and temporarily incapable of discharging the Constitutional powers and duties of the office of the President of the United States. After consultation with my counsel and the Attorney General, I am mindful of the provisions of Section 3 of the 25th Amendment to the Constitution and of the uncertainties of its application to such brief and temporary periods of incapacity.... [C]onsistent with my long-standing arrangement with Vice President George Bush, ... I have determined and it is my intention and direction that Vice President George Bush should discharge those powers and duties in my stead commencing with the administration of anesthesia to me in this instance.[67]

The procedure commenced at 11:48 a.m. A surgical team consisting of Drs. Dale Oller, John Hutton, Lee Smith, and Bimal Ghosh performed a right hemicolectomy (removal of the right part of the colon, including the cecum where the tumor was located) and connected the small bowel to the divided portion of the colon by an "end-to-end" ileocolostomy. They also examined the entire abdominal cavity carefully, in particular the liver and tissues harboring lymph nodes close to the intestine (the mesentery) to make certain there was no indication of spread of the cancer outside the colon (which there was not). After the procedure, Reagan's surgeons reported that the president "had the insides of a 40 year old."[68] The surgery went smoothly, with a blood loss of only 150 milliliters, and lasted just under three hours.

Even though from the surgeons' standpoint the president had a "smooth and uneventful" postoperative course,[69] from the patient's perspective the experience was less than happy. In his diary, Reagan remembered that he "was in a lot of discomfort

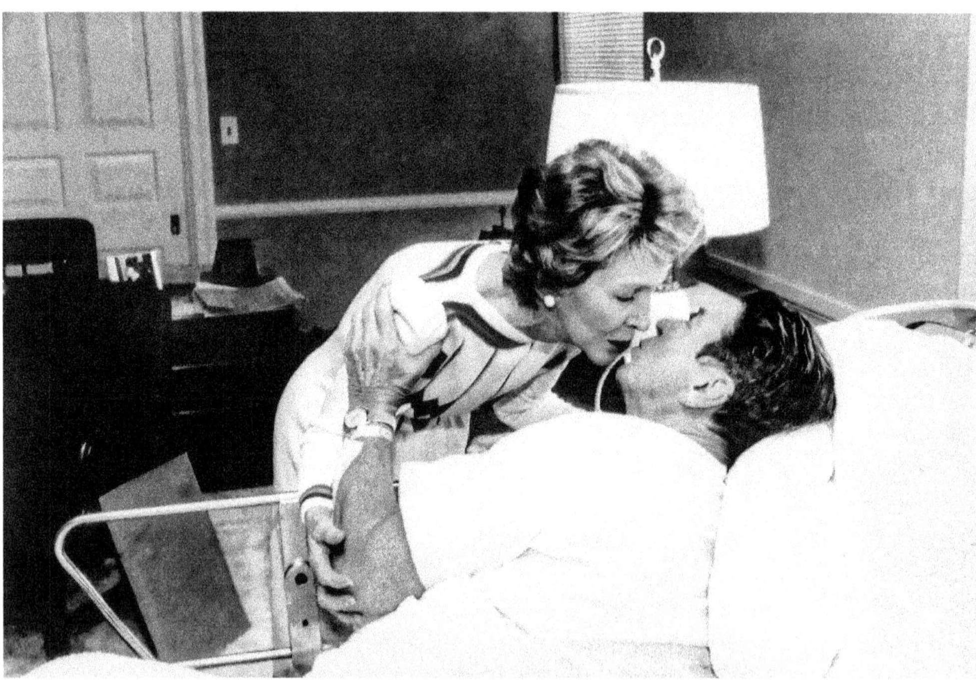

Mrs. Reagan visiting with her husband on the morning of July 14, 1985, the day after his surgery for colon cancer. Alamy Stock Photo. Credit: Gainew Gallery.

through the weekend and didn't get much sleep."[70] Despite the pain, Reagan did not lose his sense of humor. Recalling William Claude (W.C.) Field's famous line about being in Philadelphia, Reagan thought to himself, "All in all, I'd rather be at Camp David."[71]

The misery would last for another couple of days. On Monday Nancy commented, "Still not a good night for Ronnie." She then added something that shows the disconnect that sometimes exists between how physicians perceive patients' experience and how patients really feel: "but the doctors say he is doing remarkably well."[72] The patient himself entered in his biography that "Monday night was miserable. I kept waking up and felt I had no good sleep at all."[73] Then things started to turn around. On Tuesday, July 16, Mrs. Reagan commented, "Ronnie had a good day. Last night he stayed up late and watched a movie on television with Bogart and Bacall" and added that "he is reading a biography of Calvin Coolidge."[74] On Wednesday Reagan could report that he felt better, "although I still knew I'd been through something." He was also gradually starting to get back into government business and was visited by his chief of staff and vice president to discuss "our latest battles with Congress over the budget."[75] In his next note Reagan was jubilant (although tongue in cheek), "Miracles of miracles, I had my first food by mouth.... A cup of tea." The doctors promised they would remove the feeding tube the next day.

Finally, the day of discharge arrived. On Friday, Mrs. Reagan wrote in her diary, "This morning they made it official—he goes home tomorrow. Whoopee!" Before being discharged, the president was scheduled to deliver his weekly radio broadcast from the hospital, and "then we'll leave. I can't wait!"[76] With his wife at his side, President Reagan addressed the nation and gave yet another example of why he was called the "Great Communicator." After first expressing his gratitude to the hospital personnel and doctors, he went on to educate the listeners about the importance of taking care of one's health and keeping up with medical appointments: "It's important to have a checkup if you think something isn't right. So if you are listening to this right now and it reminds you of something that that you've been putting out of your mind, pick up the phone, call your doctor or local hospital and talk to somebody." And of course, Reagan couldn't help himself and quipped, "Just tell them Dr. Reagan sent you."

And then the president went on with the final part of the address, a quite emotional thank-you to the only live audience he had, his wife. He said,

> I'd like to indulge myself for a moment here. There is something I want to say, and I wanted to say it with Nancy at my side, as she is right now, as she always has been. First ladies aren't elected and they don't receive a salary. They've mostly been private persons forced to live public lives. Abigail Adams helped invent America. Dolley Madison helped protect it. Eleanor Roosevelt was FDR's eyes and ears. Nancy Reagan is my everything.
>
> When I look back at these days, Nancy, I'll remember your radiance and your strength, your support, and your taking part in the business of this nation. I say for myself, but also on behalf of the nation, thank you, partner, thanks for everything.[77]

Finally, Reagan couldn't resist making another joke: "By the way, are you doing anything this evening?" As Mrs. Reagan commented, "It's a good thing this was radio and not television, because I was sitting there with tears streaming down my face."[78]

And then it was time to head back to the White House. The president had had a remarkable recovery. Some members of the media suspected that the reports about

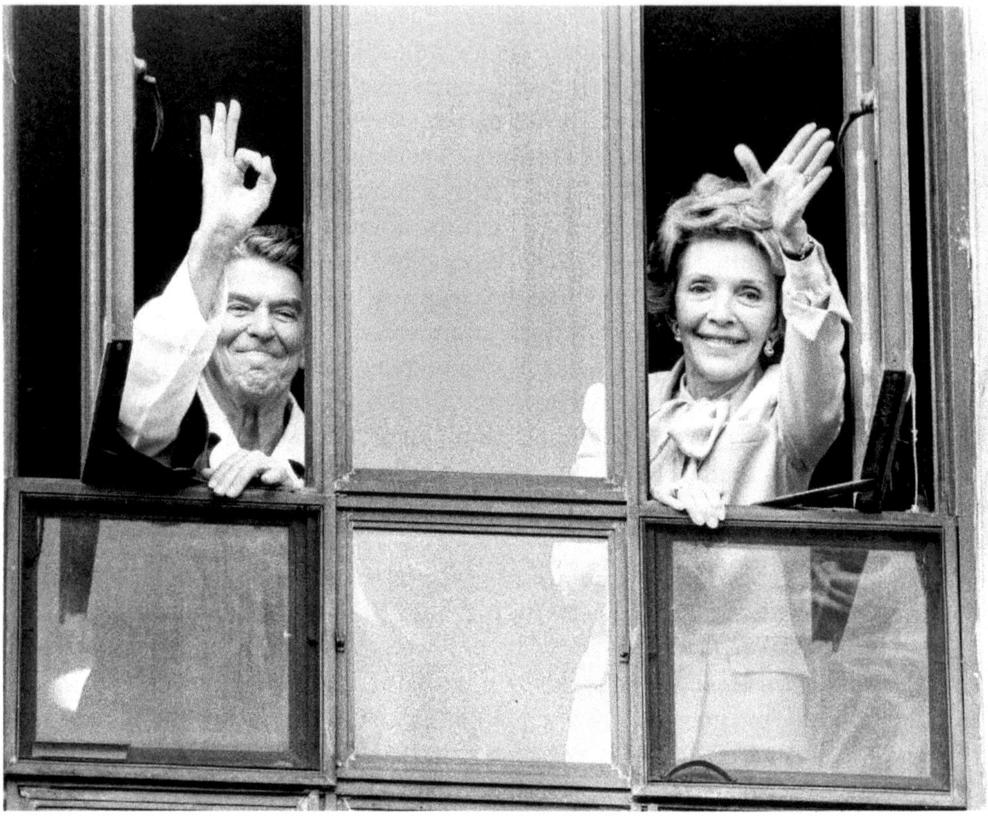

President Reagan and his wife waving from the windows of the Bethesda Naval Hospital on the afternoon of July 18, 1985. As always, Reagan was upbeat. "That's Ronnie, my beloved optimist," Nancy Reagan said. Photograph taken by Diana Walker on July 18, 1985. National Museum of American History and the Smithsonian Institution.

his recuperation had been doctored to make him look better than he was. But as Speakes wrote in the narrative of his White House years, "Not so. We told the whole truth—no vanish, no hype. He was indeed Superman."[79]

Despite the excitement and celebratory feelings caused by being released from the hospital, there was a dark cloud on the horizon: the president was told by his surgeons he could not continue to eat popcorn! He disappointedly entered in his diary that "during my colon operation, the surgeons found evidence of diverticulitis, an inflammation of the intestine that can be easily irritated by small particles of food, and they said: No more peanuts and popcorn."[80] He of course had vented his frustration to his wife, who wrote in her biography that "Ronnie's worst moment came when they told him he could no longer eat popcorn. You would have thought his whole world had come to an end."[81]

The Pathology Report

The pathologist performed a careful examination of the surgical specimen. The tissue that had been removed during the surgery comprised the terminal part of the

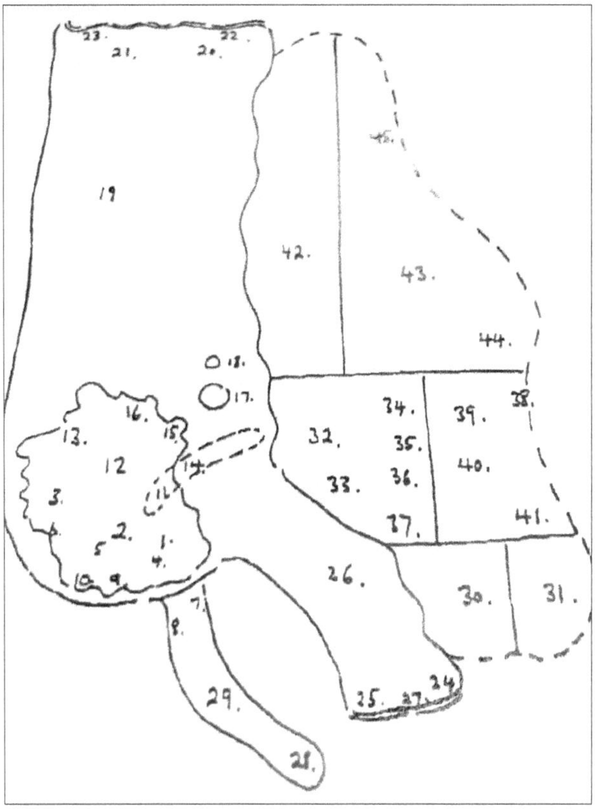

The pathologist's diagram of the surgical specimen removed during Reagan's operation on July 13, 1985. The numbers indicate the areas that were examined microscopically. The irregular area (with the numbers 1–6, 9, 10, 12, 13, 15, and 16) denotes the actual tumor. Reprinted from Beahrs, "The Medical History of President Reagan," with permission of the *Journal of the American College of Surgeons*, formerly *Surgery, Gynecology and Obstetrics*.

ileum (the most distal part of the small intestine), the appendix, the cecum, and the right (ascending) colon. In addition, tissue close to the intestine (the mesentery) containing lymph nodes was removed. The tumor, located in the cecum, measured five centimeters. The pathologist numbered the several areas that were examined microscopically, including multiple lymph nodes in the mesentery.

The pathology report was discussed with the media at a press conference two days after the surgery. It was reported that the tumor was a "villous adenoma that contained a moderately differentiated adenocarcinoma that had not involved blood vessels, nerves, the margins of the resection, or 15 lymph nodes."[82] Although there was some controversy in the literature as to whether the cancer should be classified as Dukes A, B, or B1, the bottom line was that the pathology report was favorable, showing no evidence of extension of the tumor beyond the bowel wall and no lymph node metastases, providing for a good prognosis. No radiation or chemotherapy would be needed. The favorable staging was also supported by the findings during the operation and by a CAT scan performed the evening before surgery, showing "nothing suspicious in his liver or his lungs."[83]

The interaction with the news outlets by the medical team regarding the president's tumor drew some criticism in the medical literature. One pathologist was upset that the pathology findings were reported by the surgeons without the participation of the pathologists during the initial news conference. This use of "intermediary clinical personnel to interpret the pathology data was a mistake,"[84] and explained some of the confusion over the staging of Reagan's cancer and his prognosis. Although this may seem like an academic dispute only, it was pointed out that "medical history requires that its [the President's tumor] examination, diagnosis, staging, and prognosis be accurate."[85]

History would prove that Reagan had an excellent prognosis following his cancer surgery. He would live for almost an additional two decades without the cancer coming back.

Was It "Has" or "Had?"

While Reagan was still in the hospital, Dr. Steven Rosenberg, the chief of surgery at the National Cancer Institute in Bethesda, informed the news media that "the President has cancer." The president was not pleased with that statement and pointed out that he did not have cancer but rather, "in fact, the president had cancer."[86] He went on to explain why he felt it was important to clarify why he thought "has" cancer was an inappropriate statement: "Yes, doctors found an object in my body that was cancerous. But they removed it" and "they learned that no cancer cells had entered the rest of my body at all; there was no cancer beyond the polyp, and it was removed."

It may of course be debated whether the president's comment reflected denial or was an expression of his famous optimism. His wife favored the latter when she commented on the issue: "That's Ronnie, my beloved optimist."[87] Others were astonished by Reagan's ability to dismiss bad news and just move on. "It was as though he had had a wart removed from his finger," and "his attitude was, Well, the trifle is taken care of, let's forget about it."[88]

Unsurprisingly, the difference between "has" and "had" became a hot topic in the media, dominating the headlines for days. For example, the *Los Angeles Times* found it worthy of a screamer: "Doctors Have a Tense Debate: Reagan 'Has' or 'Had' Cancer?"[89] The media also engaged many "experts," often surgeons who were remote from the care of the president but still happily provided their opinions. This behavior by professionals upset the first lady more than her husband. Mrs. Reagan commented, "I am so mad at the doctors who have nothing to do with this case, rushing to go on television with their diagnoses and explanations! I'm just furious about it."[90] She went on to describe one occasion when she was watching the news together with her husband and a doctor came on and stated, "He probably has about four years to live." Mrs. Reagan was furious, but the president just said, "What do you think about that? Ridiculous!"[91]

"Delayed" Surgery and Astrology

It was no secret that Nancy Reagan and Donald Regan, now the White House chief of staff, were not the best of friends. "Don was not my favorite person in the White House. And he wasn't exactly cuckoo about me, either."[92] In his biography, published 1988, Regan painted a less than favorable picture of the first lady, which prompted her to counter with her own memoir, *My Turn*, one year later.

There were two issues surrounding Reagan's cancer surgery in July 1985 that soured the relationship between the president's wife and Regan. The first source of disagreement was the timing of the surgery. When Mrs. Reagan called Regan the afternoon of Friday, July 12, to inform him that the president would need surgery, the timing of the operation was discussed. The decision had been made to go ahead with the procedure the following morning, but, according to Nancy Reagan, Regan felt that was an inappropriate delay and was concerned about the reason for the delay.

During much of the time in the White House, Mrs. Reagan relied on the advice of a "friend" (astrologer) in San Francisco who would predict when a day was "good" or "bad" for certain activities (such as the president giving an important speech, traveling, or meeting with foreign leaders). Regan recalled in his biography that "virtually every major move and decision the Reagans made during my time as White House Chief of Staff was cleared in advance with a woman in San Francisco who drew up horoscopes to make certain that the planets were in a favorable alignment for the enterprise."[93] He was concerned that the postponement of the surgery until the following day was the result of the astrologer's recommendation.

Nancy Reagan vehemently disagreed and wrote in her book that "Don evidently [thought] that the reason the surgery was scheduled for the next morning—or, as he wrote, was 'delayed for a day and a half'—had something to do with astrology." She then added, "That's not true. There was no delay. Ronnie went in on Friday and had the operation the next morning. Astrology had nothing to do with it."[94]

From a surgeon's perspective, the president's surgery was performed expeditiously and, absent the need for an emergency procedure, was done without any delay. It may be speculated that Mrs. Reagan in her conversation with Regan on that Friday afternoon had mentioned that a "delay" of the surgery until Monday morning (after a weekend at Camp David) had been considered as an option, explaining the comment by Regan that "the operation might be delayed for a day and a half."[95]

The other source of contention between the first lady and Regan was the pace of resumption of presidential activities, in particular how soon after the surgery government officials would be allowed to see the president. Whereas Mrs. Reagan was quite protective of her husband and wanted to shield him from tiring in personal meetings, his chief of staff was eager to allow access to the president by what he considered essential officials, including the vice president and National Security Advisor Robert "Bud" McFarlane. This dispute became a story in the media, of course, with strong and sometimes ugly sentiments about who was in charge, Mrs. Reagan or Donald Regan, and with the animosity between the parties being blown up into bold headlines.

Mrs. Reagan finally approved visits by George Bush and Bud McFarlane. McFarlane's meeting with the president took place on Thursday, July 18, five days after the surgery, a meeting that would play a significant role for the rest of Reagan's presidency. On the day before McFarlane came to see him, the president recalled that "unaware at the time where it would lead to, I recorded an event that was to mark the beginning of what became known as the Iran-Contra affair.... Some strange soundings are coming from some Iranians. Bud M. will be here tomorrow to talk about it. It could be a breakthrough on getting our seven kidnap victims back."[96]

Reagan's Colon Cancer and the Iran-Contra Scandal

How might the president's surgery for colon cancer have had anything to do with the Iran-Contra affair? Before we try to answer that question, let's first remind ourselves about some of the details surrounding a series of events that almost derailed Reagan's presidency. Of course, a reader can find much more extensive information about this event elsewhere; numerous books, newspaper articles, and published papers have dealt with Iran-Contra. The *Tower Commission Report* itself was more than five hundred pages long.

The Iran-Contra affair had some of its origin in Hezbollah's taking of American hostages in Lebanon in 1984. Increasing the "value" of the victims from the hostage takers standpoint, the Central Intelligence Agency chief in Beirut, William Buckley, was among the seven captured. The hostage situation weighed heavily on Reagan's shoulders. The Contra connection refers to the fact that some of the proceeds from the sale of arms to Iran allegedly were used to fund the Contras in Nicaragua who were fighting the communist Sandinista regime. Both the arms sale to Iran, which was under a U.S. arms embargo, and the diversion of funds to the Contras, seem to have violated the law. The main question became how much the president knew about the dealings and how much he had approved. A key factor for this question was a twenty-three–minute meeting in Reagan's hospital room at Bethesda Naval Hospital on Thursday, July 18, 1985, when the president was still recovering from major surgery.

On that fateful day, Nancy Reagan had finally given approval for Bud McFarlane to meet with the president. Regan was present at the meeting as well. The three participants of the meeting reported differing recollections of the encounter. In December 1986, the president told the Tower Commission that he "had no recollection of a meeting in the hospital in July with McFarland and that he had no notes which would show such a meeting."[97] This statement seemed to have been contradicted by Reagan himself, who in his autobiography 1990 stated that "during Bud McFarlane's visit to Bethesda Naval Hospital and in following meetings, he informed me … [about] … information from a group of moderate politically influential Iranians."[98]

Regan and McFarlane never denied their recollection of the meeting with the president on July 18 but had different memories of the issues that had been deliberated. McFarlane acknowledged that the sale of weapons to Iran had indeed been discussed but also stated that "Reagan did not explicitly approve of U.S. arms going … to Iran." McFarlane, however, felt that some of the president's comments had been an indirect blessing and an approval in general and quoted the president as saying "Go ahead, open it up."[99]

Donald Regan also remembered that the encounter had taken place but stated that he had "no recollection whatsoever of arms sale being discussed by the President and his national security adviser at the Bethesda Naval Hospital meeting," adding that "there is nothing in my notes or in my memory to suggest that the idea of swapping arms for hostages was mentioned by either man on this occasion."[100] Regan in his biography also mentioned that at a later occasion "I told the President that I had no recollection of his authorizing the sales of arms when McFarlane visited him at Bethesda Naval Hospital after his cancer surgery."[101]

Some historians have tried to explain Reagan's lack of memory of the meeting with McFarlane and Regan by his recent colon surgery and speculated that Reagan's recent major operation and his cancer diagnosis may have resulted in "flawed and irrational" decision-making and impaired judgment and memory.[102] Hangover effects of anesthesia and drugs used to relieve postoperative pain may also have played a role. It has also been speculated that early manifestations of Alzheimer's disease influenced the president's recollection of events that took place during his recovery from surgery.[103] Although it is possible that these health-related factors may have contributed to the president's inability (or unwillingness) to remember his encounter with McFarlane and Regan on July 18, others, not surprisingly, have felt convinced that political considerations were most important when Reagan on some occasions denied any recollection of the meeting.

Regardless of the details of the meeting in Reagan's hospital room and of the potential motives either man may have had not to be completely honest about what they remembered, it seems well established that an important meeting between Reagan and two of his most essential officials occurred only five days after Reagan's major surgery and only three days after he had been informed about the final diagnosis. It was an encounter that became an important factor in the events that led up to "the Iran-Contra disaster that most seriously threatened the Reagan legacy."[104]

Skin Cancer on the Nose

Frustrated, Reagan commented in his autobiography that "it happened again barely ten days later, shortly after I left Bethesda."[105] Another cancer had been detected, this one a skin cancer on his nose.

Reagan was and had always been an outdoor person. He loved to bask in the sun. "From the day I started those summers working as a lifeguard, I'd enjoyed being outside and getting a tan."[106] He remembered that during his time in Hollywood, "I *had* to stay tanned." The many years in California and at the ranch gave Reagan a lot of exposure to the sun.

Reagan had noticed "a tiny bump" on his nose for years. When he returned from Bethesda Naval Hospital after his colon surgery, the area on the nose looked reddened. A dermatologist was concerned and performed a small superficial biopsy. The microscopic examination showed that the lesion was a basal cell carcinoma.

The president underwent removal of the basal cell carcinoma on July 30, 1985, with a Mohs procedure. The technique, named after one of the doctors who developed the method, Frederic E. Mohs, is a minor surgical procedure typically performed under local anesthesia, with the lesion being cut out in stages and with microscopic examination of the edges performed while the patient is waiting to make certain that all cancer tissue is removed. People around Reagan, in particular his wife, felt it was important to conceal the true nature of the skin lesion on the president's nose. They were afraid that admission of the cancerous nature of the "pimple" on the nose would make the nation concerned that their president was "cancer prone." Bowing to pressure from the first lady, the White House Office of the Press Secretary issued a statement: "On Tuesday, July 30, a small area of irritated skin on the right side of the President's nose was removed. The irritation had recently been aggravated by the adhesive tape used [to hold down a nasogastric tube] while the President was in the hospital. It was submitted for routine studies for infection, and it was determined that no further treatment is necessary."[107] The statement obviously did not provide the whole truth, something that caused reporters to question the credibility of White House spokesperson Larry Speakes.

The president himself was not particularly concerned about the diagnosis but hated its consequences. "The doctors told me, either I had to stay out of the sun or button up and wear a hat when I did go out."[108] He continued by lamenting the ensuing misery. "First I have to give up popcorn and now sunbathing."

Even though the Mohs procedure was developed to reduce the risk for the cancer to come back,[109] Reagan's basal cell carcinoma did return. Almost exactly two years after the first operation, Reagan had another surgery for the cancer on his nose. There was again time for a highly visible bandage. When a group of visitors to the Oval Office noticed the bandage, the president commented that that it was just a "billboard" that said "Stay out of the sun."[110]

The Prostate Operation and Its Political Aftermath

On January 5, 1987, Reagan underwent a "transurethral prostatectomy" (removal of part of an enlarged prostate gland through the urethra, avoiding skin incisions). Reagan's most troubling symptom had been difficulty voiding. In addition, he had noticed blood in his urine. He had undergone a similar procedure twenty years prior.[111]

The operation was done under spinal anesthesia at Bethesda Naval Hospital, with the president awake during the surgery. The procedure "took 50 minutes. Blood loss was 350 milliliters and 23½ grams of tissue were removed."[112] The patient had a smooth postoperative course and returned to the White House on January 8. Microscopic examination of the tissue that had been removed revealed "prostatic hypertrophy with some inflammatory reaction, but no evidence of cancer."[113]

Notwithstanding that the president had undergone a routine operation with a favorable postoperative course and could be discharged from the hospital after three days, he was advised to delay his State of the Union address to Congress, scheduled for January 20. Reagan did not like that idea and went ahead and gave the speech without postponement. He "presented the address in style as he had all previous talks."[114]

Reagan's recuperation time after the prostate surgery became a new source of conflict between Donald Regan and Mrs. Reagan, similar to the situation after the president's colon surgery in 1985. Regan wanted the president to resume at least some of his duties sooner than Nancy Reagan would approve. Regan pointed out that the president had not held a press conference since November and suggested, "What about having one on January twentieth?" The first lady (according to Regan) adamantly said "No" and added, "No press conference for at least three months."[115]

Nancy Reagan, in her memoirs, discussed the new conflict with Regan and, not surprisingly, painted a different picture of their interactions. She was of the opinion that "the standard six-week recuperation period after an operation applies to *any* kind of major surgery."[116] To that she added, "And this [her husband] was a man in his late seventies, who had already been shot, who had undergone a cancer operation, and who was now under enormous political pressure [for the Iran-Contra affair]." Against Mrs. Reagan's wish, Regan announced in February that the president "would hold a press conference at the end of the month." The first lady commented, "I was furious and we had a heated argument about it on the telephone."[117] The conversation soon went ugly and turned into a shouting match. When the president's wife realized that she would not be able to change Regan's mind, she said, "Okay, have your damn press conference!" To this Regan replied, "You bet I will! ... Whereupon Don Regan hung up on me."[118]

To have one of his officials hang up on his wife was too much for Reagan; he finally gave in to the idea of letting Regan go. Regan resigned from his position a couple of weeks later. Regan described the circumstances around these events differently. He again raised the issue of astrology. When Nancy Reagan strongly objected to a press conference in January, Regan commented, "I did not ask the reason for this decision. It was obvious that Mrs. Reagan's protective instincts were fully aroused, and I assumed, too, that she had been talking to her Friend, the astrologer."[119] A couple of paragraphs later Regan added, "Mrs. Reagan's Friend had told her that January was a bad month for the President—any activity might produce unhappy results. This prognostication had the effect of immobilizing the President."

The president commented on some of these events in his autobiography. Although he "had always liked Don and enjoyed his Irish humor," he had started to realize that "many people—staff members, cabinet members, and congressional leaders—felt that Don had an oversized ego that made him difficult to deal with."[120] When Mrs. Reagan finally told her husband how Regan had hung up on her during a phone conversation about the president's schedule, Reagan realized that it was time to think about Donald Regan's exit. "I was troubled by this kind of temperamental outburst, especially towards Nancy, who had always had only my best interest at heart."[121] Reagan concluded that this "wasn't the way I wanted to run the store." On February 27, 1987, the president accepted Regan's resignation.

Hand Surgery

Getting ready to leave the White House after his two-term presidency, Reagan had his last surgery as president on January 7, 1989, when he underwent a procedure for Dupuytren's contracture of his left ring finger.[122] The condition is caused by thickening of fibrous tissue in the palm of the hand, resulting in one or more fingers—more commonly the ring finger and little finger—staying in a bent position, with inability to straighten them. Dupuytren's contracture occurs most frequently in men above middle age. If the condition impairs the function of the hand, surgery may be recommended. The procedure is typically done under regional anesthesia (blockade of the nerves running down the arm and into the hand).

The president had his procedure at Walter Reed Army Medical Center. After the operation, Dr. Hutton proclaimed that "the President is comfortable and completed the operation with flying colors" and added that "he was alert and responsive throughout the process."[123] A team of orthopedic and plastic surgeons made an incision from the tip of the patient's left ring finger to the wrist and removed the thickened fibrous tissue. The hand was sutured and bandaged. The president stayed overnight at Walter Reed and returned to the White House the following morning with his arm in a sling.

Head Injury and Removal of a Subdural Hematoma

When Reagan left office, he had undergone six surgeries as president (thoracotomy for removal of the bullet after the attempted assassination, colectomy for colon cancer, prostate surgery, two surgeries for basal cell carcinoma on the nose, and surgery for Dupuytren's contracture). But there was more to come.

Six months after moving out of the White House, the Reagans vacationed at a friend's ranch in Mexico. On July 4 while horseback riding, Reagan "was thrown high in the air 15 feet over another horse and fell on rocky ground, hitting his head."[124] He was unconscious for a short time. When he was taken to an army hospital in Arizona (just a short flight away), he complained about dizziness but was otherwise doing well. When he returned to California, further studies revealed a small subdural hematoma,[125] a small accumulation of blood outside the brain but under one of the membranes enveloping the brain. Because the now former president was doing well and showed no neurological signs of symptoms, no further measures were considered necessary at that time.

When Mr. and Mrs. Reagan were flying to Minnesota for their routine annual checkups at the Mayo Clinic, Reagan bumped his head when getting out of his seat. On arrival to the Mayo Clinic, he underwent a CT scan and an MRI of his head, which showed that the subdural hematoma diagnosed in July had grown in size. Despite having no symptoms, the findings were concerning, and Reagan was recommended to have the hematoma removed. On September 8, 1989, he underwent evacuation of the hematoma. Neurosurgeons burred a hole about the size of a dime in the skull bone covering the blood collection and removed it. Before burring the hole, Reagan's scalp was shaved on the right side, and a skin incision was made, creating a scalp flap to provide access to the bone.

A spokesperson for the ex-president was quoted as reporting that "the procedure, which was performed under general anesthesia, lasted slightly over one hour and was without complications."[126] After the surgery, "the president did exceedingly well without complications" and would be discharged home after a week.[127]

Reagan's Final Surgery After Falling and Breaking His Right Hip

On January 12, 2001, Reagan fell in his home in the Bel Air section of Los Angeles and fractured his right hip. He was taken by ambulance to St. John's Health

Center in Santa Monica and underwent surgery the following day. At the time, Reagan was less than a month from turning ninety.

The surgeon performing the procedure explained that "the various parts of the fracture were put together with a series of implants [including a metal plate]—pins and screws and then the fracture heals in that position."[128] The operation took just over one hour. After the procedure, the surgeon commented that "the condition of the president's tissue, specifically the muscle and bone, was that of a much younger man, which obviously helps substantially with his recovery."[129]

As always when Reagan needed surgery, his wife was with him. Except during X-rays and during surgery, Mrs. Reagan was at her husband's side. Reagan's spokesperson commented that "Mrs. Reagan is glued to his side."[130] The surgeon in charge also noticed Mrs. Reagan's devotion to her husband and how much it seemed to mean to the former president. "He's with Mrs. Reagan. He's very calm with Mrs. Reagan. And she feels he's back to himself. So she is happy at this point in time."[131]

Nancy Reagan's heart was warmed by an outpouring of love and support from a multitude of well-wishers. The list of people calling or sending messages contained many of the who's who in American and global politics. Outgoing president Bill Clinton made a statement: "Hillary and I are relieved that President Reagan's treatment for his injury appears to have been successful." He added, "Our thoughts and prayers are with the president, his wife Nancy, and the entire Reagan family during this difficult period. We join all Americans in wishing him a speedy recovery." Mrs. Reagan also heard from president-elect George W. Bush; his father, former president George H.W. Bush; former president Gerald Ford; Senator and Mrs. John McCain; Lady Margaret Thatcher; Prince Charles; former Canadian prime minister and Mrs. Brian Mulroney; former Japanese prime minister Nakasone; and the Reverend Billy Graham.[132]

Unfortunately, Reagan himself was probably never aware of the hundreds of phone calls and messages arriving from all corners of America and around the world. In 1994 the former president had announced in a handwritten farewell letter to the American people that he was suffering from Alzheimer's disease. During the seven years that had passed since his announcement, his mental status had continued deteriorating, and he was now at a stage when he did not recognize his family members any longer. The farewell letter by Reagan softened the heart of his daughter, Patti Davis, who had not always had a good relationship with her father. She moved back to California from New York City to be closer and assist in her father's care. In a recent interview, Ms. Davis mentioned how sad it was to see her father in such mental decline. She explained that "the former president ... wondered why people knew his name."[133]

Despite Alzheimer's disease and other health challenges, the former president went on to live for another three and a half years after his hip surgery. Reagan died on June 5, 2004, at the age of ninety-three. He was survived by his beloved Nancy for almost twelve years.

Summary and Conclusions

Medical and Political Implications

The health of U.S. presidents has always been of great interest to the public. This, of course, reflects the important role played by the presidents both nationally and internationally. The realization that any problem with a president's well-being may have wide political and economic consequences makes the president's health particularly newsworthy.

In addition, citizens' awareness of presidents' health also reflects people's curiosity in general when it comes to celebrities. In countries with a king or queen, there is often an industry built around the monarch and his or her family, supporting vast numbers of books, glitzy and gossipy magazines, and numerous clicks on the internet and certainly also helping the bottom line of many journalists.

Although America's founders primarily wanted to break away from England to stop taxation without representation, they were also fed up with the king's power and arrogance and the pomp and circumstance surrounding the royals. This was one of the reasons there were heated discussions about the title to be used when addressing the early presidents. George Washington was often referred to as "His Excellency" during the American Revolutionary War, but once he was elected leader of the country, he preferred to simply be called "Mr. President." He did not like any of the titles proposed by John Adams, including "His Elective Majesty" and "His Mightiness."[1] The third president preferred the more humble "Mr. Jefferson" over "Mr. President."[2] Today, we seem to have forgotten that a certain amount of modesty was supposed to be part of the executive branch during the early years of the nation. Many ceremonies and rituals surrounding today's American presidents are at least as pompous as those seen around monarchs in some countries nowadays.

Even if security reasons are typically given to explain why U.S. presidents are isolated from and unapproachable by the population, with the White House being protected by roadblocks, fences, and armed guards, one sometimes has to wonder if the modern presidents enjoy being so important that they need all the surrounding grandeur. It is understandable that making the entrance at a reception or state dinner to the tune of "Hail to the Chief" may tickle anyone's ego. Even as he leaves his dwellings, the president's image is certainly reinforced by arrival on the huge *Air Force One*, then, surrounded by secret service agents, by taking part in motorcades with dozens of large luxury vans with tinted glass.

This book covers nine presidents who had surgery at some point during their time in office. Some of the surgeries were minor, some major and dramatic. Sometimes the presidential surgeries were great successes and even lifesaving, whereas on other occasions the interventions by surgeons were embarrassing failures that, if anything, contributed to a president's death. Some of the failures were caused by surgeons' ignorance but also reflected the general state of medicine at the time with poor (or no) understanding of the role of bacteria and the importance of antisepsis—and even cleanliness—in surgery.

In several cases the surgeries were kept secret, and deceptions and outright lies were used to keep people in the dark. The cover-ups often reflected political considerations and were ordered by the patient. On other occasions, the issue of the patient's privacy was a factor, although, now it is commonly agreed by both presidents and ordinary citizens that the commander in chief has no right to privacy when it comes to health and medical or surgical treatment. This is understandable considering the ramifications of having the most powerful person in the world incapacitated by illness and the rumors and conspiracy theories that may be created by a lack of transparency.

That the president has a tough and demanding job is without doubt. To constantly be in the limelight and be scrutinized for any action causes tremendous stress. The burden of having to make decisions that may affect the well-being and even lives of huge numbers of people weighs heavy on the shoulders of the country's leader.

It is a common phenomenon, visible to all, to see presidents age in the office. Statistics suggest that presidents die prematurely even when assassinations are excluded from such calculations.[3] There are many testimonies that the presidents' responsibilities are "literally a killing job"[4] and that "always there is the burden of office which takes its toll on the health and well-being of the incumbent."[5] The weight of the office is almost inhuman, giving "the President more work than a man can do, more responsibilities than a man should take, more pressure than a man can bear."[6] If the president is struck by a health problem, an accident, or an assassination attempt that requires surgery, the sensational aspect escalates, and the headlines grow even bolder.

The surgeries described here have had both medical and political ramifications. In this section of the book, I will summarize presidents' surgeries and highlight some of their medical implications. I will also try to answer the question of how the medical care of a president may have been different today than at the time it happened and whether complications caused by the surgeries could have been avoided. In addition, I will discuss and summarize some of the political fallouts of surgeries on presidents and describe considerations going into the decisions to keep the presidents' surgeries away from the public eye.

George Washington

The need for presidential surgery arose early in the nation's history. Shortly after George Washington was inaugurated as the first president of the United States, his life was saved by a surgeon. If a patient has a large abscess with threatening sepsis (as Washington did), the treatment even today (like almost 250 years ago) is to cut it open and drain the pus, a procedure that surgeons typically call "incision and drainage." And this is exactly what Dr. Samuel Bard, cheered on by his father, John, did in the summer of 1789.

Already in those days, people were curious about the president's health and became nervous if something did not look right. After Washington had been operated on by the younger Dr. Bard, the newly minted president was hauled around in a wagon to let New Yorkers see with their own eyes that Washington was indeed alive and well enough to be able to wave to them and continue as their leader. People were even more anxious a year later when Washington suffered a severe case of influenza, possibly complicated by pneumonia. At that time, his condition was severe enough to make Thomas Jefferson comment that "we have been very near losing the President."[7]

Curiously, about a decade after his life was saved by a surgeon, Washington was denied surgery, resulting in a terrible death caused by what many medical historians believe was acute epiglottitis. The former president was choked to death but could probably have been saved by a tracheotomy (the surgical opening of the windpipe below the obstruction caused by the inflamed and swollen epiglottis), as proposed by one of the doctors attending Washington during his final illness. Instead of listening to their younger colleague, the more senior doctors balked at the idea of slicing the neck of such a famous patient as Washington and instead continued the treatments that were common in those days, bleeding, cupping, and purging. This, if anything, probably hastened Washington's demise.

Notwithstanding the fact that tracheotomies had been described thousands of years earlier,[8] they were considered too risky for centuries. Hippocrates had warned against the procedure because of the complications involved. During Washington lifetime, tracheotomies had begun to be acceptable in Europe in situations of compromised airways caused by inflammation or a foreign body stuck in the trachea. In addition to epiglottitis, diphtheria and peritonsillar abscesses were conditions that could be treated with tracheotomy to save lives.

It is uncertain whether a tracheotomy had ever been performed in America at the time of Washington's final illness. However, the concept of a tracheotomy to open the airway in a patient unable to breath and fighting for his life was known at least by Dr. Dick.

Nowadays, epiglottitis is an uncommon disorder. We have learned that the cause is an infection, most commonly inflicted by *Haemophilus influenzae,* although other bacteria may be involved as well. Vaccines and antibiotics have made the need for a tracheotomy in patients with epiglottitis extremely rare.[9]

Although it is possible that all three doctors caring for Washington during his final hours had heard about the procedure, it was only Dr. Dick who had the guts to propose the operation. His senior colleagues did not have the courage to follow the younger surgeon's advice, so they were all standing helplessly around Washington's deathbed to see him being choked to death.

Andrew Jackson

During his time in office, Andrew Jackson had three encounters with surgeons. Even though Jackson was billed (and paid his surgeon) for two hydrocele "operations," the procedures most likely were what we today would call "drainage and scarification" of the hydrocele. Surgery for hydrocele now most often consists of removal of the fluid-filled sac surrounding the testicle. It is of course reassuring that Jackson's surgeon did not take advantage of the situation to overcharge his famous patient but, as we have seen, billed the president appropriately.

The third time Jackson had to enlist the service of a surgeon was related to Jackson's wild life in his younger years when his character "spelled combat whatever the odds."[10] A bullet lodged in Jackson's left arm was finally removed twenty-nine years after the barroom brawl in Nashville. Of course, the surgeon cut out the bullet without anesthesia, so Old Hickory had to grit his teeth, hold on to his walking stick, and tell his surgeon to just go ahead.

Curiously, a surgery that would probably have benefited Jackson the most never occurred. There was a bullet lodged deep in his chest since the Dickinson duel in 1806. The symptoms of recurrent coughing spells, sometimes bloody, combined with fevers and foul-smelling sputa were probably due to a chronic lung abscess caused by the bullet. Thoracotomies did not become part of surgeons' armamentarium until the end of the 1800s and the beginning of the 1900s. Most likely, many of Jackson's pulmonary symptoms would have had a chance to improve if the abscess had been effectively drained (and perhaps the bullet removed) and if he had received antibiotics.

James Garfield

Seventy-nine agonizing days after being shot, James Garfield died from severe infections caused by the dirty fingers of his surgeons. The individual who arguably best personifies the medical implications of Garfield's failed surgical care was the English surgeon Joseph Lister. Had the American colleagues listened to Lister's advice and learned from his overwhelming evidence for the germ theory, our twentieth president would probably have been able to occupy the White House much longer than six months. Because of the existential role Lister's work played in the development of modern surgery (together with the introduction of anesthesia), Lister's story and his interactions with some of Garfield's surgeons deserve to be told here.

Lister was born into a wealthy and highly educated Quaker family in 1827 in the village of Upton, just outside London. His father, Joseph Jackson Lister, played an essential role in his son's education. The father was himself an acclaimed scientist whose main legacy was the improvement of the modern microscope. This led to Joseph's lifelong love for histology and pathology but was also essential for his discovery of "strange" organisms in infected tissues.

The younger Lister grew up a shy boy suffering from a stutter. This did not prevent him from excelling in school and earning multiple honorary awards during his school years. He would certainly have qualified for the Oxford University or Cambridge University, but Quakers were not allowed to attend either of these institutions at the time. Lister instead enlisted at the University College London, and in 1849, after finishing his undergraduate studies, he registered at the Medical School of that institution. During a two-year rotation as a medical student on the wards of the University College Hospital, Lister became particularly interested in surgery. He initially trained as a dresser but soon advanced to house surgeon.

Several factors contributed to the path that Lister would take during his career and make him famous around the world for his work on antiseptic surgery. He had a long-standing research interest in wounds and wound healing and had good use of the microscope his father had given him when going to University College London. When Lister started his clinical rotation at the University College Hospital in 1851, he arrived with his father's microscope in his luggage. It was said about Lister that he had "a better microscope than any man in college."[11]

Lister's experiences with patients who had severe infections further enhanced his efforts to understand the nature of infections and their prevention and treatment. Early in 1851, he saw an epidemic of erysipelas. The infection, which we now know is caused by streptococci, typically enters the body where the skin has been cut. At a time when antibiotics were not available, the infection could turn aggressive and even become life-threatening. The epidemic that spread like wildfire on the male ward, which had been free from infections for a long time, started with a patient who was already infected when admitted. Within a little more than a week, twelve patients had been infected, and four of them had died.[12]

At the time, a predominant theory was that infections spread through miasma (noxious "bad air") and that the miasma was the cause of the erysipelas outbreak on the male ward. Lister's supervisor, Dr. John Eric Erichsen, was a miasmist who was convinced that the epidemic was caused by bad air. Lister, however, was skeptical and believed that there was something in the infected wounds that caused the epidemics. Lister's suspicion was strengthened when he observed the autopsy of a boy who had died from pyaemia (sepsis). Lister understood that the youngster's infection that had originated in an elbow had spread to the lungs and a knee joint via the bloodstream, thus refuting the theory that the infection had spread via noxious air.

On another occasion, Lister had been provided with tissue from a gangrenous extremity that Erichsen had amputated. When Lister examined the dead and infected tissue under his microscope, he noticed "peculiar objects" the nature of which he did not understand but speculated that they may be "some kind of fungus."[13] He contemplated "the possibility of a minute living organism as the local cause of the disease."[14]

Obviously, Lister was already on to something but did not yet understand the enormous implications of his observations. It would be more than a decade before Lister's initial interest in infected wounds and tissues would translate into the system of aseptic surgery.

Lister graduated with a bachelor of medicine degree from University College Medical School in 1852. During the following eight years he practiced surgery at

Edinburgh, working closely with and being mentored by Dr. James Syme. Syme was the chairman of clinical surgery at Edinburgh University and was considered one of the leading surgeons in Europe at the time. Lister and Syme became close lifelong friends, and Lister was a frequent guest in Syme's home. Lister married Syme's daughter, Agnes, in 1856.

During the years in Edinburgh, Lister developed his skills as not only a surgeon but also a surgical scientist. He conducted laboratory research, much of which took advantage of his unique expertise in microscopy. Among the different areas that fascinated him, he considered his studies on inflammation to be the most important. Later in life he commented, "If my works are read when I am gone, these [the studies on inflammation] will be the ones most highly thought of."[15]

Lister's eight years in Edinburg were followed by nine years as professor of surgery at the University of Glasgow starting in 1860. During his time in Glasgow, he read with fascination some of the papers published by Louis Pasteur introducing evidence that fermentation and putrefaction were caused by "organized particles," strengthening Lister's suspicion that wound infections were caused by something present in the wounds.

It was during his time at Glasgow that Lister successfully treated two patients with open leg fractures with carbolic acid (phenol). By applying he compound to the injuries, not only did the wounds heal without becoming infected, but the fractures also healed. The patients in this way escaped what was the standard treatment of compound fractures: amputation

In 1869 Lister returned to Edinburgh, succeeding his father-in-law as professor of surgery. During the next eight years, Lister continued his experiments using carbolic acid applied to the skin of patients who were to undergo surgery and also put it directly into the surgical wounds. In addition, he made sure the surgeons washed their hands and instruments in carbolic acid solution and sprayed a mist of the solution into the air in the operating room. When Lister was offered a professorship in surgery at King's College in London in 1877, he saw it as an opportunity to widen his audience and increase the impact of aseptic surgery worldwide.

Lister's persistent application of his aseptic system and the dramatic results of reduced surgical infections earned him increasing respect and fame in Europe. When traveling on the continent, he was treated as a true hero. His antiseptic techniques were adopted with great enthusiasm, in particular by German surgeons. The experience would be dramatically different when he tried to expand his teaching to this side of the Atlantic.

When Lister attended the International Medical Congress in Philadelphia 1876, he was one of the most famous foreign surgeons participating in the centennial anniversary of the United States. He was enthusiastically received by many of the about five hundred doctors attending the conference, but some of the most influential surgeons in the crowd were skeptical about his aseptic techniques. Detailed lectures and even a patient demonstration did not sway the opinion of colleagues who refused to accept Lister's ideas. The doctors who were unconvinced by Lister included surgeons who would take care of Garfield five years later. Some of them made less than friendly comments about the English surgeon's theories. For example, Dr. Hamilton commented that "a large proportion of American surgeons seem not to have adopted the practice, whether from a lack of confidence or for other reasons I cannot say."[16] Dr. Samuel Gross, a groundbreaking figure in American surgery and the president of the International Medical Congress, offered even harsher words about Lister and his work: "Little if any faith is placed by any enlightened or experienced surgeon on this side of the Atlantic in the so-called carbolic acid treatment of Professor Lister."[17] Dr. Bliss was never a believer in Lister's technique, but when it was time to deal with the aftermath of Garfield's death, he still claimed that "most approved antiseptic dressings were used during the entire progress of the case."[18]

Although it must have been frustrating for Lister to realize that many prominent American surgeons refused to accept his evidence for the value of antiseptic surgery, he was not dissuaded. He was not there only to get acclaim and acceptance. After having made the effort to cross the Atlantic, he and his wife wanted to take the opportunity to travel the vast American continent. With the completion of the transcontinental railroad being less than a decade earlier, Joseph and Agnes traveled by train all the way to San Francisco and returned east via Salt Lake City and Chicago. In Boston, Lister finally met colleagues who were willing to wholeheartedly embrace his teaching. He knew John Collins Warren from 1869 when Warren had studied with him in Glasgow. Warren, together with the famous Boston surgeon Henry Jacob Bigelow, became strong supporters of Lister.

Despite the mixed receptions by the American colleagues, Lister enjoyed his visit to America immensely "and was glad he had undertaken it."[19]

An obvious medical implication of Garfield's failed treatment is that sometimes the views of established surgical authorities can stand in the way of lifesaving discoveries and treatments. Had influential surgeons such as Agnew, Hamilton, Bliss, and Gross been willing to adopt the new theories advocated by Lister, the outcome of President Garfield's shooting would probably have been different.

Grover Cleveland

A huge political implication of Grover Cleveland's crazy (but successful) surgery aboard the *Oneida* on July 1, 1893, was the ultimate repeal of the Sherman Silver Purchase Act.

On June 30, 1893, President Cleveland called a special session of Congress for August 7. One day later he boarded the *Oneida* for the secret surgery of his mouth tumor. At the special session, Cleveland planned to deliver a message to the legislative body about the dire economic situation in the country. The Panic of 1893 was holding a strong grip on the nation, with disastrous consequences for the country's financial markets and for the protesting, hungry, and angry masses of jobless citizens. Because the president was convinced that the major factor behind the crisis was the Silver Act of July 14, 1890, it would be essential to convince Congress to repeal that law.

Cleveland needed to be back in Washington when the special session was assembled, and he needed to look healthy and robust. On August 4, with Cleveland only a little more than a month into his convalescence after the daring surgery for his mouth tumor, he took off from Buzzards Bay and headed to Washington on a grueling two-day trip. The travel took him on "a carriage to Woods Hole, a train to Newport, a ferry to New York, a carriage across to Jersey City, a train to Washington, and, finally, a carriage to the White House."[20] Although the journey must have been exhausting, people who got a chance to see the president along the way thought he was "looking well and not the least weary" and that he "seemed to be in perfect health."[21] His recent surgery was still a secret; it would be another three and a half weeks before the news of Cleveland's operation exploded on the front page of the *Philadelphia Press.*

The special session of Congress was scheduled for August 7, but because other proceedings took longer than expected, the president had to wait for his turn until the following day. Cleveland's message would finally be delivered to the legislators on August 8. The message, 2,076 words long, was read at one o'clock by clerks in each chamber rather than by the president himself, as was the tradition at the time.[22]

The transcript of the special session message has been preserved for history.[23] In the message, Cleveland started out by providing the background of the "alarming and extraordinary business situation, involving the welfare and prosperity of all our people." He then expressed his surprise to see how the sudden "financial distrust and fear have sprung up on every side" despite what should be quite a stable situation, with "plenteous crops, with abundant promise of remunerative production and manufacture, with unusual invitation to safe investment, and with satisfactory assurance to business enterprise."

Cleveland then did not spare his words and put the blame squarely on Congress: "I believe these things are principally chargeable to Congressional legislation," referring to the Sherman Silver Purchase Act passed three years prior. He then went into detail explaining why he thought the Silver Act was a disaster: it had resulted in falling price of silver and depletion of the nation's gold reserve, with distrust of the currency as a consequence. Cleveland did not hide his disgust over what the congressmen were doing to the citizens: "The very man of all others who has the deepest interest in a sound currency and who suffers most by mischievous legislation in money matters is the man who earns his daily bread by his daily toil." Cleveland ended his message by stating that "I earnestly recommend the prompt repeal of the provisions of the act passed July 14, 1890."[24]

The special session message was extensively covered in the nation's newspapers. Interestingly, there were no comments regarding the president's health and the big surgery he had undergone recently. The secrecy and deceptions were still holding up. And of course, the mustache was still in place.

The reception of Cleveland's message was mixed. Comments made by congressmen were reported in detail by the journalists, revealing a political divide not unlike what we see nowadays. One House member commented that he "was not very favorably impressed by the message." He added that the message contains "a number of Grover Cleveland's platitudes. Mr. Cleveland never goes to the root of the evil."[25] In the same article, Representative Jerry Simpson of Kansas was quoted as saying that "it is the weakest message ever presented to the country. Weak as dish water does not express it."

The opposite side of the political spectrum also had strong opinions.

Representative Benton McMillan of Tennessee said, "The message was a particularly strong presentation of the case in the President's well-known terse and forceful manner of expression. It meets my hearty approval."[26]

Unsurprisingly, the opposing political views resulted in long and heated debates in Congress. It took the House three weeks before Cleveland's supporters could defeat the Silverites and vote to repeal the Silver Act by a margin of 239 to 109. The debate in the Senate was even more contentious, and not until a record-breaking sixty-two-day filibuster was over did the vote to repeal win by 48 to 37. On November 1, President Cleveland signed into law the decision to repeal the Silver Purchase Act.

The outcome was described in the press as "a great personal victory for President Cleveland."[27] Unfortunately, the victory would not have the positive effects Cleveland had been hoping for. The financial problems and the lack of confidence in the nation's economy would continue to cast a shadow on the president during the remainder of his time in the White House. Regardless, the fact that Cleveland would be able to push a significant legislative win through Congress only about a month after a big and risky surgical operation was indeed remarkable.

William McKinley

The shooting of President William McKinley and his unsuccessful surgery had at least two important political consequences and one medical implication.

Leon Czolgosz's deed brought the threat of anarchism to the doorstep of America. The concerns for violence in society became apparent. It had only been twenty years since President James Garfield had been shot and twenty-six years since President Abraham Lincoln had been killed by a bullet to his head.

The other political implication of McKinley's assassination—and this of course was a huge consequence of the event—can be summarized as Theodore Roosevelt. Had McKinley not died from his injury, Roosevelt, arguably one of the most influential chief executives in the history of the United States, may never have risen to the pinnacle of the presidency.

An important medical implication of McKinley's surgery was that surgeons were reminded of the importance of draining the abdomen after injury has been sustained to various organs, in particular the pancreas. Nowadays, most surgeons treating a patient with an injury to the pancreas would probably drain the abdomen with a tube or other device inserted close to the damaged organ to evacuate fluids and reduce the risk for infectious complications. This was not a given at the time of McKinley's operation but became an issue of controversy among the surgeons. A medical historian concluded that "a critical fault in the conduct of his surgical procedure was the absence of drainage to divert the pancreatic secretions from the abdominal cavity."[28]

Franklin Delano Roosevelt

Many mysteries remain surrounding Franklin D. Roosevelt's health. Even the diagnosis of polio as a cause of his paralysis has been questioned in recent writings.

An intriguing question is whether Roosevelt underwent surgery for a malignant melanoma located above his left eyebrow and whether his ultimate stroke was just a garden-variety apoplexy or a bleeding into a brain metastasis from a melanoma. Because most of Roosevelt's medical charts disappeared shortly after his death, many of the questions surrounding his health will most likely never be resolved. The fact that it is not known how and why his medical records were lost only increases the uncertainties about his health and his surgeries.

That Roosevelt's health declined for a long time before his sudden death on April 12, 1945, is an undisputed fact. What remains controversial is whether his reduced health was a factor during the Yalta Conference between the "Big Three" in February 1945. Images from the meeting portray a Roosevelt who had lost weight, looked distraught and tired, and was unfocused despite the fact that "the worst photographs" had been "suppressed by the White House, and only the kindest appeared in print."[29] Foreign observers at the meeting were concerned. For example, Winston Churchill's physician reported that Roosevelt had "all the symptoms of hardening of the arteries of the brain in an advanced stage" and added, "So I give him only a few months to live."[30] Even Joseph Stalin, in an uncharacteristic moment of softness, indicated that "had he known he [Roosevelt] was so ill, he would have been willing to hold the conference at a more convenient location for the American President."[31]

The important question is whether Roosevelt's condition affected his ability to negotiate with Stalin and Churchill at Yalta. Although different views of that question have been expressed over the years, many historians seem to agree that at Yalta the president "performed well."[32] Churchill commented that Roosevelt's mind "moved quickly and acutely over the great range of problems that the Conference considered."[33] Thus, it seems likely that Roosevelt's poor health did not influence his ability to make decisions.

Dwight D. Eisenhower

President Dwight Eisenhower had some rough years during the mid–1950s. His heart attack in 1955 (and possibly one in 1953), followed by major abdominal surgery in 1956 and a stroke in 1957, all left their marks. In particular, the heart attack and the surgery resulted in long periods of convalescence and times away from the Oval Office. There were significant political implications of Eisenhower's health problems on many fronts.

The president's heart attack in 1955 would become an important factor in his decision to run for a second term. In addition, his long convalescence after the heart attack would test the ability of his cabinet to govern the country in his absence.

As president, Eisenhower had always liked the idea of team (or committee) government. He preferred his cabinet members to be experts in their areas of responsibility but also wanted them to have enough knowledge about what was going on in the other departments. He thought that was important to make the cabinet members able to provide insightful opinions on a variety of subjects. As one historian explained, "Eisenhower intended for his administration to be a genuine group effort, rather than a one-man-show."[34] These aspects of governance would be especially important during Eisenhower's illnesses in the 1950s.

Although in general the cabinet members wanted to give the country the impression of a unified government that functioned well during the president's struggles with his health, there were (as expected) some members of the administration who had greater influence than the others. In addition, some individuals were fighting behind the scene for more influence and being able to stay close to the president. An "élite group,"[35] consisting of Vice President Richard Nixon, Secretary of State John Foster Dulles, Secretary of the Treasury George Humphrey, Attorney General Herbert Brownell, Chief of Staff Sherman Adams, and Deputy Chief of Staff Wilton B. Persons, met regularly to carry out the official operations of the government.

Having access to the president was a sign of status and prominence and, of course, influence and power. When Eisenhower remained in Denver for six weeks after his myocardial infarction, the question of who would go to Denver to be with the president and who would stay in Washington became issues of contention. Adams stayed close to Eisenhower in Colorado, whereas Nixon and Dulles rained in the capital. With the president being absent, Nixon's political prominence grew; he frequently chaired the cabinet and National Security Council meetings. Dulles acted in the foreign policy arena with increasing independency, something that would ultimately lead to a less than desirable outcome in the Middle East.

Thus, Eisenhower's struggle with illnesses, including the consequences of his heart attack in 1955 and major surgery in 1956, set the stage for Dulles's more or less independent decisions as secretary of state, resulting in a "major foreign policy debacle" in the Middle East and pushing the United States and the Soviet Union toward a direct confrontation, with potentially disastrous consequences.[36]

Experiencing significant health problems in the 1950s, Eisenhower understood the significance of having rules in place for transfer of power in case the president dies or otherwise becomes incapacitated. He ordered his attorney general to work on a constitutional amendment to address the issue. Together with a team of legal researchers and high-ranking politicians, the Brownell Commission submitted to Congress in 1957 proposed policies that could be included in an amendment. It would take years, but the proposals would be the foundation of the 25th Amendment signed into law by Lyndon Johnson in 1967.

Lyndon Baines Johnson

Like Eisenhower, Johnson had his heart problems. Both were heavy smokers and, of course, had one of the most demanding and stressful jobs there is, two significant risk factors for cardiac disease. Some historians have quoted Johnson's heart attack in 1955 (the same year Eisenhower had his major heart attack) as a reason he was a workaholic, was always impatient, and was easily angered if his will wasn't done. One of Johnson's biographers opined that "his heart attack had only made Lyndon Johnson feel more impatient, as though he now feared that he might be felled by another before he could achieve his goals."[37] Johnson's impatience and demands on people around him created resentment and was a reason why some considered him "a bully, sadist, lout and egotist."[38]

Understanding that "death might overtake him at an early age,"[39] Johnson pushed himself constantly to accomplish his goals. "There was, after all, so much that he wanted to do and only limited time in which to do it." Thus, it was like Johnson was in a vicious cycle: on the one hand, his stressful schedule and impatience increased the risk for cardiac disease, and on the other hand, his heart attack resulted in more stress and impatience to get things done in time.

Even though Johnson's cardiac problems may have actually increased his stressful behavior, he also listened to his body and understood the risks he was subjecting himself to, an insight that would have significant political implications. One historian has argued that one reason why Johnson withdrew from the presidential race in March 1968 was that he was afraid "that he could not survive four more years of presidential tensions."[40] Of course, Johnson's realization that he could lose the election because of the nationwide protests against the Vietnam War may have been the most important reason why he decided not to run again.

In addition to the heart attack in 1955, Johnson's gallbladder surgery in 1965 also had its political implications. We have already seen how he was mocked in the press for exposing the abdominal scar created by his surgeon, a scar that a cartoonist made look like a map of Vietnam. A major reason for Johnson to show off his scar was to prove to the public that he had not had surgery for cancer; he had been informed by his surgeon that surgery for abdominal cancer would require another type of incision. In addition, the scar that Johnson so happily displayed would prove that he had been in the hospital for a surgical procedure and not for another heart attack.

During Johnson's stay in the hospital after the cholecystectomy, the House of Representatives unexpectedly voted down a program supported by the president to subsidize rents paid by low-income families. This political defeat has been ascribed to the absence of Johnson's personal lobbying during his convalescence and time away from the White House. His inability to give resistant congressmen the "Johnson treatment" slowed down some of his political agenda and increased his frustration.

Johnson's own experience of significant health problems, including the need for surgery, made him sensitive to the health care of his fellow Americans and can explain at least in part why forty health-related measures were passed by Congress during Johnson's presidency, "more than in all preceding 175 years of the Republic's history."[41] The Medicare and Medicaid Act, signed into law on July 30, 1965, was one of the crown jewels of Johnson's administration.

An additional consequence of Johnson's own experiences of illnesses—and, importantly, the circumstances surrounding his ascendance to the presidency in 1963—made him realize the importance of having laws in place regulating the transfer of power in case the president would die or become otherwise incapacitated. In February 1967, Johnson signed into law the 25th Amendment, building on proposals put forward by the Eisenhower administration and prompted by President John F. Kennedy's assassination in November 1963.

Ronald Reagan

Arguably, the chief executive who had surgeries resulting in the most tangible political consequences and the most dramatic effects on the president's life was the fortieth president of the country. Ronald Reagan's lifesaving thoracotomy after the shooting outside the Washington Hilton Hotel merely a couple of months into his first term should make any surgeon proud of his profession and colleagues. Reagan was bleeding heavily from a blood vessel in his chest severed by a bullet fired only minutes before he entered the emergency room of George Washington University Hospital. Without the emergency thoracotomy, he would almost certainly have died. Even though this dramatic surgery was performed more than forty years ago, I think it is safe to say that Reagan's surgeons took care of him in a way that would meet the standards even of today's trauma care.

The attempted assassination of Reagan on March 30, 1981, had several significant political ramifications. The president's miraculous survival boosted his popularity dramatically. From the lowest approval ratings of any president since public opinion polling was begun, after the shooting, Reagan's approval rate quickly soared to 67 percent.[42]

When Reagan survived the attempt on his life, he became the first president in American history who was saved after being shot while in office. To many, Reagan mythically seemed to have conquered death and have "risen above mortality."[43] Others commented that it seemed "almost impossible to dislike" the Gipper.[44]

The fact that Reagan kept his sense of humor even after being near death and that his strong physical condition helped him recover quickly—even to the point of being able to appear before Congress to deliver a forceful speech appealing for approval of his economic program less than a month after the attempt on his life—increased the awe for him. Even the president's political opponents could not help but admire him. For example, Democratic senator from New York Daniel Patrick Moynihan wrote, "In the history of the office has any man ever so triumphed over danger and pain and near death? We are surely proud of him."[45]

The press, otherwise not well known for treating presidents kindly, in particular not Republican presidents, handled Reagan with silk gloves. Reagan and his advisers took advantage of the president's popularity and pushed through legislation that otherwise may not have been passed by Congress. Major parts of Reagan's economic recovery program, including significant tax cuts, were approved during his first term.

Another political implication of the attempt on Reagan's life was the "government by troika" and the growing influence of moderate Republicans. During Reagan's hospitalization after the shooting, three individuals became particularly influential. Michael Deaver was an assistant to the president in charge of scheduling, travel, and, importantly, the first lady's office. Deaver and Nancy Reagan worked closely together and seemed to be in constant contact. Their friendship was described as a "critical axis of power."[46]

Edwin Meese was an old friend of Reagan and had been his associate in California. Meese was an important member of Reagan's team from the start of the administration and served as counselor to the president. The White House chief of staff, James Baker, was more of an outsider and a newcomer to the Reagan team. Baker provided political balance to the administration by being a moderate Republican. The troika of Deaver, Meese, and Baker started meeting regularly and took control of the administration shortly after the shooting. They formally met with the president on a daily basis as soon as the first lady lifted the restrictions about seeing her husband. Although the troika went to see the president in the hospital on a frequent basis, they wanted to spare him from what they considered unnecessary and tiring details and most of the time dealt with those issues during meetings "in the hospital cafeteria, quietly keeping the government going."[47]

Of course, everyone knew—or would soon learn—that the most powerful person in the White House may have been the president's wife. Mrs. Reagan would make the final decisions when it came to having access to the president. Deaver's close relationship with Nancy Reagan gave him a powerful position in the troika. It would not be long before Deaver and Baker started to work together more closely and sidestep Meese. Like three kids playing in a sandbox, the two started to outmaneuver the third. The alliance between Deaver and Baker (and in the background Nancy) "slowly but surely eroded Ed Meese's power and influence within the administration."[48] This resulted in reduced influence of strong conservatives and "strengthened the hand of the pragmatists in charting the administration's direction during the first term."[49]

Thus, the shooting of Reagan and his dramatic survival thanks to the emergency thoracotomy on March 30, 1981, boosted his popularity, allowing for legislative victories during the first term, increased the influence of moderate Republicans, and cemented the role of the first lady as a power broker in her husband's administration.

Reagan's next major surgery took place during his second term. In July 1985, he underwent a colectomy for a cancer of the large bowel. Although the procedure itself was never controversial, the timing of the operation (one day after the diagnosis of the tumor rather than "immediately") resulted in dissension, mainly between Nancy Reagan and White House chief of staff Donald Regan, a controversy that would escalate into a war between them and Regan's ultimate resignation. He would leave the White House a bitter and angry man in large part because of the conflicts with the first lady.

From a surgical standpoint, the technique used at Reagan's right hemicolectomy (an open procedure via a large abdominal incision) would most likely be different today, when minimally invasive surgery, even performed with a robotic approach, is becoming the predominant technique to perform colon surgery. This would have resulted in less postoperative pain and a shorter stay in the hospital than Reagan had. The extent of the surgery, however, would be the same today, with removal of the right (ascending) colon, including the cecum, and the surrounding lymph node–bearing tissues. The success of Reagan's surgery was supported by the fact that he lived for another almost forty years without any evidence of recurrent disease.

From the perspective of Reagan's political career and legacy, the most serious implication of the president's surgery for colon cancer was the Iran-Contra scandal. Historians have blamed Reagan's apparent mismanagement of that affair and his inability (or unwillingness?) to remember what had been said or not said during his meeting with McFarland and Regan in the hospital room only five days after his surgery on a number of factors related to the operation. Those factors include the treatment of the president with strong pain medication and sedatives, potentially affecting his memory and other cognitive functions. In addition, Reagan had just been informed that the tumor that had been removed from his large bowel was cancerous, and although the stage of the cancer was favorable and associated with an excellent prognosis, the information that he had had cancer was upsetting to him and distressed him profoundly. The fact that Reagan at the time was seventy-four years old did not help.

Regardless of the reasons Reagan allowed himself to become entangled in problematic political decisions, "the effects of the Iran-Contra scandal on the country were explosive."[50] His approval rating fell like a sinking rock from 67 percent to 46 percent, "the sharpest one-month decline since such polling had begun fifty years before."[51] Reagan, who had always been considered a man "who said what he meant and meant what he said," was no longer enjoying that assessment by people. His presidency seemed to be collapsing, and his legacy was threatened.

As a nonpolitician and a nonhistorian, I find it remarkable that Reagan was able to save his presidency. This happened mainly through his performance on the world stage. It was only about a year after the Iran-Contra scandal that Reagan met with Mikhail Gorbachev at Reykjavik in Iceland. Their growing friendship and respect for each other would help thaw the Cold War and pull the world back from the brink of a catastrophic conflict.

Irrespective of one's political views, it seems to me that Reagan's achievement of being instrumental in saving the world from a disastrous great power, likely nuclear, conflict would make it easy to forgive any flaws he may have had as president. I also think it is sad to see how politicians have squandered the opportunities we had for a peaceful and safe world shortly after Reagan left office and brought us back to a political and military world situation that, at the time of this writing, seems to be as dangerous as the one we saw at the height of the Cold War.

Conclusions

In this book, we have seen successes, failures, and deceptions when it comes to presidential surgeries. In my opinion, the greatest success story is how the thoracic surgeons saved President Reagan's life shortly after he was shot in his chest. Had the doctors not acted rapidly and opened his chest to stop the bleeding, Reagan would surely have died on that frightening day in March 1981.

Among the failures, the surgeons' treatment of James Garfield and his death from severe infections stand out. The outcome would have been different if the surgeons had listened to Dr. Joseph Lister's message of antisepsis and the essential role of cleanliness. The unwillingness among the surgeons to wash their hands cost the president his life.

The circumstances around Grover Cleveland's daring surgery take the prize for deceptions and outright lies, although it may be argued that his demand for secrecy paid off politically. He did indeed manage to get the Silver Act repealed. Cleveland's surgery would also qualify for being counted among the successes. Although crazy and approaching the level of malpractice, the surgeons managed to get the tumor out of Cleveland's mouth without leaving any visible traces behind—and without killing the president!

Chapter Notes

Introduction

1. Achenbach and Cunningham, 2016.
2. Annas, pp. 945–49.
3. Rotondi, "What Happens When a President Becomes Ill or Incapacitated While in Office?"; and "What Is the 25th Amendment and When Has It Been Invoked?"
4. Feerick, "Presidential Succession and Inability"; and Feerick, *The Twenty-Fifth Amendment.*
5. Algeo, p. 12.

Chapter One

1. Heidler and Heidler, p. 72.
2. George Washington to the president of Congress, July 20, 1775, quoted in Nagy, p. 88; and Gillett, p. 22.
3. *Law of 27 July 1775,* cited as Appendix B in Gillett, p. 200.
4. Abbe, p. 10; and Eichner, pp. 25–32.
5. Pennsylvania Hospital History: Historical Timeline, 1751–1800, https://www.uphs.upenn.edu.
6. Warren, p. 99.
7. Avery, "The Story of Valley Forge."
8. Ellis, pp. 9–10.
9. Upham, p. 33.
10. Sparks, *The Writings of George Washington,* p. 88.
11. Rutkow, "Moments in Surgical History," p. 1213.
12. Di Spigna, p. 64.
13. Fenn, p. 4.
14. Drury and Clavin, p. 265.
15. Hasselgren, p. 291.
16. Gilbert, "Presidential Disability and the Twenty-Fifth Amendment," p. 848.
17. Widmer, p. C5.
18. Boudreau and Bleimann, p. 101.
19. Lossing, p. 398.
20. Ellis, p. 190.
21. Heidler and Heidler, p. 72.
22. Frost, p. 509.
23. Ibid.
24. McVickar, pp. 136–37.
25. Ibid., pp. 6–7.
26. Fothergill, pp. 369–72.
27. Hasselgren, p. 205.
28. John Bard to Samuel Bard, September 18, 1761, quoted in McVickar, pp. 14–15.
29. Samuel Bard to John Bard, July 9, 1762, quoted in McVickar, p. 25.
30. Lossing, p. 398.
31. Frost, p. 509.
32. Thomas Jefferson to James Madison, July 24, 1791, *Founders Online,* National Archives https://founders.archives.gov/documents/Madison/01-14-02-0045.
33. Ibid.
34. Hasselgren, p. 250.
35. Mease, p. 33.
36. Ellis, p. 190.
37. Fitzgerald, *The Diaries of George Washington,* quoted in Scheidemandel, p. 519.
38. Sparks, *The Life of George Washington,* p. 400.
39. Ibid.
40. Ibid., p. 401.
41. Ibid.
42. Ibid., p. 403.
43. Ibid., p. 404.
44. Washington's last words, as recorded by Tobias Lear in his journal, Saturday December 14, 1799.
45. Morens, p. 1847.
46. Borman and Davidson, p. 388.
47. Abou-Foul, p. 1000.
48. Morens, p. 1847.
49. Dick, p. 253.
50. Abou-Foul, p. 1001.
51. Morens, p. 1845.
52. *Alexandria Times,* December 19, 1799, quoted in Scheidemandel, pp. 519–20.
53. Scheidemandel, p. 520.
54. Ford, *The True George Washington,* quoted in Scheidemandel, p. 520.
55. Scheidemandel, pp. 519–21; Stavrakis, pp. 539–40; and Abou-Foul, pp. 1000–1002.
56. Scheidemandel, p. 520.
57. Richman, p. 53.
58. Wiedeman, "Presidential Operations: Medical Fact or Urban Legend?" p. 1132.

Chapter Two

1. James, Marquis, p. 17.
2. Ibid.

3. Ibid.
4. Bumgarner, p. 44.
5. Parton, p. 95.
6. Remini, p. 44.
7. James, Marquis, p. 107.
8. Ibid., p. 115.
9. Ibid., p. 107.
10. Remini, p. 53.
11. Rosenberg, p. 723.
12. James, Marquis, p. 113; and Remini, p. 53.
13. James, Marquis, p. 115.
14. Parton, p. 297.
15. Gardner, pp. 405–11, quoted in Rosenberg, p. 723.
16. Parton, p. 298.
17. James, Marquis, p. 116.
18. Rosenberg, p. 723; and Marx, p. 102–3.
19. James, Marquis, p. 118.
20. Parton, p. 299.
21. Ibid., p. 301.
22. Ibid., p. 300.
23. Remini, p. 68.
24. Ibid., p. 64.
25. Ibid.
26. Ibid., p. 65.
27. Ibid., p. 67.
28. Parton, pp. 386–87.
29. Ibid., p. 387.
30. Ibid., p. 388.
31. Remini, p. 69.
32. Parton, p. 388.
33. James, Marquis, p. 152.
34. Remini, p. 69.
35. James, Marquis, p. 152.
36. Remini, p. 69.
37. Letter from Thomas Hart Benton to Jackson, July 25, 1813, quoted in Remini, p. 69.
38. Remini, p. 69.
39. For the locations of the Nashville Inn, the City Hotel, and the post office at the downtown Court House Square of Nashville as well as the open ground beside the inn, "where cocks were accustomed to display their prowess, and tear one another to pieces for the entertainment of some of the citizens," see the map in Parton, p. 392.
40. Parton, p. 392.
41. Ibid., p. 393.
42. Ibid.
43. Ibid.
44. Remini, p. 70.
45. Parton, p. 395.
46. Ibid.
47. Ibid.
48. Ibid., p. 394.
49. Ibid.
50. Ibid., p. 395.
51. Remini, p. 71.
52. Ibid., pp. 71–72.
53. Remini, p. 72.
54. Ibid.
55. James, Marquis, p. 154.
56. General Order, September 24, 1813, Library of Congress, quoted in James, Marquis, p. 154.
57. James, Marquis, p. 154.
58. Remini, p. 73.
59. James, Marquis, p. 159.
60. Remini, p. 73.
61. Ibid.
62. Ibid.
63. Ibid.
64. Parton, pp. 439–40.
65. Ibid., p. 440.
66. AJ to Rachel, April 1, 1814, quoted in James, Marquis, p. 171.
67. James, Marquis, p. 171.
68. Remini, p. 86.
69. Ibid., p. 88.
70. Remini, p. 84.
71. Ibid.
72. Bumgarner, p. 47.
73. Ibid., p. 46.
74. Gardner, p. 408–9; and Bumgarner, p. 49.
75. Bumgarner, p. 50.
76. Remini, p. 89.
77. AJ to Rachel, November 15, 1814, Miscellaneous Jackson Papers, Harvard University Library, and AJ to Rachel, November 17, 1814, Jackson Papers, Missouri Historical Society, quoted in Remini, p. 89.
78. Holmes M. Alexander, p. 112, quoted in Bumgarner, p. 48.
79. Remini, p. 89.
80. Ibid., p. 91.
81. Ibid., p. 101.
82. Ibid., p. 51.
83. Ibid., p. 52.
84. Ibid., p. 92.
85. Whitney, p. 57.
86. "Rachel Donelson Robards Jackson (1767–1828)."
87. Remini, p. 169.
88. James, Marquis, p. 478.
89. Ibid., p. 479.
90. Boller, p. 46.
91. Rosenberg, p. 724; and Wong, pp. 19–20.
92. Brokaw, p. 110, quoted in Wong, p. 21.
93. Palmer, p. 462.
94. Ibid., p. 476.
95. Wong, pp. 21–22.
96. Ibid., p. 19.
97. Rosenberg, p. 724.
98. Remini, p. 84.
99. AJ to Rachel, September 22, 1814, Jackson Papers, Huntington Library, quoted in Remini, p. 84.
100. James, Marquis, p. 590.
101. Rosenberg, p. 725.
102. James, Marquis, p. 598.
103. Remini, p. 224.
104. Ibid.
105. Ibid.
106. James, Marquis, p. 591.
107. Deppisch, pp. 569–71.
108. Ibid., p. 571.
109. Shabani, pp. 134–42; and Yeng, pp. 335–40.
110. Deppisch, p. 570.

111. Ibid., p. 571.
112. Remini, p. 354.
113. Marx, p. 118.
114. Parton, p. 305.
115. Bumgarner, p. 53.
116. Gardner, pp. 405–11; Bumgarner, p. 54; and Remini, p. 358.
117. Gardner, p. 411, quoted in Bumgarner, p. 54.
118. Remini, p. 358.
119. Ibid.
120. Ibid.

Chapter Three

1. Peskin, p. 13.
2. Alger.
3. Bundy, p. 13.
4. Smith, p. 5.
5. Bumgarner, p. 122.
6. Rutkow, *James A. Garfield*, p. 5.
7. Whitney, p. 165, quoted in Bumgarner, p. 122.
8. Smith, p. 39.
9. Rutkow, *James A. Garfield*, pp. 6–7.
10. Ibid., p. 7.
11. Brown and Williams, pp. 1:149–50, quoted in Rutkow, *James A. Garfield*, p. 7.
12. Rutkow, *James A. Garfield*, p. 7.
13. Bundy, p. 33.
14. Brown and Williams, 1967 edition, p. 367.
15. Ibid., p. 273.
16. Ibid., p. 259.
17. Taylor, p. 65.
18. Rutkow, *James A. Garfield*, p. 16.
19. Bates, p. 25.
20. Smith, p. 238.
21. Ibid., p. 310.
22. Ibid., p. 356.
23. Rutkow, *James A. Garfield*, p. 29.
24. Balch, p. 122.
25. Rutkow, *James A. Garfield*, p. 26.
26. Smith, p. 376.
27. Ibid., p. 266.
28. Rutkow, *James A. Garfield*, p. 27.
29. Ibid.
30. Shaw, p. 218.
31. Smith, p. 425.
32. Ibid., p. 426.
33. Brown and Williams, p. 138.
34. Smith, p. 548.
35. Ibid.
36. Conwell, p. 312.
37. Smith, p. 567.
38. Rutkow, *James A. Garfield*, p. 43.
39. Shaw, p. 237.
40. Rosen, p. 152.
41. Ibid.
42. Brown and Williams, p. 250.
43. Rutkow, *James A. Garfield*, p. 43.
44. Ibid., p. 42.
45. Smith, p. 953.
46. Rutkow, *James A. Garfield*, p. 59.
47. Sherman, p. 789.
48. Caldwell, p. 330.
49. Rutkow, *James A. Garfield*, p. 70.
50. Brown and Williams, p. 555.
51. Alexander, Henry H., p. 172.
52. Hayes and Hayes, p. 43, quoted in Rutkow, *James A. Garfield*, pp. 80–81.
53. Rutkow, *James A. Garfield*, p. 83.
54. Paulson, p. 80.
55. *New York Times*, July 3, 1881, quoted in Rutkow, *James A. Garfield*, p. 83.
56. Alexander, Henry H., p. 47.
57. Ibid., p. 49.
58. Ogilvie, p. 34, quoted in Rutkow, *James A. Garfield*, p. 84.
59. Miller, Joseph M., p. 114.
60. Rutkow, *James A. Garfield*, p. 84.
61. Weiner, p. E184.
62. Ehrhardt et al., p. 1713.
63. Rutkow, *James A. Garfield*, p. 85.
64. Ibid.
65. Bliss, "The Story of President Garfield's Illness," p. 299.
66. Herndon, p. 74.
67. Bliss, "Report of the Case of President Garfield," p. 393.
68. Alexander, Henry H., p. 44.
69. Rutkow, *James A. Garfield*, p. 88.
70. Ibid., p. 89.
71. Miller, Joseph M., p. 114.
72. Herr, p. 458.
73. Ackerman, Kenneth D., pp. 402–3.
74. Ibid., p. 403.
75. *New York Times*, July 5, 1881, quoted in Rutkow, *James A. Garfield*, p. 93.
76. Bliss, "The Story of President Garfield's Illness," p. 305.
77. Rutkow, *James A. Garfield*, p. 95.
78. *New York Times*, July 5, 1881, quoted in Rutkow, *James A. Garfield*, p. 95.
79. Rutkow, *James A. Garfield*, p. 98.
80. Ibid., p. 101.
81. Anonymous, "Remarks on Medical Fees," p. 25, quoted in Rutkow, *James A. Garfield*, p. 99.
82. Anonymous, "The Evidence," quoted in Rutkow, *James A. Garfield*, p. 104.
83. *New York Sun*, July 16, 1881, quoted in Rutkow, *James A. Garfield*, p. 103.
84. Boynton, p. 493.
85. Peskin, p. 601.
86. Rutkow, *James A. Garfield*, p. 117.
87. Longmore, p. 751.
88. Ibid.
89. Ibid., p. 752.
90. McCabe, pp. 563–64.
91. Peskin, p. 601.
92. Rutkow, *James A. Garfield*, p. 120.
93. Reyburn, p. 549.
94. Rutkow, *James A. Garfield*, p. 115.
95. Ibid., p. 114.
96. Ridpath, p. 562.
97. Rutkow, *James A. Garfield*, p. 119.
98. Ibid., p. 120.

99. Ibid., pp. 119–20.
100. Reyburn, pp. 581–82.
101. Bates, p. 348.
102. Ibid., p. 348.
103. Rutkow, *James A. Garfield*, p. 125.
104. Bates, p. 348.
105. Ibid.
106. Leech and Brown, p. 247.
107. Reyburn, p. 622.
108. Ridpath, p. 627.
109. Rutkow, *James A. Garfield*, p. 126.
110. McCabe, p. 685.
111. Reyburn, p. 665.
112. Rutkow, *James A. Garfield*, p. 128.
113. Hamilton, p. 619; Pappas and Joharifard, p. 616; Ehrhardt et al., p. 1714; Miller, Joseph M., p. 116; Weiner, p. E185; and Paulson, p. 87.
114. Alexander, Henry H., p. 204.
115. Ibid., p. 237.
116. Kozol, p. 760.
117. Weiner, p. E185.
118. Bliss, "Report of the Case of President Garfield," p. 401.
119. Paulson, p. 87.
120. Rutkow, *James A. Garfield*, p. 128.
121. Esmarch, pp. 234–37.
122. Paulson, p. 87.
123. "Assassin and Avenger," p. 1; and Pappas and Joharifard, p. 617.
124. "The Question of Malpractice in the Case of the Late President Garfield," pp. 600–601.
125. Turnipseed, pp. 620–24.
126. Pappas and Joharifard, pp. 613–18.
127. Quoted in Pappas and Joharifard, p. 616, from the original autopsy report.
128. Pappas and Joharifard, p. 617.
129. The Oneida Community was a religious communal society founded in 1848 near Oneida, New York. The community believed that Christ had already returned in 70 AD. The members of the community practiced communalism with regard to property and possessions, group marriage, and male sexual continence. The Oneida Community dissolved in 1881.
130. Bates, p. 334.
131. Ibid.
132. Ibid.
133. Alexander, Henry H., p. 52.
134. Ibid., p. 46.
135. Ibid., p. 120.
136. Ibid., p. 119.
137. Ibid., p. 165.
138. Ibid.
139. Ibid., p. 166.
140. Ibid., p. 6.
141. Ibid., p. 138.
142. Ibid., p. 228.
143. Ibid., p. 81.
144. Ibid., p. 82.
145. Ibid.
146. Ibid., p. 111.
147. Ibid., p. 112.
148. Ibid., p. 123.
149. Ibid., p. 213.
150. Ibid., p. 227.
151. Ibid., p. 157.
152. Ibid., p. 190.
153. Ibid., pp. 501–2.
154. Ibid., p. 564.
155. Ibid., p. 579.
156. Ibid., p. 124.
157. Ibid., p. 845.
158. Miller, Joseph M., p. 116.
159. Feis, p. 94.
160. Herr, p. 460.
161. Anonymous, "The President's Wound, and the Management of the Case," editorial, p. 309, quoted in Rutkow, *James A. Garfield*, p. 133.
162. Bliss, "Report of the Case of President Garfield," p. 399.
163. Rutkow, *James A. Garfield*, p. 134.
164. Ibid.
165. Getien, "The Inept Doctor."
166. Herndon, p. 74.
167. Rutkow, *James A. Garfield*. p. 94.
168. Ibid., p. 134.
169. Reyburn, pp. 411–17, quoted in Weiner, p. E186.
170. Sims, pp. 594–601, quoted in Weiner, p. E186.
171. Hamilton, p. 620.
172. Kozol, p. 760.

Chapter Four

1. Algeo, p. 19.
2. Ibid., p. 23.
3. Bumgarner, p. 136.
4. Ibid., p. 137.
5. Ibid., p. 136.
6. MacMahon and Curry, p. 38.
7. Nevins, p. 11.
8. Bumgarner, p. 137.
9. Marx, p. 266.
10. Algeo, p. 21.
11. Ibid.
12. Ibid., p. 26.
13. Ibid., p. 27.
14. Ibid.
15. Ibid.
16. Nevins, quoted in Algeo, p. 30.
17. Graff, pp. 60–63.
18. Nevins, p. 448.
19. Graff, pp. 104–5; and Nevins, pp. 467–68.
20. Algeo, p. 6.
21. Parker, p. 141.
22. Algeo, p. 12.
23. Ibid., p. 8.
24. Marx, p. 254.
25. Ibid., p. 15.
26. MacMahon and Curry, p. 38.
27. Ibid.
28. Letter from O'Reilly to Bryant, June 25, 1893, quoted in Keen, *The Surgical Operations on President Cleveland in 1893* by Morreels, p. 543.

29. MacMahon and Curry, p. 39.
30. Ibid., p. 40.
31. Algeo, p. 17.
32. MacMahon and Curry, p. 41; and Algeo, p. 17.
33. Algeo, p. 17.
34. Ibid., p. 75.
35. Ibid., p. 72.
36. MacMahon and Curry, p. 45.
37. Bumgarner, p. 138.
38. MacMahon and Curry, p. 46.
39. Ibid.
40. Algeo, p. 48.
41. MacMahon and Curry, p. 44.
42. Ibid.
43. Bryant, pp. 305–18.
44. Ibid., p. 306.
45. Ibid., p. 306.
46. Ibid., p. 308.
47. Ibid., p. 309.
48. Ibid., p. 312.
49. Ibid., p. 317.
50. Algeo, p. 91.
51. Ibid.
52. Bumgarner, p. 138.
53. Renehan and Lowry, p. 379.
54. Keen, *The Surgical Operations on President Cleveland in 1893*, p. 40.
55. Algeo, p. 95.
56. Ibid., p. 96.
57. MacMahon and Curry, p. 50.
58. Morreels, p. 547.
59. MacMahon and Curry, p. 50.
60. Algeo, p. 127.
61. Ibid., p. 105.
62. MacMahon and Curry, p. 48; and Nelson, p. 10.
63. Beck, pp. 10–11; and Algeo, pp. 106–7.
64. Algeo, p. 144.
65. Ibid., pp. 159–60.
66. McElroy, pp. 30–31, quoted in Bumgarner, p. 139.
67. Bumgarner, p. 40.
68. Crispell and Gomez, p. 261.
69. Graff, pp. 131–33; and Nevins, pp. 730–35.
70. Cleveland, *Ladies Home Journal*, pp. 7–8.
71. Marx, p. 267.
72. Algeo, p. 197.
73. Jeffers, p. 340; and Graff, p. 135.
74. Keen, *Saturday Evening Post*, 1917.
75. Keen, *The Surgical Operations on President Cleveland in 1893*.
76. Algeo, p. 224.
77. Ibid., pp. 224–26.
78. Ackerman, pp. 670–78.
79. Friedell and Rosenthal, pp. 2130–35.
80. Renehan and Lowry, p. 382.

Chapter Five

1. Morgan, p. 404.
2. Yenne, p. 117.
3. Ibid., p. 119.
4. Miller, Scott, pp. 289–90.
5. Adler, p. 121.
6. Miller, Scott, pp. 298–300; and Gould, Lewis L., pp. 250–51.
7. Adler, p. 121.
8. Ibid., p. 118.
9. U.S. Inflation Calculator, www.inflationcalculator.com.
10. Gould, *William McKinley: Last Speech*, p. 3.
11. "Leon Czolgosz."
12. Leech, p. 584.
13. Ibid.
14. Ibid., pp. 584–85.
15. Ibid., pp. 594–95.
16. Olcott, p. 316, quoted in Bumgarner, p. 148.
17. Merry, p. 480; and Miller, Scott, p. 302.
18. Rixey, p. 271.
19. Adler, p. 121.
20. Ibid., p. 122.
21. Ibid., p. 123.
22. Marx, p. 275.
23. Rixey, p. 273.
24. Ibid., 272–3.
25. Ibid, p. 274.
26. Ibid.
27. Ibid.; and Marx, p. 276.
28. Adler, p. 124.
29. Rixey, p. 275.
30. Ibid.
31. Ibid.
32. Adler, p. 123.
33. Rixey, p. 275.
34. Ibid.
35. Ibid., p. 272.
36. Park, pp. 375–81, quoted in Pappas and Swanson, pp. 1107.
37. Pappas and Swanson, p. 1106.
38. Adler, p. 125.
39. Rixey, p. 279.
40. Adler, p. 126.
41. Marx, p. 278.
42. Ibid., p. 279.
43. Adler, p. 127.
44. Rixey, p. 282.
45. Ibid.
46. Ibid.
47. Ibid., 283.
48. Ibid.
49. Adler, p. 128.
50. Leech, p. 600; and Miller, Scott, pp. 319–20.
51. Miller, Scott, pp. 319–20.
52. Rixey, p. 284.
53. Pappas and Swanson, p. 1111.
54. Ibid., p. 1112.
55. Rixey, p. 291.
56. Rixey, p. 290; Adler, p. 128; and Pappas and Swanson, p. 1111.
57. Pappas and Swanson, p. 1111.
58. Rixey, p. 287.
59. Ibid.
60. Adler, p. 130.
61. Rixey, p. 286.

62. Ibid., p. 289.
63. Ibid., p. 287.
64. Adler, p. 124.
65. Ibid., p. 128.
66. Ibid., p. 130.
67. Goldman, *Living My Life*, pp. 289–90.
68. Everett, chap. 5.
69. Taylerson, p. 60; and Wesley, p. 97.
70. Goldman, "The Tragedy at Buffalo."
71. Briggs, p. 260.
72. "Leon Czolgosz."
73. MacDonald, pp. 179–94.
74. "Anarchism," Wikipedia.
75. Levy and Adams, p. 104.
76. "Anarchism," Britannica, www.britannica.com/topic/anarchism/English-anarchist-thought.
77. Ibid.
78. Jensen, p. 191; Kemp, p. 61; and Pernicone & Ottanelli, p. 144.
79. Pernicone & Ottanelli, p. 145.
80. Kemp, p. 62.
81. "Emma Goldman," Wikipedia.
82. Goldman, *Living My Life*, p. 11.
83. Ibid., p. 12.
84. Chalberg, p. 27.
85. Wexler, p. 63.
86. Chalberg, p. 76.
87. Ibid., p. 78.
88. Falk, p. 461.
89. Goldman, *Living My Life*, p. 318.
90. Ibid., p. 384.
91. Brands, p. 411.
92. Ibid., pp. 411–12.
93. Ibid., p. 412.
94. Ibid., p. 413.
95. Ibid., p. 414.
96. Renehan, p. 48.

Chapter Six

1. Bumgarner, p. 205.
2. Ibid., p. 208.
3. Ditunno and Herbison, p. 558.
4. Goldman, et al., "What Was the Cause of Franklin Delano Roosevelt's Paralytic Illness?," p. 232.
5. Tobin, pp. 57–58.
6. Ditunno and Herbison, p. 558.
7. Lomazow and Fettmann, p. 26.
8. Bumgarner, p. 209; and Ditunno and Herbison, p. 558.
9. Lomazow and Fettmann, p. 26.
10. Tobin, pp. 69–70.
11. Ibid., pp. 75–76.
12. Lomazow and Fettmann, p. 28.
13. Ibid., p. 31.
14. Gunther, *Roosevelt in Retrospect*, p. 239; and Lomazow and Fettman, p. 60.
15. Bumgarner, p. 208; and Miller, Nathan, p. 126.
16. Fabricant, p. 349.
17. Wyatt, pp. 547–56.
18. Ibid., p. 554.
19. Guillain, Barré, and Strohl, pp. 1462–70.
20. Landry, pp. 472–74.
21. Waclawik, p. 162; and Petch, p. 380.
22. Lovett, 1916; and Draper, 1917.
23. Goldman et al., "What Was the Cause of Franklin Delano Roosevelt's Paralytic Illness?," pp. 232–40.
24. Ibid., p. 232.
25. Goldman, *Prisoners of Time*, p. 250.
26. Lomazow and Fettmann, p. 27.
27. Goldman et al., "What Was the Cause of Franklin Delano Roosevelt's Paralytic Illness?," p. 238.
28. Ibid.; Goldman, *Prisoners of Time*.
29. Ditunno et al., p. 892.
30. Ibid., p. 883.
31. Ibid., p. 890.
32. Ibid., p. 891.
33. Lomazow and Fettmann, p. 53.
34. McIntire and Creel, p. 57, quoted in Lomazow and Fettmann, p. 53.
35. Lomazow and Fettmann, p. 53.
36. Perkins, p. 4, quoted in Goldsmith, "Unanswered Mysteries in the Death of Franklin D. Roosevelt," p. 900.
37. Lomazow and Fettmann, p. 52.
38. Bruenn, p. 580.
39. Bumgarner, p. 217.
40. McIntire and Creel, p. 17.
41. Lomazow and Fettmann, p. 196.
42. Ibid., p. 192.
43. Ruben, p. 6.
44. Lomazow and Fettmann, p. 121.
45. Ibid., p. 56.
46. Farley, p. 108, quoted in Lomazow and Fettmann, p. 56.
47. Franklin D. Roosevelt, press conference, December 5, 1937, Franklin D. Roosevelt Library, Hyde Park, New York, quoted in Lomazow and Fettmann, p. 57.
48. Lomazow and Fettmann, p. 94.
49. Goldsmith, *A Conspiracy of Silence*, pp. 51–52.
50. Lomazow and Fettmann, p. 94.
51. Suckley diary, February 2, 1944, quoted in Lamozow and Fettmann, p. 95.
52. Lomazow and Fettmann, p. 94.
53. Ibid., p. 96.
54. Ibid.
55. *New York Times*, February 5, 1944.
56. *Washington Post*, February 5, 1944.
57. Tully, p. 274, quoted in Goldsmith, *A Conspiracy of Silence*, p. 34.
58. Bruenn, p. 579.
59. Ibid., p. 580.
60. Ibid.
61. Lomazow and Fettmann, p. 102.
62. Bruenn, p. 581.
63. Lomazow and Fettmann, p. 105.
64. Ibid., p. 104.
65. Goldsmith, *A Conspiracy of Silence*, p. 35.
66. Bruenn, p. 590.

67. James Paullin to Ross McIntire, 1946, McIntire Papers, Franklin D. Roosevelt Library, Hyde Park, New York, quoted in Lomazow and Fettmann, p. 180.
68. McIntire and Creel, p. 242, quoted in Lomazow and Fettmann, p. 180.
69. Goldsmith, "Unanswered Mysteries in the Death of Franklin D. Roosevelt."
70. Ibid., p. 899.
71. Ibid.
72. Ibid.
73. Goldsmith, *A Conspiracy of Silence*, p. 6.
74. Goldsmith, "Unanswered Mysteries in the Death of Franklin D. Roosevelt," p. 900.
75. Ibid.
76. Bruenn, p. 579.
77. Goldsmith, "Unanswered Mysteries in the Death of Franklin D. Roosevelt," p. 900.
78. Ibid.
79. Bruenn, p. 591; and Goldsmith, "Unanswered Mysteries in the Death of Franklin D. Roosevelt," p. 908.
80. Bruenn, p. 591.
81. Goldsmith, "Unanswered Mysteries in the Death of Franklin D. Roosevelt," p. 901.
82. Goldsmith, *A Conspiracy of Silence*, p. 115.
83. Ibid.
84. Ibid., p. 114.
85. Goldsmith, "Unanswered Mysteries in the Death of Franklin D. Roosevelt," p. 900.
86. Lomazow and Fettmann, p. 91.
87. Ibid.
88. Moran, p. 150, quoted in Lomazow and Fettmann, p. 91.
89. James A. Farley, letter to the editor, *New York Times*, March 6, 1951, quoted in Goldsmith, "Unanswered Mysteries in the Death of Franklin D. Roosevelt," p. 906.
90. Goldsmith, "Unanswered Mysteries in the Death of Franklin D. Roosevelt," p. 899.
91. Ibid., p. 902.
92. Bruenn, p. 587.
93. Goldsmith, "Unanswered Mysteries in the Death of Franklin D. Roosevelt," p. 902.
94. Perkins, p. 4, quoted in Goldsmith, "Unanswered Mysteries in the Death of Franklin D. Roosevelt," p. 902.
95. Goldsmith, "Unanswered Mysteries in the Death of Franklin D. Roosevelt," p. 903.
96. Lomazow and Fettmann, p. 162.
97. Ibid., p. 166.
98. Moran, p. 242, quoted in Lomazow and Fettmann, p. 166.
99. Lomazow and Fettmann, p. 2.
100. Ibid., p. 3.
101. Goldsmith, "Unanswered Mysteries in the Death of Franklin D. Roosevelt," p. 899.
102. Lomazow and Fettmann, p. 119; and Goldsmith, *A Conspiracy of Silence*, chap. 17–20.
103. Goldsmith, *A Conspiracy of Silence*, p. 171.
104. Ibid., pp. 171–72; and Lomazow and Fettmann, pp. 119–20.
105. Goldsmith, "Unanswered Mysteries in the Death of Franklin D. Roosevelt," p. 899.
106. Goldsmith, *A Conspiracy of Silence*, p. 171; and Lomazow and Fettmann, p. 120.
107. Lomazow and Fettmann, p. 121.
108. Ibid., p. 122.
109. MacArthur, p. 199, quoted in Lomazow and Fettmann, p. 131.
110. Roosevelt and Libby, p. 283.
111. Goldsmith, "Unanswered Mysteries in the Death of Franklin D. Roosevelt," p. 904.
112. L'Etang, p. 95.
113. Ibid.
114. Lomazow and Fettmann, p. 63.
115. Ibid., p. 73.
116. Ibid., p. 74.
117. Ibid., p. 75.
118. Ackerman and Lomazow, p. 530.
119. Farrell, pp. 110–24; and Lomazow and Fettmann, p. 64.
120. Chiarion-Sileni et al., pp. 170–82.
121. Rishi and Yu, p. 45.
122. Bauer-Nilsen et al., pp. 83–88.
123. Lomazow and Fettmann, pp. 63–75.
124. Holmberg, pp. 123–31.
125. Lomazow and Fettmann, p. 130.
126. Goldsmith, "Unanswered Mysteries in the Death of Franklin D. Roosevelt," p. 905.
127. Ibid.
128. L'Etang, p. 95.
129. Wiedeman, "Presidential Operations: Medical Fact or Urban Legend?," p. 1135; and Goldsmith, "Presidential Operations," p. 546.
130. L'Etang, p. 95.
131. Lomazow and Fettmann, p. 205.
132. Ibid., pp. 79–81, 84.
133. Bruenn, pp. 579–91.
134. Marx, p. 366; McConnell, pp. 110–18; and Lomazow and Fettmann, p. 204.
135. Lomazow and Fettmann, p. 206.
136. Goldsmith, *A Conspiracy of Silence*, p. 49.
137. Goldsmith, "Introduction of Chemotherapy by Omentum for a Glioblastoma WHO-IV," p. 59.
138. Goldsmith, "Unanswered Mysteries in the Death of Franklin D. Roosevelt," p. 904.
139. Goldsmith, "Presidential Operations," p. 546.
140. Goldsmith, "Unanswered Mysteries in the Death of Franklin D. Roosevelt," p. 899.
141. Ibid.
142. Ibid., p. 904.
143. Goldsmith, *A Conspiracy of Silence*.
144. Ibid., p. 9.
145. Goldsmith, "Unanswered Mysteries in the Death of Franklin D. Roosevelt," p. 907.
146. Goldsmith, "Presidential Operations," p. 546.
147. Wiedeman, "Reply," p. 547.

Chapter Seven

1. Bumgarner, p. 225.
2. Ambrose, *Eisenhower: Soldier, General of the Army, President-Elect (1893–1952)*, p. 25.

3. Burk, p. 4.
4. Reeves, 1999.
5. Eisenhower, Dwight D., p. 76.
6. Bumgarner, p. 225.
7. Ibid.
8. Gilbert, *The Mortal Presidency*, p. 74.
9. Bumgarner, p. 226.
10. Richardson, Elmo, p. 3.
11. Gilbert, *The Mortal Presidency*, p. 87.
12. Eisenhower, John, p. 184.
13. Gilbert, *The Mortal Presidency*, p. 94.
14. Ibid.
15. Ambrose, *Eisenhower: The President (1952–1969)*, p. 43.
16. Bumgarner, p. 228.
17. D'Este, p. 303.
18. Ibid.
19. Ibid., p. 420.
20. Ibid., p. 419.
21. Dwight Eisenhower to Mamie Eisenhower, June 12, 1943, quoted in D'Este, p. 420.
22. David and David, 1983.
23. D'Este, p. 419.
24. Gilbert, *The Mortal Presidency*, p. 94.
25. "President Dwight D. Eisenhower's Farewell Address (1961)."
26. Summersby, Kay, *Eisenhower Was My Boss* p. 29.
27. Gunther, *Eisenhower, the Man and the Symbol*p. 29.
28. Ambrose, *Eisenhower: Soldier, General of the Army, President-Elect (1893–1952)*, p. 488.
29. Thomas, p. 175.
30. Gilbert, *The Mortal Presidency*, p. 89.
31. Brendon, p. 313.
32. Brown, p. 88.
33. Gilbert, *The Mortal Presidency*, p. 91.
34. Kucharski, p. 123.
35. Williams, p. 345; and Shephard, p. 785.
36. Summersby, Kay, *Eisenhower Was My Boss*, p. 29.
37. D'Este, p. 171.
38. Endnote 35, chap. 14, D'Este, p. 732.
39. Heaton, p. 662.
40. D'Este, p. 171.
41. Ibid.
42. Ibid.
43. Gilbert, *The Mortal Presidency*, p. 80.
44. Pillsbury, pp. 631–32.
45. Ibid., pp. 631–32.
46. Ibid., p. 632.
47. Ibid.
48. Ibid.
49. D'Este, p. 247.
50. Eisenhower medical records, 1910–1945, Snyder Papers, box 2, Dwight D. Eisenhower Library, Abilene, Kansas, quoted in D'Este, p. 247.
51. Regional enteritis was described in Crohn, Ginzburg, and Oppenheimer, "Regional Ileitis." Because the first author of the paper was Burrill B. Crohn, a gastroenterologist at Mount Sinai Hospital in New York City, the disease soon became known as Crohn's disease. The disease is a chronic inflammatory disorder that can affect any part of the gastrointestinal tract. The small bowel is the organ most often affected, and the inflammation can occur as a single lesion or multiple lesions separated by areas of normal bowel, so-called skipped lesions. One outcome of Crohn's disease can be scar formation in the intestinal wall, resulting in narrowing of the bowel that may ultimately cause an obstruction. The cause of Crohn's disease remains unknown. Treatments include medication and surgery. Surgery is typically performed to correct a complication of the disease, such as an obstruction.
52. Heaton, p. 662.
53. Ibid.
54. Figure 2 in Heaton, p. 663.
55. Pappas, p. 192.
56. Heaton, p. 663.
57. Ibid., p. 664.
58. Gilbert, *The Mortal Presidency*, p. 102.
59. Eisenhower, John, p. 186, quoted in Gilbert, *The Mortal Presidency*, p. 102.
60. *The Daily Press*, Saturday, June 9, 1956.
61. Cranethe, p. 1.
62. Editorials, *Daily Press*, June 9, 1956, p. 4.
63. Heaton, p. 665.
64. Ibid.
65. Ibid.
66. Ibid., pp. 661–66.
67. Marston, pp. 237–39.
68. Messerli, p. 1327.
69. Barr and Pappas.
70. Ravdin Papers 1912–1972, box 14, folder 7, University of Pennsylvania Archives and Records Center, quoted in Barr and Pappas, 2017.
71. Telegram to the American College of Surgeons from President Eisenhower, October 5, 1956, Ravdin Papers 1912–1972, box 12, folder 6, University of Pennsylvania Archives and Records Center, quoted in Barr and Pappas.
72. Hughes, p. 795.
73. Ibid.
74. Ibid.
75. Ibid, p. 794.
76. Ibid., p. 796.
77. Ibid., p. 797.
78. Ibid., p. 798.
79. United States Department of Defense, Armed Forces Institute of Pathology, Walter Reed Army Hospital, Autopsy protocol, Dwight D. Eisenhower (WRGH A-69-000), Washington, District of Columbia: Walter Reed Hospital, 1969.
80. Gilbert, *The Mortal Presidency*, p. 86.
81. Messerli, p. 1325.
82. Ibid.
83. Ibid., p. 1329.
84. Loughlin.
85. Letter from John Eisenhower to Dr. Kevin R. Loughlin, October 20, 2005, copy of entire letter included in Loughlin.
86. Lasby, 1997, quoted in Messerli, p. 1328.
87. Ibid.

Chapter Eight

1. Gilbert, *The Mortal Presidency*, p. 176.
2. Ibid., p. 177.
3. Dallek, p. 38.
4. Barber, p. 129.
5. Dallek, p. 39.
6. Miller, Merle, pp. 20–22.
7. Caro, *The Years of Lyndon Johnson: Means of Ascent*, p. 139.
8. Bumgarner, p. 252.
9. Johnson, *My Brother Lyndon*, p. 97.
10. Bumgarner p. 251.
11. Ibid.
12. Caro, *The Years of Lyndon Johnson: The Path to Power*, p. 434.
13. Bumgarner, p. 251.
14. Prud'homme, p. 213.
15. Ibid.
16. Ibid.
17. Ibid., p. 212.
18. Anthony Bourdain, quoted in Prud'homme, p. vii.
19. Prud'homme, p. 214.
20. Ibid.
21. Ibid.
22. Ibid.
23. Caro, *The Years of Lyndon Johnson: Means of Ascent*, p. 194.
24. Ibid.
25. Bumgarner, p. 252.
26. Caro, *The Years of Lyndon Johnson: Means of Ascent*, p. 194; and Bumgarner p. 252.
27. Gilbert, *The Mortal Presidency*, p. 178.
28. Caro, *The Years of Lyndon Johnson: Means of Ascent*, p. 195.
29. Ibid.
30. Bumgarner, p. 254.
31. Miller, Merle, p. 236.
32. Bumgarner, p. 251.
33. Mirkin.
34. Rosenthal, "Johnson's Washington Recalled as Time of Restless Volubility," p. 34.
35. Reedy, p. 157.
36. Gilbert, *The Mortal Presidency*, p. 203.
37. Evans and Novak, p. 90.
38. Mirkin, 2019.
39. Gilbert, *The Mortal Presidency*, p. 184.
40. Bumgarner p. 255.
41. Gilbert, *The Mortal Presidency*, p. 184.
42. Pappas and Mulvihill, p. 160.
43. Gilbert, *The Mortal Presidency*, p. 193.
44. Coccolini et al., pp. 755–63.
45. Johnson, "Statement by the President Announcing That He Would Undergo Surgery," quoted in Pappas and Mulvihill, p. 162.
46. Pappas and Mulvihill, pp. 160–66.
47. Ibid., p. 163.
48. Ibid., p. 162.
49. Ibid., p. 164.
50. Ibid.
51. Ibid.
52. Ibid.
53. Lomazow, "The Truth About Lyndon Johnson's Gallbladder Scar."
54. Ibid.
55. Pappas and Mulvihill p. 164.
56. Lomazow, "The Truth About Lyndon Johnson's Gallbladder Scar," 2011.
57. Cain, "Transcript, Oral History Interview I."
58. Ibid., p. I-15.
59. Ibid., p. I-17.
60. Ibid., p. I-18.
61. "Lyndon B. Johnson: The President's News Conference, November 3, 1966."
62. https://www.presidency.ucsb.edu/documents/the-presidents-news-conference-1179.
63. Pappas and Mulvihill, p. 165.
64. Rosenthal, "Johnson's Washington Recalled as Time of Restless Volubility," p. 34.
65. Ibid.
66. Altman, "Navy Confirms Johnson Had Surgery for Skin Cancer."
67. Ibid.
68. Ibid.
69. Bumgarner, p. 257.
70. Gilbert, *The Mortal Presidency*, p. 201.
71. Bumgarner, p. 257.
72. Mirkin.
73. Ibid.
74. Gilbert, *The Mortal Presidency*, p. 201.
75. Kearns Goodwin, p. 16.
76. Mirkin.
77. Cunningham, p. 304.

Chapter Nine

1. Bumgarner, p. 281.
2. Reagan, Ronald, p. 21.
3. Ibid.
4. Bumgarner, p. 281.
5. Reagan, Ronald, p. 262.
6. Aaron and Rockoff, p. 1689.
7. Reagan, Ronald, p. 259.
8. Ibid; and Aaron and Rockoff, p. 1689.
9. Beahrs, p. 88.
10. Morris, p. 428.
11. Reagan, Ronald, p. 259.
12. Ibid., p. 260; and Aaron and Rockoff, p. 1689.
13. Reagan, Ronald, p. 260.
14. Ibid.
15. Aaron and Rockoff, p. 1689.
16. Beahrs, p. 88.
17. Aaron and Rockoff, pp. 1689–93.
18. Reagan, Ronald, p. 262.
19. Ibid., p. 260.
20. Reagan, Nancy, p. 6.
21. Reagan, Ronald, p. 261.
22. Ibid.; and Aaron and Rockoff, p. 1690.
23. Beahrs, p. 89.
24. When peritoneal lavage is performed, clear fluid is infused through a catheter into the abdominal cavity, and the return fluid is then examined;

if blood is noted in the return fluid, this may indicate bleeding from an injured abdominal organ.

25. Reagan, Nancy, p. 9.
26. Ibid.
27. Ibid.
28. Ibid., p. 11.
29. Aaron and Rockoff, p. 1692.
30. Reagan, Nancy, p. 12.
31. Ibid., p. 15; and Aaron and Rockoff, p. 1692.
32. Reagan, Ronald, p. 264.
33. Aaron and Rockoff, p. 1692.
34. Ibid.
35. Morris, p. 443.
36. Ibid.
37. Ibid., p. 429.
38. Ibid.
39. Aaron and Rockoff, p. 1693.
40. Reagan, Nancy, p. 12.
41. Letter written to Jodi Foster by John Hinckley, Jr., quoted in "John Hinkley, Jr."
42. Reagan, Nancy, p. 18.
43. Reagan, Ronald, p. 261.
44. Reagan, Nancy, p. 242.
45. Ibid.
46. Reagan, Ronald, p. 270.
47. Speakes, p. 8.
48. Regan, p. 167.
49. Speakes, p. xi.
50. Reagan, Ronald, p. 271.
51. Reagan, Nancy, p. 242.
52. Regan, p. 167.
53. Speakes, p. xi.
54. Regan, p. 167.
55. Speakes, p. xi.
56. Reagan, Ronald, p. 499.
57. Morris, p. 516.
58. Reagan, Ronald, p. 500.
59. Speakes, p. 186.
60. Reagan, Nancy, p. 272.
61. Ibid.
62. Reagan, Ronald, p. 500.
63. Reagan, Nancy, p. 272.
64. Ibid.
65. Reagan, Ronald, p. 500.
66. Reagan, Nancy, p. 275.
67. *Public Papers of the Presidents: Ronald Reagan, 1985*, p. 919.
68. Wiedeman, p. 1136.
69. Beahrs, p. 92.
70. Reagan, Ronald, p. 500.
71. Ibid., p. 501.
72. Reagan, Nancy, p. 276.
73. Reagan, Ronald, p. 501.
74. Reagan, Nancy, p. 277.
75. Reagan, Ronald, p. 501.
76. Reagan, Nancy, p. 278.
77. The parts of the president's address presented here were quoted in Reagan, Nancy, pp. 278–79.
78. Reagan, Nancy, p. 279.
79. Speakes, p. 195.
80. Reagan, Ronald, p. 502.
81. Reagan, Nancy, p. 278.
82. Kyriakos, p. 1063.
83. Reagan, Nancy, p. 274.
84. Kyriakos, p. 1065.
85. Ibid., p. 1063.
86. Reagan, Ronald, p. 502.
87. Reagan, Nancy, p. 273.
88. Regan, p. 15.
89. "Doctors Have a Tense Debate: Reagan 'Has' or 'Had' Cancer?," quoted in Sorensen, p. 705.
90. Reagan, Nancy, pp. 277–78.
91. Ibid., p. 278.
92. Ibid., p. 312.
93. Regan, p. 3.
94. Reagan, Nancy, p. 275.
95. Regan, p. 3.
96. Reagan, Ronald, pp. 501–2.
97. *The Tower Commission Report*, p. 129, quoted in Gilbert, *The Mortal Presidency*, p. 65.
98. Reagan, Ronald, p. 504.
99. DiClerico, p. 322; and Gilbert, *The Mortal Presidency*, p. 65.
100. Gilbert, *The Mortal Presidency*, p. 65.
101. Regan, p. 83.
102. Gilbert, *The Mortal Presidency*, p. 67.
103. Ibid., p. 69.
104. Hess, p. 143.
105. Reagan, Ronald, p. 502.
106. Ibid.
107. Speakes, p. 198.
108. Reagan, Ronald, 502.
109. Etzkorn and Alam, p. 716.
110. Boffey, "Reagan to Have Surgery on Nose for Skin Cancer."
111. Beahrs, p. 92.
112. Ibid., p. 96.
113. Ibid., p. 94.
114. Ibid.
115. Regan, p. 68.
116. Reagan, Nancy, p. 325.
117. Ibid., p. 326.
118. Ibid.
119. Regan, p. 68.
120. Reagan, Ronald, p. 536.
121. Ibid., p. 537.
122. The condition is named after Baron Guillaume Dupuytren, a French military surgeon who described the condition in the 1830s. Dupuytren also became famous for treating Napoleon's hemorrhoids.
123. Johnson, "Reagan in 'Good Spirits' after Hand Surgery."
124. Beahrs, p. 94.
125. Ibid.
126. "Caused by Fall Off Horse: Reagan Survives Brain Surgery to Remove Fluid."
127. Beahrs, p. 94.
128. "Former President Reagan Recovering after Hip Surgery."
129. "Reagan Undergoes Surgery after Breaking Right Hip in a Fall."
130. "Reagan Recovering from Hip Surgery. Wife Nancy Remains at His Side."
131. "Former President Reagan Recovering after Hip Surgery."

132. "Reagan Recovering from Hip Surgery. Wife Nancy Remains at His Side."
133. Bobrow, p. C6.

Summary and Conclusions

1. Ellis, p. 193.
2. Prud'homme, p. 37.
3. Gilbert, *The Mortal Presidency*, pp. 4–11.
4. James, Dorothy Buckton, p. 104.
5. Pious, p. 12.
6. Cronin, pp. 1, 379.
7. Hasselgren, p. 262.
8. Pahor, pp. 677–87.
9. Naples, pp. 462–65.
10. James, Marquis, p. 17.
11. Fisher, p. 49.
12. Richardson, "Joseph Lister's Domestic Science."
13. Wrench, p. 33.
14. Ibid., p. 34.
15. Fisher, p. 89.
16. Rutkow, "Joseph Lister and His 1876 Tour of America."
17. Ibid.
18. Bliss, "Report of the Case of President Garfield," p. 399.
19. Cameron, p. 117.
20. Algeo, p. 123.
21. Ibid.
22. "The Message," quoted in Murray et al., pp. e1–e6.
23. "August 8, 1893: Message Regarding Economic Crisis."
24. https://millercenter.org/the-presidency/presidential-speeches/august-8-1893-special-session-message.
25. "The President's Message," *St. Louis Globe–Democrat*, August 9, 1893.
26. Ibid.
27. Algeo, p. 184.
28. Bumgarner, p. 132.
29. Gilbert, *The Mortal Presidency*, p. 62.
30. Bishop, pp. 294–95.
31. Gilbert, *The Mortal Presidency*, p. 61.
32. Ibid., p. 68.
33. Burns, p. 469.
34. Gilbert, *The Mortal Presidency*, p. 119.
35. Ibid.
36. Ibid., p. 129.
37. Clifford, p. 388.
38. Reedy, p. 157.
39. Gilbert, *The Mortal Presidency*, p. 203.
40. Ibid.
41. Ibid., p. 206.
42. Mervin, p. 113; and Gilbert, *The Mortal Presidency*, pp. 244–45.
43. Blumenthal, p. 308.
44. Mayer and McManus, p. 13.
45. Moynihan, p. 10.
46. Van Damm, p. 196.
47. Mayer and McManus, p. 113.
48. Gilbert, *The Mortal Presidency*, p. 250.
49. Ibid.
50. Ibid., p. 256.
51. Ibid.; and Karp, p. 243.

Bibliography

Books

Ackerman, Kenneth D. *Dark Horse: The Surprise Election and Political Murder of President James A. Garfield*. New York: Carroll & Graf, 2003.

Alexander, Henry H. *The Life of Guiteau and the Official History of the Most Exciting Case on Record: Being the Trial of Guiteau for Assassinating Pres. Garfield*. Philadelphia: National Publishing Company, 1882. Reprinted as part of the collection *Making of the Modern Law: Trials, 1600–1926*, Harvard Law School Library.

Alexander, Holmes M. *The American Talleyrand*. New York: Harper, 1935.

Algeo, Matthew. *The President Is a Sick Man*. Chicago: Chicago Review Press, 2011.

Alger, Horatio. *From Canal Boy to President, or the Boyhood and Manhood of James A. Garfield*. Boston: De Wolfe, Fiske, & Co., Publishers, 1881.

Ambrose, Stephen. *Eisenhower: Soldier, General of the Army, President-Elect (1893–1952)*, Vol. 1. New York: Simon & Schuster, 1983.

Ambrose, Stephen. *Eisenhower: The President (1952–1969)*, Vol. 2. New York: Simon & Schuster, 1984.

Balch, William R. *The Life of James Abram Garfield, Late President of the United States*. Philadelphia: Hubbard Brothers, 1881.

Barber, James David. *The Presidential Character*. Englewood Cliffs, NJ: Prentice-Hall, 1977.

Bates, Richard O. *The Gentleman from Ohio: An Introduction to Garfield*. Durham, NC: Moore Publishing, 1973.

Beck, Glenn. *Dreamers and Deceivers: True and Untold Stories of the Heroes and Villains Who Made America*. New York: Treshold Editions, 2014.

Berger-Knorr, Lawrence. *The Pennsylvania Relations of Dwight D. Eisenhower*. New Kingstown, PA: Sunbury, 2005.

Bishop, Jim. *FDR's Last Year*. New York: William Morrow, 1974.

Blumenthal, Sidney. *Our Long National Daydream*. New York: Harper & Row, 1988.

Boller, Paul F. *Presidential Campaigns: From George Washington to George W. Bush*. New York: Oxford University Press, 2004.

Boudreau, Allan, and Alexander Bleimann. *George Washington in New York*. New York: American Lodge of Research, 1989.

Brands, H.W. *T.R.: The Last Romantic*. New York: Basic Books, 1997.

Brendon, Piers. *Ike*. New York: Harper & Row, 1986.

Briggs, L. Vernon. *The Manner of Man That Kills: Spencer, Czolgosz, Richeson*. Charleston, SC: BiblioLife 2009. Originally published by Richard G. Badger, Boston, MA, 1921.

Brown, Harry J., and Frederick D. Williams, eds. *The Diary of James A. Garfield, 1848–1871*. East Lansing: Michigan State University Press, 1967, 1973, 1981.

Brown, John M. *Through These Men*. New York: Harper & Row, 1956.

Bumgarner, John R. *The Health of the Presidents*. Jefferson, NC: McFarland, 1993.

Bundy, Jonas Mills. *The Life of James Abram Garfield: With an Account of the President's Death and Funeral Obsequies*. New York: A.S. Barnes, 1881.

Burk, Robert F. *Dwight D. Eisenhower: Hero and Politician*. Boston: Twayne, 1986.

Burns, James MacGregor. *Roosevelt: The Lion and the Fox*. New York: Harcourt, Brace & World, 1956.

Caldwell, Robert G. *James Garfield, Party Chieftain*. New York: Dodd and Mead, 1931.

Cameron, Hector Charles. *Joseph Lister, the Friend of Man*. London: William Heinemann, 1948.

Caro, Robert A. *The Years of Lyndon Johnson: Means of Ascent*. New York: Knopf, 1990.

Caro, Robert A. *The Years of Lyndon Johnson: The Path to Power*. New York: Knopf, 1982.

Chalberg, John C. *Emma Goldman: American Individualist*. New York: HarperCollins, 1991.

Clifford, Clark. *Counsel to the President*. New York: Random House, 1991.

Conwell, Russell H. *The Life, Speeches, and Public Services of James A. Garfield, Including an Account of His Assassination, Lingering Pain, Death, and Burial*. Portland, ME: George Stinson, 1881.

Crispell, Kenneth R., and Carlos F. Gomez. *Hidden Illness in the White House*. Durham: Duke University Press, 1988.

Cronin, Thomas E. *The State of the Presidency*. Boston: Little, Brown, 1980.

Cunningham, Homer F. *The Presidents' Last Years: George Washington to Lyndon B. Johnson.* Jefferson, NC: McFarland, 1989.
Dallek, Robert. *Lone Star Rising.* New York: Oxford University Press, 1991.
David, Lester, and Irene David. *Ike & Mamie: The Story of the General and His Lady.* New York: Putnam, 1983.
D'Este, Carlo. *Eisenhower: A Soldier's Life.* New York: Henry Holt, 2002.
DiClerico, Robert E. *The Contemporary American President.* New York: Pearson, 2012.
Di Spigna, Christian. *Founding Martyr: The Life and Death of Dr. Joseph Warren, the American Revolution's Lost Hero.* New York: Crown, 2018.
Draper, George. *Acute Poliomyelitis.* Philadelphia: Blakiston's Son & Co., 1917.
Drury, Bob, and Tom Clavin. *Valley Forge.* New York: Simon & Schuster, 2018.
Eisenhower, Dwight D. *At Ease.* Garden City, NY: Doubleday, 1967.
Eisenhower, John S.D. *Strictly Personal.* Garden City, NY: Doubleday, 1974.
Ellis, Joseph J. *His Excellency George Washington.* New York: Knopf, 2004.
Evans, Rowland, and Robert Novak. *Lyndon B. Johnson: The Exercise of Power.* New York: New American Library, 1966.
Everett, Marshall. *Complete Life of William McKinley, and Story of His Assassination.* New York: Historical Press, 1901.
Falk, Candace. *Emma Goldman: A Documentary History of the American Years,* Vol. 1, *Made for America, 1890–1901.* Oakland: University of California Press, 2003.
Farley, James A. *Jim Farley's Story: The Roosevelt Years.* New York: Whittlesey House, 1948.
Feerick, John D. *The Twenty-Fifth Amendment: Its Complete History and Applications.* New York: Fordham University Press, 2014.
Feis, Ruth S.B. *Mollie Garfield in the White House.* Chicago: Rand McNally, 1963.
Fenn, Elizabeth A. *Pox Americana: The Great Smallpox Epidemic of 1775–82.* New York: Hill and Wang, 2001.
Ferrell, Robert H. *Ill-Advised: Presidential Health and Public Trust.* Columbia: University of Missouri Press, 1992.
Fisher, Richard B. *Joseph Lister, 1827–1912.* New York: Stein and Day, 1977.
Fitzpatrick, John C., ed. *The Diaries of George Washington,* Vol. 4. *1789–1799.* Boston: Houghton Mifflin, 1925.
Ford, Paul Leicester. *The True George Washington.* Philadelphia: J.R. Lippincott, 1896.
Fothergill, John. *Medical Observations and Inquiries of the Society of Physicians in London,* Vol. 2. London: Printed for William Johnston, in Ludgate-Street, 1762.
Frost, John. *Pictorial Life of George Washington: Embracing a Complete History of the Seven Years' War, the Revolutionary War, the Formation of the Federal Constitution, and the Administration of Washington.* Philadelphia: Thomas, Cowperthwait & Co., 1848.
Gallagher, Hugh Gregory. *FDR's Splendid Deception.* New York: Dodd, Mead, 1985.
Gilbert, Robert E. *The Mortal Presidency: Illness and Anguish in the White House.* New York: Fordham University Press, 1998.
Gillett, Mary C. *The Army Medical Department, 1775–1818: Center of Military History, United States Army.* Washington, D.C.: Books Express Publishing, 2012.
Goldman, Armond S. *Prisoners of Time: The Misdiagnosis of FDR's 1921 Paralytic Illness.* Expert Health Data Programming, Inc. Press (EHDP), 2017.
Goldman, Emma. *Living My Life.* New York: Knopf, 1931.
Goldsmith, Harry S. *A Conspiracy of Silence: The Health and Death of Franklin D Roosevelt.* Lincoln, NE: iUniverse, Inc., 2007.
Gould, Lewis L. *The Presidency of William McKinley.* Lawrence: University Press of Kansas, 1980.
Graff, Henry F. *Grover Cleveland.* New York: Times Books, 2002.
Gunther, John. *Eisenhower, the Man and the Symbol.* New York: Harper and Brothers, 1952.
Gunther, John. *Roosevelt in Retrospect.* New York: Harper and Brothers, 1950.
Hasselgren, Per-Olof. *Revolutionary Surgeons: Patriots and Loyalists on the Cutting Edge.* Nashville, TN: Knox, 2021.
Hayes, Henry Gillespie, and Charles Joseph Hayes. *A Complete History of the Trial of Guiteau, Assassin of President Garfield.* Philadelphia: Hubbard Brothers, 1882.
Heidler, David S., and Jeanne T. Heidler. *Washington's Circle: The Creation of the President.* New York: Random House, 2015.
Hess, Stephen. *Organizing the Presidency.* Washington, D.C.: Brookings Institution Press, 2002.
James, Dorothy Buckton. *The Contemporary Presidency.* New York: Pegasus, 1969.
James, Marquis. *The Life of Andrew Jackson: Complete in One Volume; Part One: The Border Captain; Part Two: Portrait of a President.* Indianapolis: Bobbs-Merrill, 1938.
Jeffers, H. Paul. *An Honest President: The Life and Presidencies of Grover Cleveland.* New York: William Morrow, 2000.
Jensen, Richard Bach. *The Assassination of Umberto I of Italy.* Cambridge: Cambridge University Press, 2014.
Johns, A. Wesley. *The Man Who Shot McKinley.* South Brunswick, NJ: A.S. Barnes, 1970.
Johnson, Sam Houston. *My Brother Lyndon.* New York: Cowles Book Co., 1969.
Karp, Walter. *Liberty Under Siege.* New York: Henry Holt, 1988.
Kearns Goodwin, Doris. *Lyndon Johnson and the American Dream.* New York: St. Martin's Griffin, 1991.

Keen, William Williams. *The Surgical Operations on President Cleveland in 1893.* Philadelphia: George W. Jacobs & Co., 1917.
Kemp, Michael. *The Cook, the Blacksmith, the King and the Weaver.* Jefferson, NC: McFarland, 2018.
Lasby, Clarence G. *Eisenhower's Heart Attack: How Ike Beat Heart Disease and Held On to the Presidency.* Lawrence: University Press of Kansas, 1997.
Lear, Tobias. "II, 14 December 1799: The Diary Account." Founders Online. https://founders.archives.gov/documents/Washington/06-04-02-0406-0002.
Leech, Margaret. *In the Days of McKinley.* New York: Harper and Brothers, 1959.
Leech, Margaret, and Harry J. Brown. *The Garfield Orbit.* New York: Harper and Row, 1978.
L'Etang, Hugh. *The Pathology of Leadership.* London: William Heinemann Medical Books, 1969.
Levy, Carl, and Matthew S. Adams. *The Palgrave Handbook of Anarchism.* New York: Palgrave Macmillan, 2018.
Lomazow, Steven, and Eric Fettmann. *FDR's Deadly Secret.* New York: PublicAffairs, 2009.
Lossing, Bensen J. *Recollections and Private Memories of Washington, by His Adopted Son, George Washington Parke Custis, with a Memoir of the Author, by His Daughter, and Illustrative and Explanatory Notes.* Philadelphia: J.W. Bradley, 48 Fourth Street, 1861.
Lovett, Robert W. *The Treatment of Infantile Paralysis.* Philadelphia: Blakiston's Son & Co., 1916.
MacArthur, Douglas. *Reminiscences.* New York: McGraw-Hill, 1964.
MacMahon, Edward B., and Leonard Curry. *Medical Cover-ups in the White House.* Washington, D.C.: Farragut Publishing, 1987.
Marx, Rudolph. *The Health of the Presidents.* New York: Putnam, 1960.
Mayer, Jane, and Doyle McManus. *Landslide: The Unmaking of the President, 1984–1988.* Boston: Houghton Mifflin, 1989.
McCabe, James D. *The Life and Public Services of Gen. James A. Garfield, Our Martyred President.* Tecumseh, MI: A.W. Mills, 1881.
McElroy, Robert. *Grover Cleveland, the Man and the Statesman,* Vol. 2. New York: Harper & Brothers, 1923.
McIntire, Ross, and George Creel. *White House Physician.* New York: Putnam, 1946.
McVickar, John. *The Life of Samuel Bard, M.D.: A Domestic Narrative.* Carlisle, MA: Applewood Books, 2010. Originally published as *Domestic Narrative of the Life of Samuel Bard, M.D. LL.D.: Late President of the College of Physicians and Surgeons of the University of the State of New York, &c* (New York: The Literary Rooms, Corner of Broadway and Pine-Street. A. Paul, Printer, 1822).
Mease, James. *The Surgical Works of the Late John Jones, M.D.... To Which Are Added, a Short Account of the Life of the Author; With Occasional Notes and Observations.* Philadelphia: Wrigley and Berriman, 1795.
Merry, Robert W. *President McKinley.* New York: Simon & Schuster, 2017.
Mervin, David. *Ronald Reagan and the American Presidency.* London: Longman, 1990.
Miller, Merle. *Lyndon. An Oral Biography.* New York: Putnam, 1980.
Miller, Nathan. *An Intimate History.* Garden City, NY: Doubleday, 1983.
Miller, Scott. *The President and the Assassin.* New York: Random House, 2011.
Moran, Lord. *Churchill: Taken from the Diaries of Lord Moran: The Struggle for Survival, 1940–1965.* Boston: Houghton Mifflin, 1966.
Morgan, H. Wayne. *William McKinley and His America.* Revised ed. Kent, OH: Kent State University Press, 2003.
Morris, Edmund. *Dutch: A Memoir of Ronald Reagan.* New York: Modern Library, 1999.
Moynihan, Daniel Patrick. *Came the Revolution: Argument in the Reagan Era.* New York: Harcourt, 1988.
Nagy, John A. *Dr. Benjamin Church, Spy: A Case of Espionage on the Eve of the American Revolution.* Yardley, PA: Westholme Publishing, 2013.
Nelson, W. Dale. *Who Speaks for the President? The White House Press Secretary from Cleveland to Clinton.* Syracuse, NY: Syracuse University Press, 1998.
Nesbitt, Lawrence. *What Reagan Couldn't Tell Us.* Bloomington, IN: iUniverse, 2011.
Nevins, Allan. *Grover Cleveland: A Study in Courage.* New York: Dodd, Mead, 1934.
Ogilvie, John S. *The Life and Death of James A. Garfield from the Tow Path to the White House.* Chicago: J.S. Ogilvie, 1881.
Olcott, Charles S. *The Life of William McKinley.* Boston: Houghton Mifflin, 1916.
Palmer, James F., ed. *The Works of John Hunter, F.R.S., in Four Volumes.* Vol. 1. London: Longman, Rees, Orme, Brown, Green, and Longman, 1835. Reprinted by Cambridge University Press, 2015.
Parker, George F. *A Life of Grover Cleveland with a Sketch of Adlai Stevenson.* New York: Cassell Publishing, 1892.
Parton, James. *Life of Andrew Jackson.* Vols. 1, 2, and 3. New York: Mason Brothers, 1859.
Pernicone, Nunzio, and Fraser M. Ottanelli. *Assassins against the Old Order: Italian Anarchist Violence in Fin De Siècle Europe.* Champaign: University of Illinois Press, 2018.
Peskin, Allan. *Garfield: A Biography.* Kent, OH: Kent State University Press, 1978.
Pious, Richard M. *The American Presidency.* New York: Basic Books, 1979.
Prud'homme, Alex. *Dinner with the President: Food, Politics, and a History of Breaking Bread at the White House.* New York: Knopf, 2023.
Public Papers of the Presidents: Ronald Reagan, 1985. Washington, D.C.: U.S. Government Printing Office, 1988.
Reagan, Nancy, with William Novak. *My Turn. The*

Memoirs of Nancy Reagan. New York: Random House, 1989.
Reagan, Ronald. *An American Life*. New York: Simon & Schuster, 1990.
Reedy, George. *Lyndon B. Johnson: A Memoir*. New York: Andrews & McMeel, 1980.
Regan, Donald T. *For the Record: From Wall Street to Washington*. Orlando, FL: Harcourt Brace Jovanovich, 1988.
Remini, Robert V. *The Life of Andrew Jackson*. New York: Harper Perennial Political Classics, 2009. Based on Robert V. Remini, *The Life of Andrew Jackson*, Vol. 1, 1977; Vol. 2, 1981; Vol. 3, 1984.
Renehan, Edward J., Jr. *The Lion's Pride: Theodore Roosevelt and His Family in Peace and War*. New York: Oxford University Press, 1998.
Richardson, Elmo. *The Presidency of Dwight D. Eisenhower*. Lawrence: Regents Press of Kansas, 1979.
Ridpath, John C. *The Life and Work of James Garfield*. Cincinnati, OH: Jones Brothers, 1881.
Roosevelt, James, and Bill Libby. *My Parents: A Differing View*. Chicago: Playboy, 1976.
Rosen, Fred. *Murdering the President: Alexander Graham Bell and the Race to Save James Garfield*. Lincoln, NE: Potomac Books, 2016.
Rosenman, Samuel I. *Working with Roosevelt*. New York: Harper & Brothers, 1952.
Rutkow, Ira. *James A. Garfield*. New York: Times Books, Henry Holt, 2006.
Shaw, John, ed. *Crete and James: Personal Letters of Lucretia and James Garfield*. East Lansing: Michigan State University Press, 1994.
Shephard, Roy J. *An Illustrated History of Health and Fitness, from Pre-History to Our Post-Modern World*. New York: Springer International Publishing, 2014.
Sherman, John. *Recollections of Forty Years in the House, Senate and Cabinet: An Autobiography*, Vol. 2. Chicago: Werner, 1895.
Smith, Theodore C. *The Life and Letters of James Abram Garfield*. New Haven, CT: Yale University Press, 1925.
Sparks, Jared. *The Life of George Washington, Commander-in-Chief of the American Armies, and First President of the United States: To Which Are Added, His Diaries and Speeches; and Various Miscellaneous Papers Relating to His Habits and Opinions; By Jared Sparks; In Two Volumes*. Vol. 2. London: Henry Colburn, Publisher, Great Marlborough Street, 1839.
Sparks, Jared. *The Writings of George Washington; Being His Correspondence, Addresses, Messages, and Other Papers, Official and Private: Selected and Published from the Original Manuscripts, with a Life of the Author, Notes, and Illustrations*, Vol. 2,. Part 1, *Comprising Official Letters Relating to the French War, and Private Letters before the American Revolution*. Boston: Russell, Odiorne, and Metcalf, and Hilliard, Gray, and Co., 1834.
Speakes, Larry. *Speaking Out: Inside the Reagan White House*. New York: Scribner, 1988.
Summersby, Kay. *Eisenhower Was My Boss*. New York: Prentice-Hall, 1948.
Summersby Morgan, Kay. *Past Forgetting: My Love Affair with Dwight D. Eisenhower*. New York: Simon & Schuster, 1977.
Taylerson, A.W.F. *The Revolver, 1889–1914*. New York: Crown, 1971.
Taylor, John M. *Garfield of Ohio: The Available Man*. New York: Norton, 1970.
Thomas, Evan. *Ike's Bluff: President Eisenhower's Secret Battle to Save the World*. Boston: Little, Brown, 2012.
Tobin, James. *The Man He Became: How FDR Defied Polio to Win the Presidency*. New York: Simon & Schuster, 2013.
The Tower Commission Report. New York: Bantam Books, 1987.
Tully, Grace. *Franklin Delano Roosevelt: My Boss*. Chicago: People's Book Club, 1949.
Upham, Charles Wentworth. *The Life of General Washington, First President of the United States: Written by Himself Comprising His Memoirs and Correspondence as Prepared by Him for Publication, Including Several Original Letters Now First Printed*. Edited by Rev. C.W. Upham in Two Volumes, Vol. 1. London: Office of the National Illustrated Library, 227 Strand, 1851.
Van Damm, Helene. *At Reagan's Side*. New York: Doubleday, 1989.
Warren, Edward. *The Life of John Warren, M.D.: Surgeon-General during the War of the Revolution, First Professor of Anatomy and Surgery in Harvard College, President of the Massachusetts Medical Society, Etc*. Boston: Noyes Holmes and Company, 1874.
Wexler, Alice. *Emma Goldman: An Intimate Life*. New York: Pantheon Books, 1984.
Whitney, David C. *The American Presidents*. Garden City, NY: Doubleday, 1985.
Williams, Charles. *Harold Macmillan*. Beverly Hills, CA: Phoenix Books, 2010.
Wilson, John. *Talking to the President: The Pragmatics of Presidential Language*. New York: Oxford University Press, 2015.
Wrench, Guy Theodore. *Lord Lister: His Life and Work*. London: T. Fisher Unwin, 1913.
Yenne, Bill. *The Complete Book of US Presidents*. Minneapolis, MN: Zenith, 2016.

Articles

Aaron, Benjamin L., and S. David Rockoff. "The Attempted Assassination of President Reagan: Medical Implications and Historical Perspectives." *Journal of the American Medical Association* 272 (1994):1689–1693.
Abbe, Truman. "The Surgery of the Revolutionary War." *Medical Record: A Weekly Journal of Medicine and Surgery* 4 (1913): 1–27.
Abou-Foul, Ahmad K. "A Lesson on Human Factors in Airway Management Learnt from the Death of George Washington." *Otolaryngology—Head and Neck Surgery* 163 (2020): 1000–1002.
Achenbach, Joel, and Lillian Cunningham. "The

Hidden History of Presidential Disease, Sickness and Secrecy." *Washington Post,* September 12, 2016.

Ackerman, A. Bernard, and Steven Lomazow. "An Inquiry into the Nature of the Pigmented Lesion above Franklin Delano Roosevelt's Left Eyebrow." *Archives of Dermatology* 144 (2008): 529–532.

Ackerman, Lauren V. "Verrucous Carcinoma of the Oral Cavity." *Surgery* 23 (1948): 670–678.

Adler, Selig. "The Operation on President McKinley." *Scientific American* 208 (1963): 118–131.

Altman, Lawrence K. "Navy Confirms Johnson Had Surgery for Skin Cancer." *New York Times,* June 29, 1977, p. 14.

Altman, Lawrence K. "White House Revises Description of Reagan Skin Cancer Removal." *New York Times,* August 8, 1985.

Annas, George J. "The Health of the President and Presidential Candidates: The Public's Right to Know." *New England Journal of Medicine* 333 (1995): 945–949.

"Assassin and Avenger: The Trial of Guiteau and His Alleged Assailant." *Washington Post,* November 21, 1881, p. 1.

Avery, Ron. "The Story of Valley Forge." Historic Valley Forge, www.ushistory.org/ValleyForge/history/vstory.html.

Barr, Justin, and Theodore N. Pappas. "President Eisenhower and His Bowel Obstruction." *Bulletin of the American College of Surgeons,* November 1, 2017.

Bauer-Nilsen, Kristine, et al. "Stereotactic Radiosurgery for Brain Metastases from Malignant Melanoma and the Impact of Hemorrhagic Metastases." *Journal of Neuro-Oncology* 140 (2018): 83–88.

Beahrs, Oliver H. "The Medical History of President Reagan." *Journal of the American College of Surgeons* 178 (1994): 86–96.

Bliss, Doctor W. "Report of the Case of President Garfield, Accompanied with a Detailed Account of the Autopsy." *Medical Record* 20 (1881): 393–402.

Bliss, Doctor W. "The Story of President Garfield's Illness." *Century Magazine* 23 (1881): 299–305.

Bobrow, Emily. "Patti Davis: The Daughter of Ronald Reagan Offers Advice for Alzheimer's Caregivers." *Wall Street Journal.* September 25–26, 2021, p. C6.

Boffey, Philip M. "Reagan to Have Surgery on Nose for Skin Cancer." *New York Times,* July 31, 1987.

Boodman, S., and S. Royner. "Reagan's Fall: Head Injury More Than Meets the Eye." *Los Angeles Times,* September 15, 1989.

Borman, J., and J.T. Davidson. "A History of Tracheostomy: *Si Spiritum Ducit Vivit* (Cicero)." *British Journal of Anaesthesia* 35 (1963): 388–390.

Boynton, Silas. "President Garfield's Care, Dr. Boynton's Statement." *American Observer Medical Monthly* 18 (1881): 492–494.

Brokaw, A.V,L. "Report of Cases." *Saint Louis Courier of Medicine* 5 (1891): 110.

Brown, Martin L., and Arnold L. Potosky. "The Presidential Effect: The Public Health Response to Media Coverage About Ronald Reagan's Colon Cancer." *Public Opinion Quarterly* 54 (1990): 317–329.

Bruenn, Howard G. "Clinical Notes on the Illness and Death of President Franklin D. Roosevelt." *Annals of Internal Medicine* 72 (1970): 579–591.

Bryant, Joseph D. "On Excision of the Superior Maxilla. A Study of Two Hundred and Fifty Cases." *Annals of Surgery* 11 (1890): 305–318.

Cain, James C. Transcript, Oral History Interview I, 2/22/70, by David G. McComb. Internet copy, LBJ Library.

Chiarion-Sileni, Vanna, et al. "Brain Metastases from Malignant Melanoma." *Forum* (Genova) 13 (2003): 170–182.

Cleveland, Grover. "Woman's Mission and Woman's Clubs." *Ladies Home Journal* 22 (October 7, 1905): 7–8.

Coccolini, Federico, et al. "Laparoscopic Cholecystectomy in Acute Cholecystitis: Refining the Best Surgical Timing Through Network Meta-analysis of Randomized Trials." *Surgical Laparoscopy Endoscopy & Percutaneous Techniques* 32 (2022): 755–763.

Cranethe, Butron. "Stock Market Surges on Doctors' Assurance That Eisenhower Is Fit; Doctors' Report Rallies Market." *New York Times,* February 16, 1956, p. 1.

Crohn, Burrill B., et al. "Regional Ileitis: A Pathological and Clinical Entity." *Journal of the American Medical Association* 99 (1932): 1323–1329.

Deppisch, L.M., et al. "Andrew Jackson's Exposure to Mercury and Lead: Poisoned President?" *Journal of the American Medical Association* 282 (1999): 569–571.

Dick, Elisha C. "Facts and Observations Relative to the Disease of Cynanche Trachealis, or Croup." *Philadelphia Medical and Physical Journal,* Suppl. 3 (1809): 242–255.

Ditunno, John F., et al. "Franklin Delano Roosevelt: The Diagnosis of Poliomyelitis Revisited." *American Academy of Physical Medicine and Rehabilitation* 8 (2016): 883–893.

Ditunno, John F., and Gerald J. Herbison. "Franklin D. Roosevelt: Diagnosis, Clinical Course, and Rehabilitation from Poliomyelitis." *American Journal of Physical and Medical Rehabilitation* 81 (2002): 557–566.

Ehrhardt, John D., et al. "'Yes, I Shot the President, but His Physicians Killed Him': The Assassination of President James A. Garfield." *American Surgeon* 84 (2018): 1711–1716.

Eichner, L.G. "The Military Practice of Medicine During the Revolutionary War." *Tredyffrin Easttown Historical Society Quarterly Archives* 41 (2004): 25–32.

Esmarch, Friedrich. "Concerning the Treatment of the Wound of President Garfield." *Boston Medical and Surgical Journal* 107 (1882): 234–237.

Etzkorn, Jeremy R., and Murad Alam. "What Is

Mohs Surgery?" *Journal of the American Medical Association, Dermatology* 156 (2020): 716.
"The Evidence." *Walsh's Retrospect* 3 (1882): 305–307.
Fabricant, Noah D. "Franklin D. Roosevelt's Tonsillectomy and Poliomyelitis." *Eye Ear Nose and Throat Monthly* 36 (1957): 348–349.
Farrell, Hubert J. "Cutaneous Melanomas with Special Reference to Prognosis." *Archives of Dermatology and Syphilology* 26 (1932): 110–124.
Feerick, John D. "Presidential Succession and Inability: Before and after the Twenty-Fifth Amendment." *Fordham Law Review* 79 (2010): 908–949.
Friedell, H.L., and L.M. Rosenthal. "The Etiologic Role of Chewing Tobacco in Cancer of the Mouth." *Journal of the American Medical Association* 116 (1941): 2130–2135.
Gardner Francis T. "The Gentleman from Tennessee." *Surgery Gynecology & Obstetrics* 88 (1949): 405–411.
Gertstenzang, J., and R. Steinbrook. "Reagan Reported 'Fine' after Prostate Surgery: Initial Tests Show No Sign of Cancer; President 'Working, Reading' in Hospital, First Lady Says." *Los Angeles Times*, January 6, 1987.
Getien, Larry. "The Inept Doctor Who killed President Garfield." *New York Post*, September 22, 2016.
Gilbert, Robert E. "The Politics of Presidential Illness: Ronald Reagan and the Iran-Contra Scandal." *Politics and the Life Sciences* 33 (2014): 58–76.
Gilbert, Robert E. "Presidential Disability and the Twenty-Fifth Amendment: The Difficulties Posed by Psychological Illness." *Fordham Law Review* 79, no. 3 (2011): 843–879.
Goldman, Armond S., et al. "Franklin Delano Roosevelt's (FDR's) (1882–1945) 1921 Neurological Disease Revisited: The Most Likely Diagnosis Remains Guillain-Barré Syndrome." *Journal of Medical Biography* 24 (2016): 452–459.
Goldman, Armond S., et al. "What Was the Cause of Franklin Delano Roosevelt's Paralytic Illness?" *Journal of Medical Biography* 11 (2003): 232–240.
Goldman, Emma. "The Tragedy at Buffalo." *Free Society*, October, 1901.
Goldsmith, Harry S. "Introduction of Chemotherapy by Omentum for a Glioblastoma WHO-IV." *Surgical Neurology International* 14 (2023): 59.
Goldsmith, Harry S. "Presidential Operations." *Journal of the American College of Surgeons* 209 (2009): 546–547.
Goldsmith, Harry S. "Unanswered Mysteries in the Death of Franklin D. Roosevelt." *Surgery Gynecology & Obstetrics* 149 (1979): 899–908.
Guillain, Georges Charles, Jean-Alexandre Barré, and André Strohl. "Sur un syndrome de radiculonévrite avec hyperalbuminose du liquide céphalo-rachidien sans réaction cellulaire: Remarques sur les caractères cliniques et graphiques des réflexes tendineux." *Bulletins et Mémoires de la Société des Médecins des Hôpitaux de Paris* 40 (1916): 1462–1470.
Hamilton, Frank Hastings. "A Review of the Late President Garfield's Case." *British Medical Journal* (October 15, 1881): 619–620.
Heaton, Leonard D., et al. "President Eisenhower's Operation for Regional Enteritis: A Footnote to History." *Annals of Surgery* 159 (1964): 661–666.
Herndon, James H. "Ignorance Is Bliss." *Harvard Orthhopaedic Journal* 15 (2013): 74–77.
Herr, Harry W. "Ignorance Is Bliss: The Listerian Revolution and Education of American Surgeons." *Journal of Urology* 177 (2007): 457–460.
Holmberg, Carl Jacob, et al. "Surgery for Gastrointestinal Metastases of Malignant Melanoma: A Retrospective Exploratory Study." *World Journal of Surgical Oncology* 17 (2019): 123–131.
Hughes, Carl W., et al. "A Review of the Late General Eisenhower's Operations: Epilog to a Footnote to History." *Annals of Surgery* 173 (1971): 793–799.
Johnson, J. "Reagan in 'Good Spirits' after Hand Surgery." *New York Times*, January 8, 1989.
Keen, William W. "The Surgical Operations on President Cleveland in 1893." *Saturday Evening Post* (September 22, 1917): 24–25.
Kozol, Robert A. "Frank Hastings Hamilton: Medical Educator and Surgeon to President Garfield." *American Journal of Surgery* 151 (1986): 759–760.
Kucharski, A. "Medical Management of Political Patients: The Case of Dwight D. Eisenhower." *Perspectives in Biology and Medicine* 22 (1978): 115–126.
Kyriakos, Michael. "The President's Cancer, the Dukes Classification, and Confusion." *Archives of Pathology and Laboratory Medicine* 109 (1985): 1063–1066.
Landry, Jean Baptiste Octave. "Note sur la paralysie ascendante aigue." *Gazette Hebdomadaire de Medicin* 6 (1859): 472–474.
Longmore, Thomas. "Remarks on the Instruments Designed for Exploring Gun-shot Wounds, with a View to Detect Bullets or Other Foreign Bodies Suspected to Be Lodged in Them." *British Medical Journal* (December 30, 1871): 751–752.
Loughlin, Kevin R. "The Search for Eisenhower's Adrenal Tumor." *Hektoen International: A Journal of Medical Humanities* (Spring 2020). https://hekint.org/2020/05/27/the-search-for-eisenhowers-adrenal-tumor/.
MacDonald, Carlos F. "The Trial, Execution, Autopsy and Mental Status of Leon F. Czolgosz, Alias Fred Nieman, the Assassin of President McKinley." *Journal of Mental Pathology* 1 (1902): 179–194.
Marston, Adrian. "Did President Eisenhower Have Crohn's Disease?" *Journal of Medical Biography* 10 (2002): 237–239.
McConnell, Ben H. "The Little Stroke: A Report on 89 cases." *Journal of the American Geriatric Society* 9 (1961): 110–118.
"The Message." *Buffalo Evening News*, August 8, 1893, p. 1.
Messerli, Franz H., et al. "The President and the

Pheochromocytoma." *American Journal of Cardiology* 99 (2007): 1325–1329.
Miller, Joseph M. "The Death of James Abram Garfield." *Surgery, Gynecology & Obstetrics* 107 (1958): 113–118.
Morens, David M. "Death of a President." *New England Journal of Medicine* 341 (1999): 1845–1849.
Morreels, Charles L. "New Historical Information on the Cleveland Operations." *Surgery* 62 (1967): 542–551.
Murray, Margaret, et al. "Maxillary Prosthetics, Speech Impairment, and Presidential Politics: How Grover Cleveland Was Able to Speak Normally after His 'secret' Operation." *Surgery Journal* 6 (2020): e1–e6.
Naples, James, et al. "Reemergence of the Natural History of Otolaryngologic Infections: Lessons Learned from 2 American Presidents." *Otolaryngology—Head and Neck Surgery* 157 (2017): 462–465.
Pahor, Ahmes L. "Ear, Nose, and Throat in Ancient Egypt." *Journal of Laryngology & Otology* 106 (1992): 773–779.
Pappas, Theodore N. "President Eisenhower's Bowel Obstruction: The Story of His Surgeons and Their Decision to Operate." *Annals of Surgery* 258 (2013): 192–197.
Pappas, Theodore N., and Sharzad Joharifard. "Did James A. Garfield Die of Cholecystitis? Revisiting the Autopsy of the 20th President of the United States." *American Journal of Surgery* 206 (2013): 613–618.
Pappas, Theodore N., and Michael S. Mulvihill. "The President's Gallbladder: A Historical Account of the Cholecystectomy of Lyndon Baines Johnson." *Surgery* 147 (2010): 160–166.
Pappas, Theodore, and Sven Swanson. "Anarchy and the Surgical Care of President William McKinley." *Journal of Trauma and Acute Care Surgery* 72 (2012): 1106–1113.
Park, Roswell. "Reminiscences of McKinley Week." In Julian Park. *Selected Papers Surgical and Scientific*, 375–81. Buffalo, NY: Subscribers, 1914.
Paulson, George. "Death of a President and His Assassin: Errors in Their Diagnosis and Autopsies." *Journal of the History of the Neurosciences* 15 (2006): 77–91.
Perkins, Jeanne. "The President's Doctor." *Life*, July 31, 1944, p. 4.
Petch, C.P. "Guillain, Barré … and Strohl?" *The Lancet* 2 (1978): 380.
Pillsbury, Donald M. "General Eisenhower's 'Melanoma.'" *Journal of the American Academy of Dermatology* 4 (1981): 631–632.
"The President's Wound, and the Management of the Case." Editorial. *Boston Medical and Surgical Journal* 105 (1881): 309.
"The Question of Malpractice in the Case of the Late President Garfield." Editorial. *Medical Record* 20 (1881): 600–601.
"Reagan Skin Cancer Is Least Risky Type." *Chicago Tribune*, August 6, 1985.
"Remarks on Medical Fees." *New York Chronicle of Medicine and Surgery*, 1824–1825: 1:25.
Renehan, Andrew, and John C. Lowry. "The Oral Tumours of Two American Presidents: What If They Were Alive Today?" *Journal of the Royal Society of Medicine* 88 (1995): 373–383.
Reyburn, Robert. "History of the Case of President Garfield." *Boston Medical and Surgical Journal* 130 (1894): 411–417, 460–464, 498–502, 545–549, 578–582, 621–624, 664–669.
Richardson, Ruth. "Joseph Lister's Domestic Science." *The Lancet* 382, no. 9898 (2013): e8–e9.
Richman, Irwin. "George Washington's Physicians (Elisha Dick)." *Pennsylvania Medicine* 69 (1966): 53–54.
Rishi, Anupam, and Hsiang-Hsuan Michael Yu. "Current Treatment of Melanoma Brain Metastasis." *Current Treatment Options in Oncology* 21 (2021): 45.
Rixey, Presley M., et al. "The Official Report on the Case of President McKinley: Special Contribution." *Buffalo Medical Journal* (October 1901): 271–293.
Rosenberg, J.C. "A Study of Andrew Jackson's Wounds and Illnesses." *American Journal of Surgery* 117 (1969): 721–725.
Rosenthal, A. "Reagan to Undergo Surgery for Finger Ailment Saturday." *New York Times*, January 4, 1989.
Rosenthal, Jack. "Johnson's Washington Recalled as Time of Restless Volubility." *New York Times*, January 25, 1973, p. 34.
Ruben, Robert J. "Dr Ross McIntire, Otolaryngologist, and His Care of President Franklin D. Roosevelt." *Otolaryngology—Head and Neck Surgery* 141 (2009): 4–6.
Rutkow, Ira. "Joseph Lister and His 1876 Tour of America." *Annals of Surgery* 257 (2013): 1181–1187.
Rutkow, Ira M. "Moments in Surgical History: Zabdiel Boylston and Smallpox Inoculation." *Archives of Surgery* 136 (2001): 1213.
Scheidemandel, Heinz H.E. "Did George Washington Die of Quincy?" *Acta Otolaryngolica* 102 (1976): 519–521.
Shabani, Mahtab, et al. "Lead Poisoning: A Neglected Potential Diagnosis in Abdominal Pain." *BMC Gastroenterology* 20 (2020): 134–142.
Sims, James Marion. "The Surgical Treatment of President Garfield." *North America Review* 133 (1881): 594–601.
Sorensen, Robert H., et al. "President Reagan's Life Saving Colectomy and Subsequent Historical Implication." *Military Medicine* 179 (2014): 704–707.
Stavrakis, Peter. "Heroic Medicine, Bloodletting, and the Sad Fate of George Washington." *Maryland Medical Journal* 46 (1997): 539–540.
Steinbrook, R. "Reagan Has Surgery for Fluid on Brain." *Los Angeles Times*, September 9, 1989.
Trunkey, Donald, and Farhood Farjah. "Medical and Surgical Care of Our Four Assassinated

Presidents." *Journal of the American College of Surgeons* 201 (2005): 976–989.

Turnipseed, E.B. "A Dissenting Voice from the Standpoints Taken by D.W. Bliss, M.D., in Regard to the Diagnosis, Prognosis, and Treatment of the Case of President Garfield." *Medical Record* 20 (1881): 620–624.

Van Hootegem, Philippe, and Simon Travis. "Is Crohn's Disease a Rightly Used Eponym?" *Journal of Crohn's and Colitis* 14 (2020): 867–871.

Waclawik, Andrew J. "The Legacy of the Seminal Publication by Guillain, Barré, and Strohl: The History behind the Eponym." *Wisconsin Medical Journal* 117 (2018): 160–163.

Weiner, Bradley K. "The Case of James A. Garfield: A Historical Perspective." *Spine* 28 (2003): E183–E186.

Widmer, Ted. "The Hushed Crises of America's Sick Presidents." *Wall Street Journal,* October 10–11, 2020, p. C5.

Wiedeman, James E. "Presidential Operations: Medical Fact or Urban Legend?" *Journal of the American College of Surgeons* 208 (2009): 1132–1137.

Wiedeman, James E. "Reply." *Journal of the American College of Surgeons* 209 (2009): 547.

Wong, Vincent J., et al. "Was President Andrew Jackson Overcharged? An Economic Evaluation of 19th Century Charges for Urologic Procedures and Their Comparison to the Modern RVU Era." *International Journal of Urologic History* 1 (2021): 19–24.

Wyatt, H.V. "Incubation of Poliomyelitis as Calculated from the Time of Entry into the Central Nervous System via the Peripheral Nerve Pathways." *Reviews of Infectious Diseases* 12 (1990): 547–556.

Yeng, Yuan, et al. "Chronic Lead Poisoning Induced Abdominal Pain and Anemia: A Case Report and Review of the Literature." *BMC Gastroenterology* 20 (2020): 335–340.

Websites and Other Sources

The American Presidency Project, https://www.presidency.ucsb.edu/.

"Anarchism." Brittanica. https://www.britannica.com/topic/anarchism.

"Anarchism." Wikipedia. https://en.wikipedia.org/wiki/Anarchism (accessed March 10, 2023).

"August 8, 1893: Message Regarding Economic Crisis." The Miller Center, https://millercenter.org/the-presidency/presidential-speeches/august-8-1893-message-regarding-economic-crisis.

"Caused by Fall Off Horse: Reagan Survives Brain Surgery to Remove Fluid." *Los Angeles Times,* September 10, 1989. www.latimes.com/archives/la-xpm-1989-09-10-mn-2561-story.html.

"Doctors Have a Tense Debate: Reagan 'Has' or 'Had' Cancer?" *Los Angeles Times,* July 20, 1985. http://articles.latimes.com/1985-07-20/news/mn-5861_1_cancer-experts.

"Emma Goldman." Wikipedia. https://en.wikipedia.org/wiki/Emma_Goldman (accessed March 15, 2023).

"English Anarchist Thought." Britannica. www.britannica.com/topic/anarchism/English-anarchist-thought (accessed March 13, 2023).

"Former President Reagan Recovering after Hip Surgery." CBS News, January 3, 2002. https://www.cbsnews.com/news/former-president-reagan-recovering-after-hip-surgery/.

Gould, Lewis. "William McKinley: Last Speech." Salem Press, https://www.salempress.com/Media/SalemPress/samples/dd_1900s_pgs.pdf (Accessed March 19, 2022).

Honke, W. "It Was a Big Moment in the History of Skin Cancer Awareness." Sun & Skin News, October 1, 2019. www.skincancer.org/blog/whats-that-on presidant-reagan-nose/.

Jefferson, Thomas. "To James Madison from Thomas Jefferson, 24 July 1791." Founders Online, https://founders.archives.gov/documents/Madison/01-14-02-0045. Original source: *The Papers of James Madison,* Vol. 14, *6 April 1791–16 March 1793,* edited by Robert A. Rutland and Thomas A. Mason, 55–56. Charlottesville: University Press of Virginia, 1983.

"John Hinckley, Jr." https://en.wikipedia.org/wiki/John_Hinckley_Jr.

Johnson, Lyndon. "Statement by the President Announcing That He Would Undergo Surgery (October 5, 1965)." American Presidency Project. https://www.presidency.ucsb.edu/documents/statement-the-president-announcing-that-he-would-undergo-surgery.

"Leon Czolgosz." Wikipedia. https://en.wikipedia.org/wiki/Leon_Czolgosz (accessed March 18, 2022).

Lomazow, Steven. "The Truth About Lyndon Johnson's Gall Bladder Scar." FDR's Deadly Secret. https://fdrsdeadlysecret.blogspot.com/2011/03/truth-about-lyndon-johnsons-gall.html.

"Lyndon B. Johnson: The President's News Conference, November 3, 1966." American Presidency Project. https://www.presidency.ucsb.edu/documents/the-presidents-news-conference-1178.

Mirkin, Gabe. "Lyndon Baines Johnson's Heart Attacks." Villages-News.com, February 6, 2019. https://www.villages-news.com/2019/02/06/lyndon-baines-johnsons-heart-attacks/.

"President Dwight D. Eisenhower's Farewell Address (1961)." National Archives, https://www.archives.gov/milestone-documents/president-dwight-d-eisenhowers-farewell-address.

"President Reagan's Medical Procedures." Ronald Reagan Presidential Library & Museum." https://www.reaganlibrary.gov/reagans/reagan-administration/president-reagans-medical-procedures.

"The President's Message." *St. Louis Globe-Democrat,* August 9, 1893.

"Rachel Donelson Robards Jackson (1767–1828)." National Women's History Museum. www.womenshistory.org (accessed June 28, 2023).

"Reagan Breaks Hip, Faces Surgery Today." SF Gate, January 13, 2001. https://www.sfgate.com/health/article/reagan-breaks-hip-faces-surgery-today-2965559.php.
"Reagan Recovering from Hip Surgery. Wife Nancy Remains at His Side." CNN, January 15, 2001. https://www.cnn.com/2001/US/01/14/reagan.03/index.html.
"Reagan Undergoes Surgery after Breaking Right Hip in a Fall." *New York Times,* January 14, 2001. https://www.nytimes.com/2001/01/14/us/reagan-undergoes-surgery-after-breaking-right-hip-in-a-fall.html.
Reeves, Thomas C. "Dwight D. Eisenhower, President of United States." Britannica, initially submitted July 28, 1999. www.britannica.com/biography/Dwight-D-Eisenhower (accessed June 7, 2021).
Rotondi, J.P. "What Happens When a President Becomes Ill or Incapacitated While in Office?" History.com, October 13, 2020. www.history.com/news/presidents-ill-25-amendment.
U.S. Inflation Calculator. https://www.usinflationcalculator.com/.
"What Is the 25th Amendment and When Has It Been Invoked?" History News Network. https://www.hnn.us/article/what-is-the-25th-amendment-and-when-has-it-been-in (accessed September 20, 2022).

Index

www.ingramcontent.com/pod-product-compliance
Ingram Content Group UK Ltd.
Pitfield, Milton Keynes, MK11 3LW, UK
UKHW051930100926
8556IPUK00022B/1469